Effect of Cancer
on
Quality of Life

Editor
David Osoba, M.D.
Head, Division of Communities Oncology
British Columbia Cancer Agency
Vancouver, British Columbia
Canada

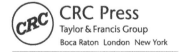

CRC Press
Taylor & Francis Group
Boca Raton London New York

CRC Press is an imprint of the
Taylor & Francis Group, an **informa** business

CRC Press
Taylor & Francis Group
6000 Broken Sound Parkway NW, Suite 300
Boca Raton, FL 33487-2742

© 1991 by Taylor & Francis Group, LLC
CRC Press is an imprint of Taylor & Francis Group, an Informa business

ISBN 13: 9780849369773 (hbk)
ISBN 13: 9780367450588 (pbk)

No claim to original U.S. Government works

This book contains information obtained from authentic and highly regarded sources. Reasonable efforts have been made to
publish reliable data and information, but the author and publisher cannot assume responsibility for the validity of all materials
or the consequences of their use. The authors and publishers have attempted to trace the copyright holders of all material reproduced in this publication and apologize to copyright holders if permission to publish in this form has not been obtained. If any
copyright material has not been acknowledged please write and let us know so we may rectify in any future reprint.

Except as permitted under U.S. Copyright Law, no part of this book may be reprinted, reproduced, transmitted, or utilized in any
form by any electronic, mechanical, or other means, now known or hereafter invented, including photocopying, microfilming,
and recording, or in any information storage or retrieval system, without written permission from the publishers.

For permission to photocopy or use material electronically from this work, please access www.copyright.com (http://www.copy-
right.com/) or contact the Copyright Clearance Center, Inc. (CCC), 222 Rosewood Drive, Danvers, MA 01923, 978-750-8400.
CCC is a not-for-profit organization that provides licenses and registration for a variety of users. For organizations that have been
granted a photocopy license by the CCC, a separate system of payment has been arranged.

Trademark Notice: Product or corporate names may be trademarks or registered trademarks, and are used only for identification and explanation without intent to infringe.

Visit the Taylor & Francis Web site at
http://www.taylorandfrancis.com

and the CRC Press Web site at
http://www.crcpress.com

PREFACE

Several recent books have dealt with quality of life in cancer as a health status endpoint. Undoubtedly, more are in the planning and writing stages at this very moment. Therefore, it seems reasonable to ask "Why this particular book on the effect of cancer on quality of life, and why at this time?".

The main reason is to provide novel perspectives on topics not usually included in other books on cancer and quality of life. For example, there is a tacit assumption that control of symptoms will automatically improve quality of life. This assumption is held widely and is probably true, but it should still be tested to determine just how much certain symptoms affect quality of life. Therefore, this book contains chapters dealing with the special challenges related to the methodology involved in improving control of symptoms such as nausea and vomiting (Morrow and Black, Willan et al., and Warr) and pain (Portenoy, Cleeland, and Bruera and MacDonald). Not only is this important for research into symptom control, but also in palliative care and hospice, for nowhere has this assumption been accepted as a fact more than in the palliative care setting. Yet, little research has actually been published which delineates to what extent the successful control of certain symptoms and the attempt to provide emotional and spiritual support have produced a measureable impact on the quality of life of the terminally ill patient and of the family. On the one hand, the benefits seem so obvious that research in this area is unnecessary but, on the other, many questions are unanswered because of the paucity of research which goes beyond assessing symptom control. Two chapters, one by Ahmedzai in the United Kingdom and the other from Masterson-Allen and Mor in the U.S., provide insights into the special challenges associated with research in palliative care.

Feeny et al. deal with the special issues associated with measuring quality of life in children, a field that poses unique conditions and challenges. There is a chapter on combining quality-of-life measurement with an economic evaluation by Goodwin — an important approach to gaining a fuller picture of the impact of cancer on society. Also, we must be aware of some of the potential abuses of quality-of-life data: a chapter by Till is devoted to this topic. These novel perspectives are timely and relevant.

The use of quality-of-life measures in clinical trials is relatively new and there are new approaches to be tried and evaluated. Jaeschke and Guyatt suggest N of 1 clinical trials — an approach that makes sense in that it is the patient who sets the normative standard for his/her own quality of life and, therefore, it is the patient who should make comparisons between the current state of quality of life and that which he/she deems normative or desirable. Mor et al. provide a novel approach to dealing with the unmet needs of patients with cancer. Also, conventional statistical methods — especially for dealing with missing data — need to be re-examined. Zee and Pater provide new insight into approaches for dealing with such problems.

Measuring quality of life in health care (whether in cancer or other diseases), although not a new idea, is gaining momentum both in clinical trials and in clinical practice. To keep pace with the changing perceptions of the purpose and place of quality-of-life measurement, the methodology, and the results of recent studies, it is necessary to publish updates in these areas. The advantage of combining these in a single volume is the convenience provided to the reader who can obtain a more global perspective of the whole field than is possible from single articles in a variety of journals.

Stjernsward and Teoh underline the enormity of the problems faced by patients on a global scale, while Ware provides conceptual insights that form the basis of health-status measures. However, the incorporation of quality-of-life measures into either clinical trials or day-to-day practice is not universally accepted by all investigators and practitioners. Dealing with the barriers that still need to be overcome is addressed by Osoba and some of the considerations relevant to clinical trials are covered by Levine. Practical advice in the form of an algorithm and relevant criteria for selecting quality-of-life measures are included in the chapter by Osoba et al.

The move from the conceptual stage to actual measurement in the clinical setting requires a rigorous scientific process involving psychometric analysis and field testing of new questionnaires. Aaronson et al. provide the latest psychometric data from field trials of the EORTC core Quality of Life Questionnaire. The use of other questionnaires, with current results from recent studies, is dealt with in chapters by Wood-Dauphinee and Williams in their review of the Quality of Life Index, by Levine who reviews studies on breast cancer, and by Lasry who writes on sexual functioning and body image in patients who have had either radical mastectomy or breast-sparing surgery for breast cancer. Regrettably, Schipper was unable to provide a chapter summarizing the recent results of using Functional Living Index-Cancer in a variety of clinical trials.

It is a quality of humankind to try to predict what the future has in store for us. In the quality-of-life arena this would translate into being able to predict the future quality of life in patients with a variety of cancers and situations from a prior knowledge of independent determinants of quality of life. Iscoe et al. provide background information which should serve as grist for the mill. May the future of quality-of-life considerations fare well, not only in cancer and other illnesses, but in all human endeavours.

ACKNOWLEDGMENTS

I wish to express my gratitude to the editors of CRC Press for choosing the subject of quality of life in cancer for one of their volumes. In particular, I owe a special debt to each of the authors who made a contribution to this book. The writing of a chapter often involves the "burning of midnight oil" with the attendant personal sacrifices, but contributing to a book also involves the giving of advice and of involvement beyond one's own specific chapter. Much of the advice that helped me in the planning of this book came at a meeting of most of the authors in April of 1989 in Montreal. At this meeting the scope of the book was planned and an attempt was made to avoid as much overlap between chapters as was reasonably possible. Each author presented an outline of his or her intended chapter and the other authors then provided advice on how the chapter might be improved and what aspects of it might be changed to avoid overlap. This meeting was extremely valuable and would not have been possible without the generous financial support of the following pharmaceutical firms. I thank them all.

Adria Laboratories of Canada Ltd.
Beecham Clinical Pharmacology (Canada)
Bristol-Myers Pharmaceutical Group, Division of Bristol-Myers Canada Inc.
Glaxo Canada Inc.
Knoll Pharmaceuticals Canada
Lederle Oncology Department, Cyanamid Canada Inc.
Pharmacia (Canada) Inc.
Purdue Frederick Inc.
Schering Canada Inc.
The Upjohn Company of Canada

Although secretarial assistance is often taken for granted since it comes as "part of the turf" when working in an institution such as mine, I am aware now more than ever that the preparation of a book with chapters written by many authors requires excellent secretarial and managerial skills. My task was lightened by Barbara Fiddler, Colleen Pelletier, Lillian Tse, Mary Naylor, Luisa Filomarino, and Fiona Buss, who each in their own way assisted greatly in bringing this work to fruition. I am very grateful to them all.

David Osoba
September, 1990

THE EDITOR

David Osoba, M.D., is a medical oncologist, Head of the Division of Communities Oncology, and Director of the Communities Oncology Program at the British Columbia Cancer Agency, and a Clinical Professor in the Department of Medicine, University of British Columbia, Vancouver, B.C.

Dr. Osoba obtained his M.D. from the University of Alberta, Edmonton, Alberta, in 1956 after obtaining a B.Sc. in 1954. Subsequently, he trained in internal medicine and hematology and became a Fellow of the Royal College of Physicians and Surgeons of Canada in 1961.

He is a member of the American Society for Clinical Oncology, the Canadian Association of Medical Oncologists (which he helped found in 1987), the Canadian Oncology Society (of which he was President in 1985-1986), the National Cancer Institute of Canada, the Clinical Trials Group of the National Cancer Institute of Canada (for which he chairs the Quality of Life Committee), and the Quality of Life Study Group of the European Organization for Research and Treatment of Cancer. He is chairman of the Medical Advisory Committee for the Canadian Cancer Society (B.C. and Yukon Division) and is a member of numerous national and international committees. His awards include the McEachern Fellowship from the Canadian Cancer Society, and the Medal of the Royal College of Physicians and Surgeons of Canada. He has been a Scholar and Associate of the Medical Research Council of Canada and a Consultant to the World Health Organization.

Dr. Osoba has been the recipient of research grants from the Medical Research Council of Canada and the Ontario Cancer Treatment and Research Foundation. He has published over 100 papers. His current major research interest is in measuring quality of life in patients with cancer who are in clinical trials, and is also interested in the development of new chemotherapy protocols for patients with cancer in the head and neck region.

CONTRIBUTORS

Neil K. Aaronson, Ph.D.
Head
Division of Psychosocial Research and
  Epidemiology
The Netherlands Cancer Institute
Amsterdam, The Netherlands

Sam Ahmedzai, M.B.Ch.B., M.R.C.P.
Medical Director
Leicestershire Hospice
Leicester, United Kingdom

Ronald D. Barr, M.D.
Professor and Chairman of Hematology
Departments of Pediatrics and Pathology
  and Medicine
McMaster University
Hamilton, Canada

Peter M. Black, M.P.H.
Research Associate
Department of Oncology
University of Rochester Medical Center
Rochester, New York

Eduardo Bruera, Ph.D.
Department of Palliative Care Unit
Edmonton General Hospital
Edmonton, Canada

Monika Bullinger, Dr. Phil.
Assistant Professor
Institute for Medical Psychology
University of Munich
Munich, Germany

Charles S. Cleeland, Ph.D.
Professor
Department of Neurology
University of Wisconsin
Madison, Wisconsin

Dirk Crabeels, M.Sc.
Project Manager
Department of Radiotherapy
The Netherlands Cancer Institute
Amsterdam, The Netherlands

C. Erlichman, M.D., F.R.C.P.C.
Staff Physician
Department of Medicine
University of Toronto
Toronto, Canada

J. Estapè, M.D.
Professor and Chairman
Department of Medical Oncology
H. Clinic
Barcelona, Spain

David Feeny, Ph.D.
Professor
Department of Clinical Epidemiology and
  Biostatistics
McMaster University
Hamilton, Canada

Antonio Filiberti, Ph.D.
Division of Diagnostic Oncology
Instituto Nacionale per lo Studio e la
  Cura dei Tumori
Milan, Italy

H. Flechtner, M.D.
Clinic for Child and Adolescent
  Psychiatry
University of Cologne
Cologne, Germany

Ulrich Frick, Ph.D.
Biometric Centre for Therapy Studies
Munich, Germany

William Furlong
Research Coordinator
Department of Clinical Epidemiology and
  Biostatistics
McMaster University
Hamilton, Canada

**Pamela J. Goodwin, M.D., F.R.C.P.C.,
  M.Sc.**
Assistant Professor
Departments of Medicine and Preventive
  Medicine and Biostatistics
Faculty of Medicine
University of Toronto
Toronto, Canada

Edward Guadagnoli, Ph.D.
Assistant Professor
Harvard Medical School
Boston, Massachusetts

Gordon H. Guyatt, M.D.
Professor
Departments of Medicine and Clinical
  Epidemiology and Biostatistics
McMaster University
Hamilton, Canada

Christoph Hürny, M.D.
Vice-Chairman
Medical Division Lory
Inselspital
Bern, Switzerland

Neill Iscoe, M.D., F.R.C.P.C.
Assistant Professor
Department of Medicine
Toronto Bayview Regional Cancer Center
Toronto, Canada

Roman Jaeschke, M.D.
Assistant Professor
Department of Medicine
McMaster University and St. Joseph's
  Hospital
Hamilton, Canada

Stein Kaasa, M.D., Ph.D.
Department of Oncology and
  Radiotherapy
Norwegian Radium Hospital
Oslo, Norway

Marianne Klee, M.D.
Research Fellow
Department of Oncology
Rigshospitalet The Finsen Institute
Copenhagen, Denmark

Jean-Claude M. Lasry, Ph.D.
Research Associate/Professor
Departments of Psychiatry and
  Psychology
Jewish General Hospital/University of
  Montreal
Montreal, Canada

Mark N. Levine, M.D.
Associate Professor
Department of Medicine and Clinical
  Epidemiology and Biostatistics
McMaster University
Head of Medicine
Ontario Cancer Foundation
Hamilton, Canada

Martin Levitt, M.D.
Associate Professor
Department of Medicine
University of Manitoba
Winnipeg, Canada

R. Neil MacDonald, M.D.
Professor
Department of Palliative Care Medicine
University of Alberta
Edmonton, Canada

Susan Masterson-Allen, M.A., A.B.D.
Research Associate
Center for Gerontology and Health Care
  Research
Brown University
Providence, Rhode Island

Miroslav Mastilica, M.A.
Assistant Professor
Department of Medical Sociology
Andrija Stampar School of Public Health
University of Zagreb
Zagreb, Yugoslavia

Vincent Mor, Ph.D.
Associate Professor
Director
Center for Gerontology Health Care
  Research
Brown University
Providence, Rhode Island

Gary R. Morrow, Ph.D.
Associate Professor
Head, Behavioral Medicine Unit
University of Rochester Cancer Center
Rochester, New York

David Osoba, M.D.
Clinical Professor
Department of Medicine
University of British Columbia
Vancouver, Canada

Joseph L. Pater, M.D.
Professor
Department of Community Health and
 Epidemiology
Queen's University
Kingston, Canada

Bettina Pfausler
University Hospital of Innsbruck
Innsbruck, Austria

Russell K. Portenoy, M.D.
Associate Attending Neurologist
Director of Analgesic Studies, Pain
 Service
Department of Neurology
Memorial Sloan-Kettering Cancer Center
New York, New York

Darius Razavi, M.D.
Head
Rehabilitation and Psycho-Oncology Unit
Institute of Jules Bordet
Brussels, Belgium

Peter B. C. Rofe, M.B.
Lecturer
Department of Psychiatry
University of Adelaide
Adelaide, Soth Australia

Rebecca B. Rosenstein, Ph.D.
Assistant Scientist
Department of Clinical Research
Eye Research Institute
Boston, Massachussetts

Simon Schraub, M.D.
Professor
Department of Radiothérapie Oncologie
Center Hospitalier de Besançon F.
Besançon, France

Jan Sternswärd, M.D.
Chief
Cancer and Palliative Care Unit
World Health Organization
Geneva, Switzerland

Marianne Sullivan, Ph.D.
Associate Professor
Department of Medicine I
Sahlgtenska Hospital
Gottenburg, Sweden

John Paul Szalai, Ph.D.
Director
Research Design and Biostatistics
Sunnybrook Health Science Center
University of Toronto
North York, Canada

Fumikazu Takeda, M.D.
Director of Hospital
Department of Neurosurgery Clinic
Saitama Cancer Center
Ina Saitama, Japan

Noreen Teoh, B.S.
Technical Officer
Cancer and Palliative Care Unit
World Health Organization
Geneva, Switzerland

James E. Till, Ph.D.
Senior Scientist
Division of Epidemiology and Statistics
The Ontario Cancer Institute/Princess
 Margaret Hospital
Toronto, Canada

George W. Torrance, Ph.D.
Professor
Department of Clinical Epidemiology and
 Biostatistics
McMaster University
Hamilton, Canada

John E. Ware, Jr., Ph.D.
Director, Senior Scientist
International Resource Center
Institute for the Improvement of Medical
  Care and Health
New England Medical Center
Boston, Massachusetts

David Warr, M.D.
Assistant Professor
Department of Medicine
Princess Margaret Hospital
Toronto, Canada

Sheila Weitzman, M.B.
Pediatric Oncologist
Department of Pediatrics
University of Toronto and Hospital for
  Sick Children
Toronto, Canada

Andrew R. Willan, Ph.D.
Associate Professor
Department of Clinical Epidemiology and
  Biostatistics
McMaster University
Hamilton, Canada

J. Ivan Williams, Ph.D.
Professor
Department of Preventive Medicine and
  Biostatistics
University of Toronto
Toronto, Canada

Sharon L. Wood-Dauphinee, Ph.D.
Associate Professor
School of Physical and Occupational
  Therapy
Department of Epidemiology and
  Biostatistics
McGill University
Montreal, Canada

Benny Zee, Ph.D.
Assistant Professor
Department of Community Health and
  Epidemiology
Queen's University
Kingston, Canada

TABLE OF CONTENTS

Chapter 1

PERSPECTIVES ON QUALITY OF LIFE AND THE GLOBAL CANCER PROBLEM

Jan Stjernswärd and Noreen Teoh

TABLE OF CONTENTS

I. INTRODUCTION

Cancer is one of the three leading causes of death for the productive age group 15 to 55 years in both developed and developing countries. The other two leading causes of death are accidents and cardiovascular diseases. Cancer is recognized as a major health problem in the developed regions of the world. However, the prevalence of communicable diseases often hides the fact that cancer is also becoming a serious problem in developing countries.

Cancer rates in developing countries are progressively approaching those in the industrialized countries, mainly because of an increase in the average age of the population, continued improvement in the control of other major health problems, and a continued increase in tobacco use. Counter measures should therefore be adopted without delay.

At present, an estimated 7,000,000 new cancer patients are diagnosed annually, of which slightly more than one half are in the developing countries. Cancer is a Third World problem too. Every year, about 5,000,000 cancer patients die of their disease.

In general, there are three approaches available for controlling a cancer: prevention, early detection, and curative therapy. In reviewing the eight most common tumors globally, it is evident that not all approaches are effective for most tumors (Table 1).

Even though about one third of cancers today are preventable, few effective national prevention programs have been implemented. Similarly, one third of today's tumors could be cured if they were diagnosed early; but again, only a limited number of countries have established both the early-detection and treatment services necessary to take advantage of the progress in medical science.[2]

II. CURRENT PERSPECTIVES IN CONTROLLING CANCER

In most countries, if one were to ask what is the national goal in cancer, the response would be "to find a cure". Indeed, the overwhelming majority of resources for cancer are allocated to precisely that — finding a cure. However, it may be that a better response to the question would be "to prevent cancer" or "to detect cancer early and cure it".

Currently, aggressive therapeutic attempts to achieve a minor prolongation of life or the act of uncomfortable dying predominate over concerns for quality of life and dignity in death in a familiar environment.[2]

Although for most cancer patients, pain relief and relief of other common symptoms is the only realistic option, few of the cancer control resources go to palliative care and generally, there is little or no training of health care professions in this type of care.

Quality of life and comfort before death could be considerably improved through the application of current knowledge for relieving cancer pain and implementing existing knowledge in palliative care. All too often, palliative care is ignored or seen as something that comes at the very end of the list of treatment options, a type of "waste-paper basket" alternative (Figure 1).

The size of the problem is big. In developed countries, 67% of male and 60% of female cancer patients will die of their disease. In developing countries, the figure is much higher. Instead, palliative care needs to be seen as an integral part of cancer care in both developed and developing countries (Figures 2 and 3). Curative care and palliative care are not mutually exclusive. For most cancer patients, however, no curative treatment exists. The quality of life in these patients would be better if they had access to palliative care from the start.[1]

III. STRATEGIES AND PRIORITIES OF THE WORLD HEALTH ORGANIZATION (WHO)

The WHO global cancer control program is based on the concept that enough knowledge

TABLE 1
Availability of Effective Strategies for the Control of the Eight Most Common Cancers Worldwide[1]

Tumor[a]	No. of cases[b]	Primary prevention	Early diagnosis	Curative therapy[c]	Palliative care
Stomach	670	+[d]	–	–	+ +
Lung	660	+ +	–	–	+ +
Breast	572	–	+ +	+ +	+ +
Colon/rectum	572	+	+	+	+ +
Cervix	466	+	+ +	+ +	+ +
Mouth/pharynx	379	+ +	+ +	+ +	+ +
Esophagus	310	–	–	–	+ +
Liver	251	+ +	–	–	+ +

[a] Listed in order of the eight most common tumors globally.
[b] Per year, in thousands.
[c] Curative for majority of cases with a realistic opportunity of finding them early.
[d] + + = effective, + = partly effective, – = not effective.

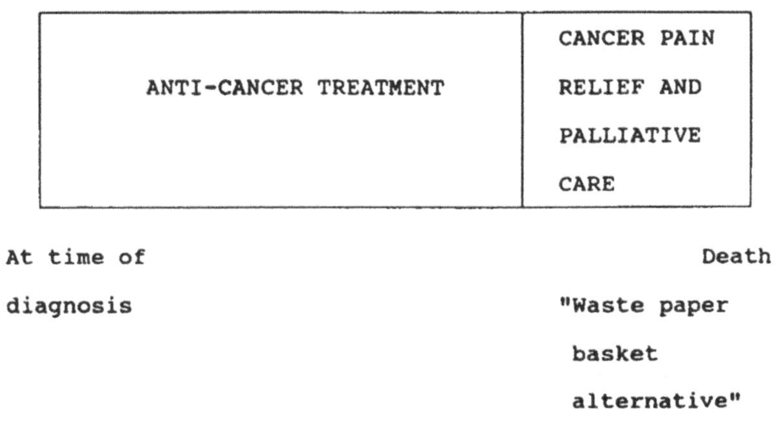

ANTI-CANCER TREATMENT
CANCER PAIN RELIEF AND PALLIATIVE CARE
At time of diagnosis
Death
"Waste paper basket alternative"

FIGURE 1. Present allocation of cancer resources.[1]

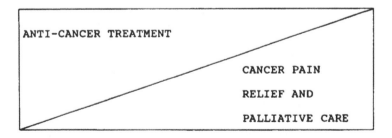

ANTI-CANCER TREATMENT
CANCER PAIN RELIEF AND PALLIATIVE CARE
At time of diagnosis
Death

FIGURE 2. Proposed allocation of cancer resources in developed countries.[1]

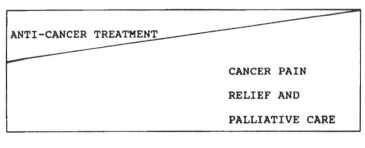

At time of   Death

diagnosis

FIGURE 3.   Proposed allocation of cancer resources in developing countries.[1]

exists today about cancer to take effective action that will significantly reduce cancer morbidity and mortality worldwide, if properly implemented.

There is an urgent need for rethinking. Global resources are limited as well as unequally distributed, and it is not realistic to expect them to increase appreciably in the near future. Setting the right priorities and strategies in a systematic way to gain maximum benefit from available resources, preferably through well-conceived national cancer control programs, has become mandatory. Without doing so, there can be little impact on cancer, especially in the less developed countries.

The WHO urges governments to strengthen or, where lacking, to consider initiating the development of cancer control measures as an integral part of national health plans. Three key priorities in a well-conceived national cancer control program include primary prevention, early detection coupled with therapy, and palliative care.

IV. CHALLENGES

A number of countries are now beginning to consider cost-effectiveness in developing national strategies to control cancer. Comparisons are being made between the extent of cancer control that can be purchased with fixed resources: prevention vs. early detection vs. therapy vs. palliative care.

In the area of primary prevention, the largest group preventable are tobacco-related cancers: lung cancer associated with tobacco smoking and oral cancer associated with tobacco chewing habits of Asia. Liver cancer is also preventable for the most part by vaccination against hepatitis B. It is important that quality-of-life investigations in cancer focus not only on the relatively small differences in quality of life between therapeutic approaches, but also consider differences in quality of life between cancer patients and individuals free of disease.

In the developing countries, approximately 80% of the cancer cases arrive at health facilities only when the disease is in an advanced and incurable stage. The purpose of early detection is to find cancer, or its precursors when they are small, localized, and comparatively easy to cure. Measurements should be made available to compare the difference between the quality of life for patients whose cancer is detected early and easily excised as opposed to patients who present themselves at health centers with diseases in an advanced stage, where there is high morbidity with treatment.

Unfortunately, the majority of the world's cancer patients fall into the large group where no effective therapy exists and only palliative treatment can be offered. There is a need for quality of life studies to investigate the appropriateness of palliative care, rather than the administration of therapies that are known to be ineffective which are often given simply because the physician feels that he must provide some therapy for every patient. Such studies could provide the physicians and the patients a suitable basis for making the most appropriate treatment decisions.

V. CONCLUSIONS

WHO provides technical support to countries in formulating and implementing national cancer policies, taking into account their cost effectiveness. Of the eight most common tumors, cancers of the lung, mouth, and liver are eligible for primary prevention.

Tumors of the cervix, breast, and mouth can be controlled in part by early detection and referral in time for effective therapy. WHO is advocating the "3-Step Analgesic" ladder approach toward relieving cancer pain and, recently, formulated methods to control other common symptoms. These are promoted as part of National Cancer Control Programs.

Further developments of methods for measuring quality of life in all the different aspects of cancer control, and not only in therapy (as is presently mostly done), will help convince policy makers to set more balanced priorities in cancer care and to establish national resource allocation. Results from reliable and valid quality-of-life measures could lead to important changes in cancer control policy.[3] A consensus needs to be drawn on a scientifically valid and reliable method for estimating quality of life; it should be practical and realistic to use, and with minor modifications, applicable cross-culturally. Can the experts agree on such a method soon? Up to now, few quality of life studies have led to changes in clinical practice. To address this problem, WHO has established Collaborating Centres at the Netherlands Cancer Institute in Amsterdam, Holland; Saitama Cancer Center in Saitama, Japan; and the St. Boniface General Hospital Research Centre in Winnipeg, Canada.

REFERENCES

1. WHO Technical Report Series, No. 804, Cancer pain relief and palliative care. Report of a WHO Expert Committee, WHO, Geneva, No. 804, 1990.
2. **Stanley, K., Stjernswärd, J., and Koroltchouk, V.,** Cancer of the stomach, lung and breast: mortality trends and control strategies, *World Health Stat. Q.,* 41, 107, 1988.
3. **Stjernswärd, J., Stanley, K., and Koroltchouk, V.,** Quality of life of cancer patients: goals and objectives, in *Assessment of Quality of Life and Cancer Treatment,* Ventafridda, V. et al., Eds., Excerpta Medica, Amsterdam 1986, 1.

Chapter 2

MEASURING FUNCTIONING, WELL-BEING, AND OTHER GENERIC HEALTH CONCEPTS

John E. Ware, Jr.

TABLE OF CONTENTS

I. INTRODUCTION

There is an increasing consensus in the health care field regarding the centrality of the patient's point of view in monitoring the quality of medical care outcomes.[1] Indeed, the goal of medical care today for most patients is the achievement of a more "effective" life[2] and the preservation of function and well-being.[3-7] The patient is the best source on the achievement of these goals. Unfortunately, however, information about patients' experiences of disease and treatment is not routinely collected in clinical research or medical practice.

We are entering a new era in which information from patients about functional status, well-being, and other important health care concepts will be routinely collected to fill major gaps in existing databases. Included are databases used to compare costs and benefits of various financial and organizational aspects of health care services, by organizational managers who try to provide the best value for health care dollars, by clinical investigators who evaluate new treatments and technologies, and by practicing physicians and other providers who try to achieve the best possible outcomes for their patients.

The primary source of this information will be from more practical standardized patient surveys derived from those that have served research well over the past decade. The most efficient way to monitor functional status and well-being for most adults is via scoring of carefully constructed sets of survey questions. Advances in assessment methods, particularly in terms of surveys of patient perspectives have facilitated this kind of data collection (see, for example, References 8 through 11), although their use on a large scale has not been practical.

It is clear that the field of cancer and health care in general very much need more cost effective ways to obtain new and better data about patient functioning, well-being and other generic health outcomes. The methods must be practical and they must satisfy the most crucial psychometric standards. The trade-off between practical considerations and psychometric standards has led to a rethinking of measurement strategy. Better measurement is measurement that has information one absolutely has to have, and no more. Towards these objectives I discuss here highly desirable trends toward increasing standardization of health-related quality of life concepts, the development of more practical assessment methods that can be used on a larger scale, and the creation of new databases that will facilitate improved understanding of how disease and treatment affect functional status, well-being, and other patient outcomes.

II. CONCEPTUAL ISSUES

At the risk of oversimplification, let us begin with the simple notion that life has two dimensions: quantity and quality. The distinction between them is well illustrated in the common greeting "may you have a long and health life." Quantity is expressed in terms of length of life, average life expectancy, mortality rates, deaths due to specific causes, and numerous other indicators.[12] In developed countries, these indicators are of little value in understanding the quality of years lived.[13] Thus, measurement of the second dimension of life requires another set of more qualitative indicators. It has become fashionable to equate health — defined comprehensively — with *quality of life*.[9,14-16] However, it is important to keep in mind that quality of life, as traditionally defined, is a much broader concept than health.[17] In addition to health, quality of life encompasses standard of living, the quality of housing and the neighborhood in which one lives, job satisfaction, and many other factors. A review of the content of survey instruments widely used in quality of life studies during the past decade underscores the importance of this distinction (e.g., References 18 and 19).

The popularity of the quality of life concept in the cancer field and in the health care literature in general is understandable, given the increasing comprehensiveness of health measures. While health used to be defined primarily in terms of death and the extent of morbidity (i.e., disease), the emerging conceptualization of health is far broader.[17,20] It encompasses how well people function in everyday life, emotional well-being, and personal evaluations of health in general. To distinguish the new conceptualization from the old, the term "quality of life" has been adopted. This practice has some utility. It provides a shorthand for making reference to a collection of concepts that are more qualitative than traditional clinical endpoints and it has facilitated discussions of these concepts in the literature on clinical trials and clinical practice (e.g., References 15 and 16).

Ultimately this use of the quality of life nomenclature is likely to cause some confusion because it is too encompassing. Jobs, housing, schools, and the neighborhood are not attributes of an individual's health and, relative to functional status and well-being, they overlap less with the purview of the health care system.[17,20]

A. DEFINING HEALTH

An important feature of health is its dimensionality. Health has distinct components, that must be measured and interpreted separately, to fully understand health at a point in time, as well as changes in health over time. What are these components? We find clues in definitions of health offered by the World Health Organization[21] as well as in dictionaries. The WHO defined health as a "state of complete physical, mental, and social well-being and not merely the absence of disease or infirmity." Dictionary definitions also identify both physical and mental dimensions of health. The former pertains to the body and bodily needs, the latter to the mind and particularly to the emotional and intellectual status of the individual. Health connotes "completeness" — nothing is missing from the person; it connotes "proper function" — all is working efficiently. The dictionary also suggests "well-being" — health includes "soundness" and "vitality." Thus, both the WHO and dictionary definitions provide clear precedents for the dimensionality of health and specifically for the distinction between physical and mental health. Empirical evidence in support of this distinction is also quite convincing.[20,22-23] Two features of these definitions are crucial; namely, the dimensionality of health and the full range of health states ranging from disease to well-being.

The range of health states assessed by a health measure is equally important. Many widely used measurement scales artificially restrict the range of individual differences in health they enumerate. Consistent with a disease orientation, most disease-specific measures emphasize the negative end of the health continuum. The result is a substantial loss of information. The situation is analogous to a scale for measuring weight that ends at 100 lb. All objects that weigh more are assigned the same score. This is satisfactory for a world where nothing weighs more than 100 lb or where differences above 100 lb are irrelevant. An important development during the past decade has been the construction of reliable scales that extend into the well-being range.

Thus, the second criterion recommended for evaluating a health status measure is the range of health levels that are defined. Scales that restrict the range of measurement, other considerations being equal, are inferior to scales that do not. Differences in health and changes in health over time will be measured more precisely, with corresponding gains in the power of hypothesis-testing, by scales that assess the full range of health states.[24] Two clues for evaluating this important feature are the distributions of scores observed in general and in patient populations, and the content of scale items. Measures that tap the full range of individual differences in health will yield distributions of scores with greater variability; fewer people will obtain the lowest or highest possible score.

III. A COMPREHENSIVE MEASUREMENT STRATEGY

Medical care providers collect data about functioning for virtually every bodily organ,

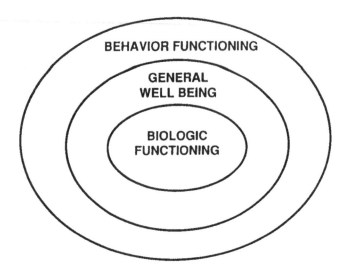

FIGURE 1.   Health status concepts.

but none of these measures tells about the function of the entire individual — which is certainly affected by disease and treatment (see Figure 1). Further, these measures of biologic phenomena cannot be used to characterize human phenomena. There simply aren't good algorithms for combining diverse biologic information to predict functioning and such algorithms are doomed to leave too much about quality of life unexplained. The most comprehensive models I have seen to date explain less than half of the reliable variance in, for example, physical functioning. Thus, biologic indicators are not adequate proxies for measures of functional status, well-being or other quality-of-life concepts or to changes in these variables over time.

A. DISEASE-SPECIFIC VS. GENERIC APPROACHES

Should we emphasize disease-specific or generic measures? Before proceeding, let me define what I mean by generic measures. Generic scales assess concepts that are relevant to everyone. They are not specific to any age, disease, or treatment group. Generic measures focus on such basic human values as the ability to function in everyday life and emotional well-being.

For most studies, the overwhelming answer to the question above is to use both generic and disease-specific measures and to analyze them together. We should not reject one database in favor of the other. We went through a period in the 1960s during which the validity of a patient rating a generic health concept was questioned when it did not agree with indicators of biologic functioning. The logic of validity has since been turned around. We are now entering an era in which the same findings are accepted as evidence for the necessity of including patient assessments in evaluations of patient outcomes. Patient assessments are necessary because the current medical record and provider judgments are not valid proxies for patient ratings of functioning, well-being, or other aspects of the quality of life.

We should not always expect assessments of different health components or clinical vs. generic measures to agree and they often don't. One example comes from a study of the effects of anti-hypertensive therapy on quality of life.[15] Therapies shown to be equally efficacious in terms of medical efficacy (i.e., blood pressure control) had significantly different quality of life profiles. In other words, it is possible to work with a patient in therapy to achieve a better quality-of-life outcome without compromising biologic function. The same logic applies to the treatment of cancer.

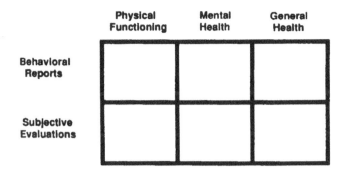

FIGURE 2.   Categories of health concepts and measures.

The greatest progress is going to occur, not by substituting one measurement or assessment strategy for another, but by mastering them in concert. We should not underestimate
the power of a database that includes measurements of biologic functioning familiar to
medical providers, measurements that they believe in because they have clinical validity,
in parallel with other measures of generic health concepts, not typically linked with such
measures in clinical practice or research. This is the most powerful strategy for analyzing
and understanding patient outcomes. Measuring disease-specific end-points, as well as a
common set of generic health outcomes for various conditions, will also contribute a new
database that will allow physicians to better inform patients about the quality-of-life trade-
offs involved in the pursuit of different clinical end-points.[25]

B. A MINIMUM SET OF GENERIC HEALTH CONCEPTS

At the risk of oversimplifying the past 40 years of health assessment research, I suggest
that most generic health measures fall into one of the six categories shown in Figure 2.
Included are three kinds of health concepts: physical functioning, mental health, and general
health perceptions. These concepts are often measured in terms of limitations in behavioral
functioning and measures or well-being or other more subjective personal evaluations. Specific examples are discussed below. Measures of physical limitations and disability due to
health focus on the more concrete, observable, tangible and objective category of health
measures. Measures in this category use a standard external to the individual, such as usual
role activity, walking at a certain rate, or customary self-care behaviors. This is the physical
function axis in a two-dimensional conceptualization of health. It is the concept that has
been preferred and best understood up until now. There are a number of well developed
measures of functioning available.

Interestingly, almost completely orthogonal to the physical functioning axis is the mental
health axis, which includes psychological distress, psychological well-being, and life satisfaction. In most populations individuals at all levels of the physical functioning axis are
observed at all levels of the mental health axis. This phenomenon is well illustrated in Figure
3, which shows a bivariate plot of physical functioning and mental health scores for 3445
patients with chronic conditions at the beginning of the Medical Outcomes Study (MOS).
(See Tarlov et al.[26] for details regarding MOS design and the characteristics of these patients.)
As illustrated in Figure 3, in most populations the correlation between physical functioning
and general mental health is relatively weak, only about 0.20 or less (assuming confounding
of measures across axes has been removed). Most people score above the midpoint on both
scales (the upper corner of Figure 3). Moving away from that corner we find people scattered
throughout the space defined by the two scales. In this range, one cannot predict the score
on one axis from the other.

The implication of Figure 3 is that one cannot know the physical and mental health

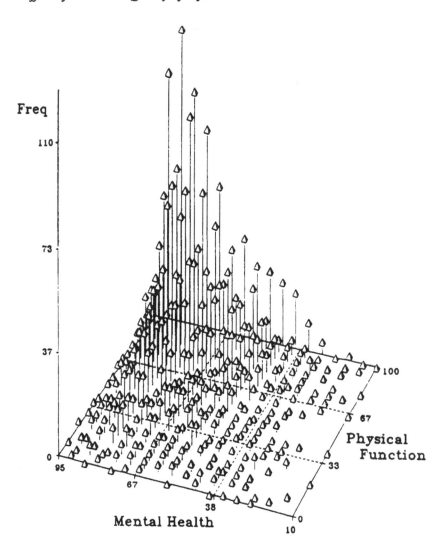

FIGURE 3.   Bivariate plot of physical functioning and mental health scores for patients
with chronic conditions at the beginning of the MOSP (see text).

benefits of treatment without measuring both. Consider two people sitting on a fencepost, for example. One may be experiencing a lot of pain and may have difficulty just sitting there. The other person may sit in ecstasy. In order to know, we have to ask them. It used to be thought that psychological distress and well-being couldn't be measured reliably. We have learned that quite reliable scores for the mental health axis can be obtained and that they add a completely different perspective to that gained from assessments of physical functioning.

Finally, there is a third concept — general health perceptions — which cuts across the physical and mental axes and introduces still another perspective. It includes measures that are personal evaluations of health, based on whatever health means to the respondent. This category of measures brings each person's own health values to the equation. He might be a mental-health oriented person or a physical-health oriented person. Health perceptions represent the third category necessary for comprehensiveness among generic health measures.

IV. THE CONTENT OF HEALTH SURVEYS

In addition to minimum standards for measurement models that claim to be comprehensive, other issues are crucial to the orderly advancement of the field of health assessment. The degree of correspondence between the words used to label health scales and indexes and the actual content of the questionnaire items from which they are constructed is also very important. We are inclined to label measures in terms of what we want them to measure.

With the goal of facilitating resolution of these issues, some of the more important and frequently measured health concepts are discussed below along with examples of specific questionnaire items from the published literature. Included are physical functioning, social and role functioning, mental health, and general health perceptions. These concepts have important features in common. First, each is generic as defined above and, thus, should be seriously considered for inclusion in studies of cancer and other conditions regardless of the treatment in question or the age of the population of interest. Second, each is distinct both conceptually and in terms of the patterns of empirical results that are generated.[22] Therefore, there is likely to be value in measuring and interpreting each concept separately prior to aggregation.

Comments about these concepts presented below are based on the author's experience in trying to measure them and on reviews of the published literature. A thorough review of the rather substantial body of literature that has accumulated about these concepts is beyond the scope of this paper. Observations about the content of published measures and empirical results are discussed elsewhere for physical and role functioning,[27] general mental health,[24] social functioning[28-29] and perceptions of health in general.[30] In addition to results discussed in these reviews, empirical evidence supporting distinctions among the five concepts includes multivariate analyses of associations among health measures[22,30] and multivariate studies that used measures of these concepts to predict consumption of general medical services[31] and mental health services,[32] and health transitions over 3- and 5-year intervals.[33-34] In all applications, independent measures of these concepts made unique contributions to the predictive models evaluated. Thus, each measure contributes information about health not captured by measures of the other concepts.

The five generic health concepts are defined below and some comments about their measurement are offered. Examples of questionnaire items that appear consistent with the definitions appear in Table 1. Items were selected to represent the full range of health states defined by each concept as well as measures of both behavioral dysfunction and more subjective evaluations of each concept.

A. PHYSICAL HEALTH

Physical health is commonly measured in terms of limitations in the performance of or ability to perform self-care activities (e.g., eating, bathing, dressing), mobility, moderate and more strenuous physical activities and bodily pain. Responses to questionnaire items in this category are generally more valid if respondents are instructed to focus on limitations due to *physical* health problems as opposed to some other cause.

The physical health items in Table 1 vary in terms of the range of differences in functioning that are assessed. For example, items that assess self-care (e.g., limitations in eating, dressing, bathing, or using the toilet) assess the negative end of the continuum, which is very important because of the consequences of these limitations. In studies of the severely ill, an extensive battery of measures focused on self-care limitations may be appropriate.[35-36] Items that measure these limitations should be used sparingly in studies of general populations, for whom self-care limitations are relatively rare.[27]

Some items assess important qualitative features of different physical health states. Others tap individual differences in level of effort, pain, difficulty, or need for assistance in per-

TABLE 1
Items Measuring Generic Health Concepts

Concepts	Definition	Abbreviated items	Ref.
Physical			
Physical limitations	Limitations in performance of self-care, mobility, and physical activities	Needs help with bathing, dressing In bed, chair, couch, for most of day Do not walk at all	Katz et al.[35] Kaplan, Bush, and Berry[61] Bergner et al.[44]
Physical abilities	Ability to perform everyday activities	Able to walk uphill, upstairs Able to participate in sports, strenuous activities	Hulka and Cassel[62] Stewart et al.[37]
Days in bed	Confinement to bed due to health problems	During past 30 days, number of days health keeps one in bed all day or most of day	NCHS[12]
Bodily pain	Ratings of the intensity, duration, and frequency of bodily pain and limitations in usual activities due to pain	During the past 3 months, how much pain have you had? How much pain interfered with things	NCHS[12] Daut, Cleeland, and Randall[63]
Physical well-being	Personal evaluation of physical condition	Ratings of physical shape or condition	Dupuy[39] Chambers et al.[64]
Social and Role			
Interpersonal contacts	Frequency of visits with friends and relatives	Number of friends visited Going out less often to visit people	Donald and Ware[28] Bergner et al.[44]
	Frequency of telephone contacts with close friends or relatives during specific period of time	How often on telephone with close friends/relatives, past month	Donald and Ware[28]
Social resources	Quantity and quality of social ties, network	Number of close friends, people to talk with	Donald and Ware[28]
Role functioning	Freedom from limitations in performance of usual role activities (e.g., work, housework, school) due to poor health	Limited in kind or amount of major role activity Working shorter hours Health causes problems at work Unable to work because of health	NCHS[12] Bergner et al.[44] Hunt[65] Stewart et al.[37]
Mental			
Anxiety/depression	Feelings of anxiety, nervousness, tenseness, depression, moodiness, downheartedness	Depressed or very unhappy Bothered by nervousness or nerves	Bradburn[66] Dupuy[39,40]
Psychological well-being	Frequency and intensity of general positive affect	Happy, pleased, satisfied with life Wake up expecting an interesting day Feel cheerful, lighthearted	Dupuy[39,40] Costello and Comrey[67] Veit and Ware[68]

TABLE 1 (continued)
Items Measuring Generic Health Concepts

Concepts	Definition	Abbreviated items	Ref.
Behavioral/emotional control	Control of behavior, thoughts, and feelings during specified period	Felt emotionally stable Lose control of behavior, thoughts, feelings Laugh or cry suddenly	Dupuy[39,40] Veit and Ware[68] Bergner et al.[44]
Cognitive functioning	Orientation to time and place, memory, attention span, and alertness	Feel confused, forget a lot, make more mistakes than usual	Bergner et al.[44]

General Health Perceptions

Concepts	Definition	Abbreviated items	Ref.
Current health	Self-rating of health at present	In general, is health excellent, good, fair, or poor? Energy, pep, vitality Been feeling bad lately	NCHS[12] Dupuy[39] Davies and Ware[30]
Health outlook	Expectations regarding health in the future	I expect to have a very health life	Ware[69]

forming physical activities.[37-38] If asked only whether they perform a given set of physical activities, two individuals may give identical responses, although they may differ substantially in responses to more qualitative measures of effort and suffering. The latter measures enhance precision. Precision for tests of hypotheses about physical health can also be enhanced by the addition of measures tapping pain, physical well-being, energy level, vitality, and satisfaction with physical shape or condition.[22,38-40]

B. SOCIAL AND ROLE FUNCTIONING

As illustrated in Table 1, social functioning includes two distinct concepts:[28-29] social contacts and other activities (e.g., visits with friends and relatives), and social ties or resources (e.g., close friends and relatives that can be relied upon for tangible and intangible support). Social contacts are the more directly observable of the two concepts. Measures of social contacts can be criticized for their failure to assess how social events are personally experienced. Counting social activities is analogous to counting feelings without reference to whether they were good or bad. Personal evaluations are therefore necessary to tap the quality of social contacts, a more relevant concept.[29]

Social resources cannot be directly observed. The quality of resources can be judged only by the individual, and that quality is best measured by asking about it directly. Measures of social resources represent personal evaluations of the adequacy of interpersonal relationships, including ties to people who will listen to personal problems and provide tangible support and needed companionship. People who are satisfied with their social resources feel "plugged in" or "connected" with others; they feel cared for, loved and wanted.[41]

Role functioning refers to the performance of or capacity to perform usual role activities; included are formal employment, school work, and housework (see Table 1). Although discussions of health concepts sometimes interchange the concepts of role and social functioning,[42-43] they are distinct and should be interpreted separately. In most populations, limitations in role performance are due to physical health problems. Effects of psychological impairment on role performance are more likely to be detected by role functioning measures that explicitly ask about limitations due to personal and emotional problems. In keeping with this argument, the measures of role functioning included in the 1990 census ask about role limitations due to both physical and emotional problems.

Role performance reflects physical health and the demands of usual role activity. Thus, the effect of disease and treatment would be expected to vary more for role functioning than for physical functioning. Role limitations are observed both in the presence and in the absence of physical limitations.[27] Pending further research, it may be best to measure and interpret measures of physical and role limitations separately. Standardized measures that distinguish the two concepts are available for this purpose.[27,44]

C. MENTAL HEALTH

While differences in physical health are often manifested in behavioral performance, mental health encompasses emotional and intellectual states that may or may not be revealed by overt behavior. For this reason, general mental health measures include subjective assessments of the frequency and intensity of symptoms of psychological distress, psychological well-being and cognitive functioning.[28,40,44] The most efficient way to assess these concepts for most people is to ask them about them directly.

The distinction between behavioral self-reports and self-ratings of the intensity and frequency of feeling states is not always great, as illustrated by a comparison of items from the Sickness Impact Profile (e.g., "act nervous") and the Mental Health Inventory (e.g., "be nervous").[28,45] Not surprisingly, these measures are substantially correlated.[46] A noteworthy feature of comprehensive general measures of mental health is the range of differences they tap throughout the mental health continuum and specifically the inclusion of items assessing psychological well-being.[28,39,45,47-49]

Most measures published prior to 1970[50-52] were insensitive to differences in levels of well-being among those free of psychological distress.[45] Clinically and socially relevant changes in mental health are not always captured by measures of psychological distress. The impact of cancer and other conditions may be to "take the top off" of a person's life. Life becomes less enjoyable or less interesting; there is less about which to be happy and cheerful. Capturing this effect among those who are otherwise free of psychological distress requires items that assess psychological well-being.

General mental health items such as those in Table 1 may not be appropriate for diagnosing specific mental disorders, although some scales with similar item content have proven useful in screening.[49,53] Interview schedules designed to standardize the diagnosis of selected mental disorders including the Diagnostic Interview Schedule[54] and the Schedule for Affective Disorders and Schizophrenia[55] are also appropriate for this purpose.

The third important mental health concept illustrated in Table 1 is cognitive functioning. This concept includes orientation with respect to time and place and such mental processes as memory, comprehension, abstract reasoning, and problem solving.[56-57] Kane and Kane[36] have reviewed available measures of cognitive functioning.

D. GENERAL HEALTH PERCEPTIONS

Self-ratings of health in general are among the most commonly used measures of health.[30] Almost everyone has been asked to provide a rating of his health as "excellent," "very good," "good," "fair," or "poor".[2] These measures are based on the notion that your health is what you think it is. They are considered *ratings* because they reflect individual differences in the evaluation of information people have about their health. They are considered measures of *general* health because they do not focus on a specific dimension of health, and because they have been linked empirically to all of the four health concepts defined above.[30]

There are two good reasons to measure general health perceptions with items such as those in the fifth section of Table 1. First, personal evaluations of health experiences are not completely captured by items in the other four sections. For example, reports of behavioral performance do not capture important subjective manifestations of differences in health such as health outlook, worry, and concern about health. Second, because measures of limitations or behavioral dysfunctions are inherently negative, they do not extend measurement into the well-being range. Thus, to satisfy the second criterion of content validity — measuring the full range of health status — measures of general health perceptions that include self-assessments of health, feelings of well-being, energy level, and vitality are required.

V. STANDARDS FOR EVALUATING MORE PRACTICAL MEASURES

With support from the Kaiser Family Foundation, my colleagues and I are now comparing the briefest forms of measurement, e.g., the best single-item measure, with longer but still short multi-item scales, and with some of the best full-length research versions of those scales. Our question is how well does a more brief measure work relative to much longer measures used in research? Not surprisingly, preliminary findings indicate that longer measures do better. However, the question should be: "Do shorter measures do well enough?" The answer is very important because the most psychometrically elegant instrument is useless if it is impractical to use. Thus, we should be very interested in how briefer measures do in these comparisons.

On what basis should measure be compared and how do we construct them in the first place? There are a number of things wrong with what we traditionally do in psychometrics; take reliability as an example. Reliability is important, but we learned quickly that while reliability is a prerequisite, there are other attributes of a score (scale) that are equally or more important. In comparing scales, most important are tests that closely approximate the intended use of the scale. Unfortunately patterns of traditional reliability and validity coefficients often bear little or no relationship to the results from actual applications of measures.

Some attributes of measures typically ignored include things like how many different scores are possible. An enumeration system that puts people into one of four levels or categories with a reliability of 0.90 isn't as valuable as is one that puts people into ten categories with the same reliability. This particular attribute of measurement may not prove critical in a cross-sectional analysis comparing things as different, as for example, Volkswagens and trucks. The latter is analogous to comparing disease groups that differ a lot. Most measures do well in that kind of comparison. When we start measuring change in health over time, however, this issue becomes crucial. How much change can occur within a given health category before the person changes to the next category? The number of levels of measurement is a very important attribute or measure. This attribute is almost never discussed in books on health assessment.

Another important and related issue is simply how many people get the lowest or the highest possible score for a given measure. If 90% of the people in a long-term care facility have the worst possible score before a cost-containment strategy is implemented, you don't have precision for showing a worsening in their condition as a result. If 80% of the people earn the highest possible score on a physical health index (as they did in the Health Insurance Experiment), and we randomly assign them to free care, we don't have much chance of determining whether there is any benefit of free care using that particular measure. Fortunately, this wasn't the only measure used in that experiment.[58] I suggest that we routinely report how many people get the lowest and the highest possible scores when measures are published as well as the number of scores possible, in addition to reliability coefficients.

The same logic should apply to results regarding validity; it is extremely important that the kind of analysis used to judge the validity of a measure approximate as closely as possible the intended use of the measure in medical practice, a clinical trial, or a policy study. One example of what I mean is the issue of whether a given questionnaire is sensitive to the extent and nature of differences in functional status and well-being across groups of patients with different chronic conditions. My colleagues and I recently reported an example of such

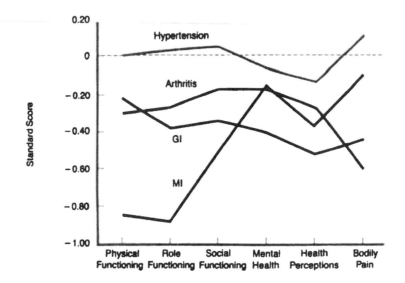

FIGURE 4.   Health profiles for patients with four conditions. Dotted line indicates patients with no chronic conditions; GI, gastrointestinal disorder; and MI, myocardial infarction.

comparisons in evaluating the validity of the 20-item MOS short-form survey.[7] Figure 4 presents examples of profiles for patients with four different chronic conditions at a point in time when the study began. Each profile is expressed as standard score deviations from the averages for well patients (represented by the horizontal dotted line). The first three data points (columns) for each disease are defined by functional status scales, the last three by well-being scales. We have connected the points across scales for each disease to help identify a particular disease profile. These are scored so that the lower the profile on the scales the worse the profile.

Figure 4 generally confirms clinical wisdom about the impact of these diseases. Not surprisingly, patients with hypertension (the top profile in Figure 4) function no differently than well patients. The only significant decrement was their score for health perceptions. Patients with hypertension tend to believe their health is worse. Arthritis has the most pain. Physical, role, and social functioning is poor for MI survivors and tends to be as bad as, if not worse than, any of the nine chronic conditions we have studied to date.

One of the lessons from this is that, on average, the patient point of view is valid. Further, even very brief measures can be used to measure differences in health across groups of patients. The questionnaire used to estimate scores in Figure 4 was administered to about 12,000 patients while waiting in a doctor's office, in about $3^{1}/_{2}$ min each.

Relative to available full-length research instruments, including our own, this short-form has one fifth to one tenth the number of questionnaire items. Yet it is valid in that it produced a pattern of results that make sense from a clinical point of view. One surprising finding (not shown in Figure 4) is the very low profile of scores for patients with depression, including those with a psychiatric diagnosis and those suffering with symptoms of depression. They scored very low on these scales relative to other chronic diseases, suggesting that the burden of depression may have been underestimated to date.[53]

Of course, other kinds of tests are necessary before conclusions are drawn about candidate measures. How well does a questionnaire distinguish differences in functional status and well-being across groups differing in severity within a diagnostic category? Research in progress within the MOS is encouraging in this regard. For example, in preliminary analyses of MOS data, average functional status scores for diabetics differing in severity (e.g., with or without renal failure) show ordinal consistency in relation to clinical severity. Thus, these measures may be sensitive to differences in severity within a diagnostic group. This kind of analysis does not prove that if treatment moved people from severity level five to level three, we would see a corresponding change in functioning. This example is based on a cross-sectional analysis. We are currently linking measures of actual change in disease severity over time with measures of change in functional status and well-being. This is another example of a validity test that more closely approximates the intended use of a measure. Again, preliminary results are encouraging.

VI. A NEW ERA OF HEALTH ASSESSMENT

The potential of generic measures of functional status, well-being, and other health-related quality of life concepts, even short forms, to be used successfully across a wide range of purposes is illustrated by the Vitality Scale used in the MOS. This four-item scale, which takes about 1 min to complete, is based on the work of Dupuy.[38] It measures a continuum of energy vs. fatigue. Its early history, which is documented-in-part elsewhere,[24] includes successful use in a general population health survey about 15 years ago,[38] the Health Insurance Experiment,[24] a more recent clinical trial comparing antihypertensive therapies,[15] and across groups of patients with very different chronic medical and psychiatric conditions in the MOS.[58] Its track record defies the notion that completely different measures are needed for different applications. This scale illustrates the potential of a standardized generic measure, in this case a 1-min vitality scale, for the purpose of describing the young and the old in the U.S. population, the sick and the well, and in measuring outcomes across homogeneous groups of patients receiving different treatments in a randomized trial.

Generic concepts and standardized measures of patient perspectives regarding health status are unifying concepts. They are common denominators, for purposes of comparisons across age, disease, and treatment groups. The health measurement dollar in this country would buy far more useful information if definitions and measurements of health concepts were more often standardized across clinical trials in the cancer field and other fields as well as in general population surveys. There is some evidence that the idea of standardization is taking hold. The 1988 health supplement for the National Center for Health Statistics (NCHS) survey for children includes some standardized psychometric scales that have been used before only in trials and other research projects. As a result, we will soon have a much better data base for purposes of comparison between data for patients and general population data. For example, if the NCHS scales were included in studies of children with cancer, the burden of the disease and the benefits of treatment could be better understood by comparing results from cancer trials against national norms.

A second major area of application of generic health assessment is in health policy evaluations. The health care system is being restructured in this country, largely in response to rising health care costs. Even those attributes of the basic structure of the health care system previously assumed to be stable are being manipulated with the goal of cost containment. Although some may claim otherwise, no one knows which features of which systems of health care delivery are essential and therefore ought to be preserved in the interest of obtaining the best possible outcomes for patients. Cost-containment strategies must be evaluated in terms of their impact on patient health outcomes. One quite tangible step in this direction is a law recently passed by the U.S. Congress — the Outcomes Assessment Research Act of 1989. This legislation created a new agency — The Agency for Health Care Policy and Research — and calls for measurement of functional status, well being, and satisfaction with care along with other end points to evaluate policies that affect patient outcomes. The budget for this effort is about $600 million over the next 5 years. Health care management is another area. The emphasis here is on how to achieve the best

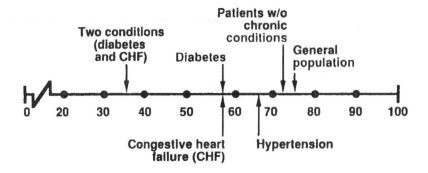

FIGURE 5.   Relative burden of chronic conditions in terms of general health perceptions.

value for each health care dollar. However, no one knows what the values are. The purchasers of health care services want to know why they can't pay less for services when someone offers to charge less. Managers could well use outcome information to help organize and set priorities more effectively. Again, this requires a new health care database with information about both the costs of care as well as patient outcomes.

There is also the opportunity to use standardized patient surveys of functional status and well-being in everyday medical practice. For me, this is one of the most promising applications of standardized patient surveys. Assuming that the central goal of medical care to get the best possible outcome for a patient, the question then becomes how can that happen without monitoring outcomes in terms that matter most to patients, namely, routine measurement of functional status and well being concepts? Seemingly, information about a patient's status on these different concepts at the outset of diagnosis or treatment, as well as along the way, would lead to a better outcome. However, physicians and other health care providers may need special training to use this information and to effectively manage patients with the goal of maximizing their functioning. With this goal in mind, The American College of Physicians[8] has asked that patients' medical histories be standardized to include routine functional status and well-being assessment.

Ideally, we would like to estimate the burden of disease and the benefits of treatment in comparable units. For example, imagine enumerating a continuum that looks something like the scale in Figure 5. This figure presents a 0 to 100 general health rating scale; 0 and 100 are the lowest and highest possible scores, respectively. This is an example of one of many functional status and well-being scales. We first indicate where the general population falls on the scale (see the right-most arrow in Figure 5), using data published elsewhere.[7] Only slightly (but significantly) lower on this scale are patients without chronic conditions who were assessed while in doctors offices. Still lower on the scale are estimates for those with hypertension, diabetes, and congestive heart failure (CHF). The combined impact of two conditions is illustrated by the left-most arrow for patients suffering from both diabetes and CHF. Of course, patients within each diagnostic group would be expected to differ substantially depending on their severity level. Other factors (comorbid conditions, age, and other sociodemographic variables) can be controlled for in making these estimates (for examples[7]).

Where do the various cancers fall along a generic continuum like that in Figure 5? Where would cancer patients score on scales defining other functional status and well-being concepts? How does the burden of the various cancers compare with each other and with that of other diseases that the cancers may have to compete with for resources in an era of cost containment? What are the benefits of various cancer therapies in these terms, relative to the therapeutic benefits possible for other conditions?

During the 1990s, clinical investigators and those in medical practice will be held increasingly accountable for knowing and justifying what they do in terms of patient outcomes — in terms of the value of a given research program as well as the value of a given treatment program. The implications of different health care policies for patient outcomes, not just expenditures, will also be judged. This era has been termed the "third revolution in medical care".[60] Our challenge is to better integrate information about the quality of life concepts that are most important to patients into clinical research and into everyday medical practice with the goal of achieving the best possible outcome for each patient and the best possible value for each health care dollar.

ACKNOWLEDGMENTS

Preparation of this chapter was supported by grants from the Henry J. Kaiser Family Foundation for the use of functional status and well-being scales in medical practice and clinical research and from the John A. Hartford Foundation of New York for the dissemination of information about how to measure the quality of health care outcomes.

The Medical Outcomes Study (MOS) has been sponsored by grants from the Henry J. Kaiser Family Foundation, the Robert Wood Johnson Foundation, the Pew Charitable Trusts, the Agency for Health Care Policy and Research, the National Institute on Aging, and the National Institute of Mental Health.

The author gratefully acknowledges the contributions of his MOS colleagues and consultants, including Sharon Arnold, Ph.D., Sandra H. Berry, M.A., M. Audrey Burnam, Ph.D., Maureen Carney, M.S., Judith Perlman, Allyson Ross Davies, Ph.D., Toshi Hayashi, Ron D. Hays, Ph.D., Willard G. Manning, Ph.D., Elizabeth McGlynn, Ph.D., Eugene C. Nelson, Sc.D., Lynn Ordway, Edward B. Perrin, Ph.D., William Rogers, Ph.D., Cathy Sherbourne, Ph.D., Anita L. Stewart, Ph.D., Alvin R. Tarlov, M.D., Kenneth B. Wells, M.D., M.P.H., and Michael Zubkoff, Ph.D. He also gratefully acknowledges the administrative support of Kathy Clark, who also assisted in preparing this manuscript.

REFERENCES

1. **Geigle, R. and Jones, S. B.,** Outcomes measurement: a report from the front, *Inquiry*, 27, 7, 1990.
2. **McDermott, W.,** Absence of indicators of the influence of physicians on a society's health, *Am. J. Med.*, 70, 833, 1981.
3. **Cluff, L. E.,** Chronic disease, function and the quality of care, *J. Chronic Dis.*, 34, 299, 1981.
4. **Tarlov, A. R.,** Shattuck Lecture: The increasing supply of physicians, the changing structure of the health-services system, and the future practice of medicine, *N. Engl. J. Med.*, 308, 1235, 1983.
5. **Shroeder, S. A.,** Outcome assessment 70 years later: are we ready?, *N. Engl. J. Med.*, 216, 160, 1987.
6. **Ellwood, P. M.,** Outcomes management: a technology of patient experience, *N. Engl. J. Med.*, 318, 1549, 1988.
7. **Stewart, A. L., Greenfield, S., Hays, R. D., et al.,** Functional status and well-being of patients with chronic conditions: results from the medical outcomes study, *JAMA*, 262, 907, 1989.
8. **American Cancer Society,** Proceedings of the working conference on methodology in behavioral and psychosocial cancer research — 1983, *Cancer*, 53 (Suppl.), 2217, 1984.
9. **Wenger, N. K., Mattson, M. E., Furberg, C. D., et al.,** *Assessment of Quality of Life in Clinical Trials of Cardiovascular Therapies*, Le Jack, New York, 1984.
10. **Lohr, K. N. and Ware, J. E.,** Advances in health assessment, special issue, *J. Chronic Dis.*, 40 (Suppl. 1), 193, 1987.
11. **Lohr, K. N.,** Advances in health status assessment: overview of the conference, *Med. Care*, 27, 1989.
12. **NCHS:** Health. United States, U.S. Dept. of Health and Human Services, 1981.
13. **Elinson, J.,** Introduction to the theme: sociomedical health indicators, in *Socio-Medical Health Indicators*, Elinson, J. and Siegmann, A. E., Eds., Baywood, Farmingdale, NY, 1979, 3.
14. **Wenger, N. K.,** The concept of quality of life, *Q. Life Cardiovasc. Care*, 1, 8, 1984.

15. Croog, S. H., Levine, S., Testa, M. A., et al., The effects of antihypertensive therapy on the quality of life, *N. Engl. J. Med.*, 314, 1657, 1986.

16. Chobanian, A. V., Editorial, antihypertensive therapy in evolution, *N. Engl. J. Med.*, 314, 1701, 1986.

17. Ware, J. E., Methodological considerations in the selection of health status assessment procedures, in *Assessment of Quality of Life in Clinical Trials of Cardiovascular Disease*, Wenger, N. K., et al., Eds., Le Jacq, New York, 1984, 87.

18. Campbell, A., Converse, P. E., and Rodgers, W. L., *The Quality of American Life*, Russell Sage Foundation, New York, 1976.

19. Andrews, F. M. and Withey, S. B., *Social Indicators of Well-Being*, Plenum Press, New York, 1976.

20. Ware, J. E., The assessment of health status, in *Applications of Social Science to Clinical Medicine and Health Policy*, Aiken, L. H. and Mechanic, D., Eds., Rutgers University Press, New Brunswick, NJ, 1986, 204.

21. World Health Organization: Constitution of World Health Organization, in *Basic Documents*, WHO, Geneva, 1948.

22. Ware, J. E., Davies-Avery, A., and Brook, R. H., *Conceptualization and Measurement of Health for Adults in the Health Insurance Study*, Vol. VI, Rand Corporation (R-1987/6-HEW), Santa Monica, CA, 1980.

23. Hays, R. D. and Stewart, A. L., The structure of self-reported health in chronic disease patients, *J. Consult. Clin. Psychol.*, 2, 1, 22, 1990.

24. Ware, J. E., Johnston, S. A., Davies-Avery, A., et al., *Conceptualization and Measurement of Health for Adults in the Health Insurance Study*, Vol. III, Rand Corporation (R-1987/3-HEW), Santa Monica, CA, 1979.

25. Fowler, F. J., Jr., Wennberg, J. E., Timothy, R. P., et al., Status and quality of life following prostatectomy, *JAMA*, 259, 3018, 1988.

26. Tarlov, A. R., Ware, J. E., Greenfield, S., et al., The medical outcomes study: an application of methods for monitoring the results of medical care, *JAMA*, 262, 7, 925, 1989.

27. Stewart, A. L., Ware, J. E., Brook, R. H., et al., *Conceptualization and Measurement of Physical Health for Adults in the Health Insurance Study*, Vol. II, Rand Corporation (R-1987/3-HEW), Santa Monica, CA, 1979.

28. Donald, C. A., Ware, J. E., Brook, R. H., et al., *Conceptualization and Measurement of Health for Adults in the Health Insurance Study*, Vol. IV, Rand Corporation (R-1987/3-HEW), Santa Monica, CA, 1978.

29. Donald, C. A. and Ware, J. E., The measurement of social support, in *Research and Community Mental Health*, Greenley, J. R., Ed., JAI Press, Greenwich, CT, 1984, 325.

30. Davies, A. R. and Ware, J. E., *Measuring Health Perceptions in the Health Insurance Experiment*, Rand Corporation (R-2711-HHS), Santa Monica, CA, 1981.

31. Manning, W. G., Newhouse, J. P., and Ware, J. E., The status of health in demand estimation; or beyond excellent, good, fair, poor, in *Economic Aspects of Health*, Fuchs, V. R., Ed., Chicago: University of Chicago Press, Chicago, 1982, 143.

32. Ware, J. E., Manning, W. G., Duan, N., et al., Health status and the use of outpatient mental health services, *Am. Psychol.*, 39, 1090, 1984.

33. Brook, R. H., Ware, J. E., Rogers, W. H., et al., *The Effect of Coinsurance on the Health of Adults*, Rand Corporation (R-30550HHS), Santa Monica, CA, 1984.

34. Ware, J. E., Brook, R. H., Rogers, W. H., et al., *Health Outcomes for Adults in Prepaid and Fee-for-Service Systems of Care: Results from the Health Insurance Experiment*, Rand Corporation (R-3459-HHS), Santa Monica, CA, in press.

35. Katz, S., Ford, A. B., Moskowitz, R. W., et al., Studies of illness in the aged, *JAMA*, 185, 94, 1963.

36. Kane, R. A. and Kane, R. L., *Assessing the Elderly*, Lexington Books, Lexington, MA, 1981.

37. Stewart, A. L., Ware, J. E., and Brook, R. H., Advances in the measurement of functional status: construction of aggregate indexes, *Med. Care*, 19, 473, 1981.

38. Jette, A. M., Functional capacity evaluation: an empirical approach, *Arch. Phys. Med. Rehabil.*, 61, 85, 1980.

39. Dupuy, H. J., The psychological section of the current Health and Nutrition Examination Survey, Proc. Public Health Conference on Records and Statistics Meeting Jointly with the National Conference on Health Statistics, National Conference on Health Statistics, Washington, D.C., 1972.

40. Dupuy, H. J., The psychological general well-being (PGWB) index, in *Assessment of Quality of Life in Clinical Trials of Cardiovascular Therapies*, Wenger, N. K. et al., Eds., Le Jacq, New York, 1984, 170.

41. Cobb, S., Social support as a moderator of life stress, *Psychosom. Med.*, 38, 300, 1976.

42. Patrick, D. L., Bush, J. W., and Chen, M. M., Methods for measuring levels of well-being for a health status index, *Health Serv. Res.*, 8, 228, 1973.

43. Reynolds, W. J., Rushing, W. A., and Miles, D. L., The validation of a functional status index, *J. Health Soc. Behav.*, 15, 271, 1974.

44. **Bergner, M., Bobbitt, R. A., Pollard, W. E., et al.**, The sickness impact profile: validation of a health status measure, *Med. Care*, 14, 57, 1976.

45. **Veit, C. T. and Ware, J. E.**, The structure of psychological distress and well-being in general populations, *J. Consult. Clin. Psychol.*, 51, 730, 1983.

46. **Hall, J.**, Personal communication, Department of Community Medicine, Westmead Center, The Paramatta Hospitals, Westmead, Australia, January 1986.

47. **Bradburn, N. M.**, *The Structure of Psychological Well-Being*, Aldine, Chicago, 1969.

48. **Radloff, L. S.**, The CES-D scale: a self-report depression scale for research in the general population, *Appl. Psychol. Meas.*, 3, 385, 1977.

49. **Goldberg, D.**, *Manual of the General Health Questionnaire*, NFER, Windsor, England, 1978.

50. **Macmillanm, A. M.**, The health opinion survey: technique for estimating prevalence of psychoneurotic and related types of disorder in communities, *Psychol. Rep.*, 3, 325, 1957.

51. **Gurin, G., Veroff, J., and Field, S.**, *Americans View Their Mental Health — A Nationwide Interview Survey*, Basic Books, New York, 1960.

52. **Langner, T. S.**, A twenty-two item screening score of psychiatric symptoms indicating impairment, *J. Health Hum. Behav.*, 3, 269, 1962.

53. **Wells, K. B., Stewart, A. L., Hays, R. D., et al.**, Detection of depressive disorder for patients receiving prepaid or fee-for-service care: results from the medical outcomes study, *JAMA*, 262(23), 3298, 1989.

54. **Robins, L. N., Helzer, J. E., Coughan, J., et al.**, National Institute of Mental Health Diagnostic Interview Schedule: its history, characteristics, and validity, *Arch. Gen. Psychiatry*, 38, 381, 1981.

55. **Endicott, J. and Spitzer, R. L.**, A diagnostic interview: the schedule for affective disorders and schizophrenia, *Arch. Gen. Psychiatry*, 35, 837, 1978.

56. **Folstein, M. F., Folstein, S., and McHugh, P. R.**, Mini-mental state: a practical method for grading the cognitive state of patients for the clinician, *J. Psychiatr. Res.*, 12, 189, 1975.

57. **Dohrenwend, B. P., Levay, I., and Shrout, P. E.**, Screening scales from the Psychiatric Epidemiology Research Interview (PERI), in *Community Surveys*, Myers, J. K. and Weissman, M. H., Eds., Rutgers University Press, New Brunswick, NJ, 1983.

58. **Brook, R. H., Ware, J. E., Rogers, W. R., et al.**, Does free care improve adults' health? Results from randomized controlled trial, *N. Engl. J. Med.*, 309(23), 1426, 1983.

59. **Stewart, A. L. and Ware, J. E.**, Eds., Measuring Functional Status and Well-Being: The Medical Outcomes Study Approach, in preparation.

60. **Relman, A. S.**, Assessment and accountability: the third revolution in medical care, *N. Engl. J. Med.*, 319, 1220, 1988.

61. **Kaplan, R. M., Bush, J. W., and Berry, C. C.**, Health status: types of validity and the index of well-being, *Health Serv. Res.*, 11, 478, 1976.

62. **Hulka, B. S. and Cassel, J. C.**, The AAFP-UNC study of the organization, utilization and assessment of primary medical care, *Am. J. Public Health*, 63, 494, 1973.

63. **Daut, R. L., Cleeland, C. S., and Flanery, R. C.**, Development of the Wisconsin brief pain questionnaire to assess pain in cancer and other disease, *Pain*, 17, 197, 1983.

64. **Chambers, L. W., MacDonald, L. A., Tugwell, P., et al.**, The McMaster Health Index Questionnaire as a measure of quality of life for patients with rheumatoid disease, *J. Rheumatol.*, 9, 780, 1982.

65. **Hunt, S. M., McEwen, J., Mckenna, S. P., et al.**, The Nottingham Health Profile: Subject health status and medical consultations, *Soc. Sci. Med.*, 15A, 221, 1981.

66. **Bradburn, N. M.**, *The Structure of Psychological Well-Being*, Aldine, Chicago, 1969.

67. **Costello, C. G. and Comrey, A. L.**, Scales for measuring depression and anxiety, *J. Psychol.*, 66, 303, 1967.

68. **Veit, C. T. and Ware, J. E.**, The structure of psychological distress and well-being in general populations, *J. Consult. Clin. Psychol.*, 51, 730, 1983.

69. **Ware, J. E.**, Scales for measuring general health perceptions, *Health Serv. Res.*, 11, 396, 1976.

Chapter 3

MEASURING THE EFFECT OF CANCER ON QUALITY OF LIFE

David Osoba

TABLE OF CONTENTS

I. THE EFFECT OF CANCER ON QUALITY OF LIFE

Diseases desperate grown
By desperate appliance are relieved,
Or not at all.

William Shakespeare[1]

Whether or not Shakespeare had cancer in mind when he penned these words, there is no doubt that cancer fits the description of diseases "desperate grown", and that present-day attempts to cure them is often "by desperate appliance" or they are "relieved . . . not at all."

The effects of cancer are felt at many levels, ranging from the global level to the national level and, most poignantly, at the level of the individual. At the national level it is estimated that one in three Canadians will develop cancer during their lifetimes and one in four will die of it.[2] These estimates are probably also true for most other economically developed countries. When added to the costs of treatment and care, the lost person-years of life with the attendant loss of productivity have an enormous impact on the economy of a nation. However, the effects on individuals and families go beyond effects measured only in economic terms. The loss of health with the resultant deficits in physical function, sense of well-being, and social interaction, often accompanied by physical, emotional, and spiritual suffering, all affect quality of life. In addition, despite improvements in survival for some forms of cancer, it is still highly feared, invoking not only the vision of the suffering associated with the disease, but also of the suffering associated with its treatment.

Before the era of surgery the major factor affecting quality of life was the disease itself, although the administration of various ineffective physics and drugs must have had "side effects" as well. With the use of surgery, followed by the introduction of radiation therapy, chemotherapy, and modern biological therapy, patients have had to deal with new and varied toxicities of these treatments. Although some of the most mutilating surgery, such as hemicorporectomy, is rarely done now, the effects of radical surgery in the head and neck region, on the breast, or on the limbs are still experienced by many patients. The side effects of chemotherapy (nausea and vomiting, hair loss, fatigue, mucositis, neuropathy, and infection to mention only a few) are a major concern and may lead to noncompliance with potentially curative therapy. Radiation therapy also produces side effects of varying severity depending on which part of the body has been treated and on the doses used. Some of these side effects may be long term in nature (e.g., dyspnea, myelopathy, fibrosis, etc.). Recent developments in immunotherapy are also more toxic than originally hoped. Thus, the alopecia and fatigue following therapy with interferon, and the side effects of interleukins and LAK cells are additional burdens in the lives of patients receiving these treatments. Even when the intent of treatment is not curative, but palliative, the toxicity associated with therapy must still be contended with. And, finally, attempts to relieve symptoms such as nausea and vomiting or pain by the use of antiemetics or analgesics may introduce new and debilitating side effects.

A large part of the total effort devoted to treating patients with cancer is spent on ameliorating the deleterious effects of the therapies themselves. To some extent these efforts are successful. Surgery is generally more organ conserving, radiation therapy is delivered more effectively and many side effects of chemotherapy and biological therapy can now be controlled. Furthermore, the psychosocial impact of cancer is being recognized and attempts to provide counseling, rehabilitation, palliative care, and assistance in the home are becoming commonplace in economically developed countries.

II. WHY MEASURE QUALITY OF LIFE?

Despite improvements in the therapy of cancer and in the control of the side effects of therapy, relatively little formal knowledge exists about the effects of the disease and of its treatment on the quality of the lives of those affected. Clinicians are likely to gather biological data such as overall survival, disease-free survival, and response rates, together with hematological and other evidence of toxicity. But, how do the symptoms of the cancer and the treatment side effects affect the emotional, spiritual, and social dimensions of patients' lives? And to what extent are effects in these dimensions experienced by patients as an increased burden of cancer? What proportion of patients with various forms of cancer experience an increased burden in any given dimension of life? It can be claimed, justifiably, that many physicians *are* concerned about the quality of each of their patients' lives in their day-to-day practices. They ask questions, make assessments, give advice, and introduce interventions which often are designed to improve quality of life. However, even when they are concerned with quality of life in their patients, physicians are more likely to be guided by intuitive and experiential paradigms than by paradigms based on results of formal scientific investigation. In part, this is because many questions have not been posed as research questions and, in part, because the tools for answering these questions have only recently become available and are not yet accepted generally as part of routine clinical practice.

It seems reasonable to predict that curing a patient's cancer will result in a return of quality of life to the precancer state. How often is this true? May not quality of life be altered permanently even though the cancer has been cured? Has this possibility been tested scientifically? We assume that relief of symptoms, e.g., nausea and vomiting or pain, must be accompanied *de facto* by an improvement in quality of life. Is it always so? To what extent is quality of life improved? Does the relief of all-engrossing pain allow other, previously unrecognized, concerns to surface? In formal clinical trials of new therapies or strategies, it is disease-free survival, overall survival and toxicity (generally assessed only physiologically) that are the major end-points. If a new treatment, A, is compared to a standard treatment, B, and survival is improved significantly by treatment A, then it is concluded that treatment A is superior. Is this always true? How valid is this conclusion if only some of the important factors, e.g., survival and toxicity, are considered and quality of life is not considered? If treatments A and B are equivalent with respect to survival and toxicity, do they have equivalent effects on quality of life? If quality of life is not assessed can we assume that our decision about which treatment to adopt is always correct? How much value (utility) do patients themselves place on survival, and at what personal cost? How much value do patients place on quality of life vs. quantity of life?

As clinicians have begun to take an interest in measuring quality of life (an exercise, until recently, entirely in the hands of social scientists) the results of some studies have been counterintuitive and thus surprising. In a study of a small sample of patients with osteosarcoma it seemed reasonable before the study to assume that patients given limb-preserving radiation therapy would have a better quality of life than patients undergoing limb amputation. However, it was found that those whose limbs were preserved had unanticipated sexual difficulties.[3] While, as pointed out by Till,[4] these results need to be interpreted with caution, they nevertheless illustrate that intuitive bias needs to be tested by scientific methodology. Another study, based on a large sample of patients involved a comparison of continuous therapy to intermittent therapy in patients receiving chemotherapy for breast cancer.[5] Prestudy bias would suggest that quality of life is more likely to be adversely affected by continuous therapy. However, the authors found that the opposite was true, likely because the intermittent therapy had a higher probability of inducing a remission in the disease than did interrupted therapy and, therefore, of ameliorating the disease-related impact on quality of life. Although this study is flawed in that not all patients in both arms completed the quality-of-life as-

TABLE 1
Clinical Value of Measuring Quality of Life

Obtaining new information for a holistic estimate of the total burden imposed by the disease and its treatment
Improving communication by providing quantitative, objective information

sessments, thus making it uncertain if the missing information would have altered the results, it does point out once again that intuitive bias can be unreliable.

Other attempts to assess quality of life, as affected by timing of therapy, are also instructive. For example, patients with limited-stage small-cell lung cancer treated by elective adjuvant ("prophylactic") cranial radiation had less physical morbidity in their remaining lives, as assessed by the Karnofsky Performance Index, than did patients whose cerebral metastases were irradiated only after clinical manifestations became evident.[6] However, survival was similar in both groups. An obvious criticism of this study is that the Karnofsky Performance Index[7] is an assessment of physical activity primarily. Perhaps, measurement of cognitive function and of psychosocial aspects of life, in addition to physical function, may have led to a different conclusion. But, once again, rather than criticizing this study because it did not go far enough in assessing quality of life, we should recognize that the effects of therapeutic strategies and of therapy itself on quality of life are not certain until they have been measured.

A. OBTAINING INFORMATION

How much should clinicians know about the effects of cancer and its treatment in their patients? Is it sufficient to know the biological and physiological effects of therapy or should clinicians know more? As stated earlier, clinicians may indeed assess effects other than biological ones — that they are concerned about each patient's quality of life and ask appropriate quality-of-life questions when caring for patients. However, it is not known how systematically clinicians ask quality-of-life questions, what questions they ask, and to what extent the answers are incorporated into treatment (management) decisions. What does seem certain is that if a formal, documented approach to assessing quality of life is lacking, (and most clinicians do not document quality of life), then clinicians will not be able to assess fully the effect of cancer and its treatment on a patient's life. Furthermore, they will not be able to communicate effectively with each other about questions related to quality of life. Lacking systematic, quantitative, widely accepted methodology results in information and communication gaps which need bridging before concerted, rational efforts can be made to improve quality of life as well as quantity of life in patients with cancer. In short, measuring quality of life provides a fuller knowledge of the effect of cancer and its treatment and, hence, the total burden imposed on the patient (Table 1). The more informed health care professionals are, the better they are able to advise their patients, whether in obtaining informed consent for clinical trials or in day-to-day clinical practice.

There are many potential clinical applications of quality-of-life measures in patients with cancer, but only a few will be discussed briefly to illustrate the variety of possible applications (Table 2).

Performing quality-of-life measures in randomized (phase III) clinical trials may provide an answer to which of two or more treatment arms is preferable, particularly when the treatment arms result in similar or equivalent biological effects, e.g., survival. Even when overall toxicity is similar biologically, the effect of the toxicity in one arm may have a less deleterious impact on quality of life because of a differing effect on emotional or social functioning.

In phase III clinical trials, patients are often stratified according to certain prognostic factors, e.g., stage of disease or performance status, in order to equally balance the assign-

TABLE 2
Examples of Clinical Applications of Quality-of-Life
Data

Clinical Trials

Choosing between treatments with equivalent biological effects
Stratification of patients entering clinical trials
Determining patient preferences (utilities)
Combining quality with quantity to estimate the benefits of therapy
 (e.g., quality-adjusted life years (QALY), and quality of time
 without symptoms and treatment (Q-TWiST)
Economic evaluations (e.g., cost-utility)

Clinical Practice

The early detection of morbidity
Quality assurance in health care institutions
Clinical decision making

ment of patients to the treatment arms. Potentially, the pretreatment state of quality of life may have prognostic significance, as suggested recently by one study.[8] Thus, quality-of-life status may be a stratification variable to be added to other known variables in the design of some clinical trials.

Measuring quality of life can be used for assessing the preferences and the values (utilities) that patients place on particular quality-of-life states. If patients in a clinical trial are asked to express a preference for a particular treatment, after having experienced the treatments being tested, the questions ascertaining preferences conceivably might be combined with a utility assessment such as a standard gamble,[9] time trade-off[10] or maximal endurable time,[11] in which patients also indicate how much risk they would be willing to experience in order to gain the preferred state.

The qualitative data (expressed quantitatively) obtained from measuring quality of life may be combined with quantitative survival data to provide a new way of expressing both quality and quantity in a single number, i.e., quality-adjusted life years (QALY) of survival.[12] Another attempt to factor quality into survival is the quality of time without symptoms or treatment (Q-TWiST).[13] These expressions of survival may be useful medically, and might also be used to obtain assessments of cost-utility when economic costs have been factored in.

Cost-utility evaluation is a relatively new method for evaluating economic costs in light of the utility a patient gives to a particular health state.[14] It may be possible to incorporate patient preferences for quality-of-life states in such evaluations.[15] If a measure of the economic cost of the treatment that is required to gain a particular quality-of-life state is carried out as part of a clinical trial, the combined information might be used to obtain cost-utility information. Such analyses previously have been applied to assessing the economic costs of particular health care interventions,[14] but could also be incorporated into measuring the costs of interventions required to attain desired quality-of-life states.

A major reason for measuring quality of life is that if the measures used are responsive to small, but clinically important,[16] changes in quality of life, then the resulting information will provide earlier detection of morbidity associated with either the cancer or its treatment. Being aware of morbidity at an earlier stage may allow the institution of earlier interventions designed to ameliorate the morbidity. As a further step, if the earliest manifestations of quality-of-life morbidity are known, and if they are predictable and preventable, appropriate preventative measures may be taken.

An important aspect of health care is quality assurance.[17] This is a process by which the results of services intended to improve care are compared with a predetermined standard or with external standards to assess whether improvements in care have actually occurred. Quality-of-life data can enhance the quality assurance process by adding information which currently is either not collected at all or not collected in a usable way.

If the results of quality-of-life assessments are incorporated into the patient's medical record, then a review of the record on subsequent patient visits could serve as a basis for rational clinical decision making. Such information can be obtained relatively early by the use of self-assessment questionnaires that are filled out while the patient is waiting to see the physician. The data would provide information in addition to the usual data collected by the physician.

Finally, studying quality of life in a systematic, scientific manner is likely to teach us about quality of life itself. This new knowledge can, in turn, be used in an iterative manner to improve our methodology and our ability to study quality of life, and may lead to as yet unforeseen changes in our views of how therapeutic strategies should be directed in the future.

A taxonomy of reasons for measuring quality of life is discussed from a different perspective in Chapter 7.[18]

B. IMPROVING COMMUNICATION

Although attention may be given to quality-of-life issues in clinical practice, documentation of these issues is either lacking or not recorded in quantitative terms. Thus, communication between health care providers is hampered because it is dependent upon the use of qualitative terms which are subject to varying interpretation. In addition, if the assessments are done by the health care provider, who uses his or her own normative standard to interpret a patient's quality of life, further variation is introduced into the material which is communicated to others.

While the use of descriptive terms to describe quality of life may be useful in the exploratory stages of studies designed to assess quality of life, they are difficult to quantify, thus making numerical expression preferable, particularly when making comparisons of quality of life either between patients (or groups of patients) or between different times in the same patient(s). It is for this reason, that the word "measurement" as opposed to "assessment" has been used in this paper. Assessment may be achieved by either measurement or by the use of descriptive terms, but measurement, by definition, is expressed only in numerical terms. A numerical approach allows summation of items in subscales into subscale scores and subscale scores into total or aggregate scores. Numbers can also express the answers to global questions, such as "How would you rate your quality of life during the past week?" Another advantage of numerical results is that they can be analyzed statistically. Thus, the numerical approach is mandatory in such settings as clinical trials. Numerical results may be perceived to be less useful when attempting to communicate the possible effects of treatment to patients because they need to be translated back into language understandable to each patient. However, this should not be construed as a valid reason for not getting the numbers in the first place, since clinicians commonly translate probabilities (expressed initially as numbers) of response or survival into terms understandable to patients.

Giving advice based on quantitative data to patients and their families is likely to be more objective and, therefore, more comprehensive than advice based only on the health care provider's subjective assessment. In time, as quantitative data on large populations of patients becomes available it will supplement individual experience as a source of advice. Thus, the use of formal, self-assessment, quality-of-life measures which provide quantitative data, should lead to improved communication not only among health care providers but also between health care providers and their patients and others.

III. DEFINING QUALITY OF LIFE

Before quality of life can be measured it needs to be defined. Conceptually, quality of life has to do with the sense of satisfaction and well-being that an individual feels about his or her life, encompassing qualities such as "the degree to which an individual succeeds in accomplishing his desires"[19] and "the extent to which a person's hopes and ambitions are matched and fulfilled by experience".[20] However, because these descriptions of quality of life are very broad, they fall short of a definition that can be operationalized into the scientific measurement of quality of life. For the definition to be operationalized, it is necessary to narrow the scope to health-related quality of life. In this context, one operationally useful definition states that quality of life "includes psychologic and social functioning as well as physical functioning and incorporates positive aspects of well-being as well as negative aspects of disease or infirmity".[21] This definition suggests that quality of life may be measured, in part, by a measurement of certain components, or dimensions, of life, i.e., physical functioning, psychological functioning, and social functioning. Others have suggested that further dimensions, such as somatic discomfort, disease symptoms, treatment side-effects, sexuality, and body image should also be included in clinical studies.[22] It may be argued that life is more than these dimensions, that the sum is greater than these parts. While this is likely to be true, the acceptance of the existence of discreet dimensions of life allows us to proceed with an assessment or measurement of factors which make up the dimensions themselves (e.g., anxiety and depression in the psychological dimension). Two well-known assessments of physical functioning in patients with cancer are the Karnofsky scale[7] and the Zubrod scale[23] (and its variants). Although both of these were intended for use by health-care workers and not as self-assessment tools, and neither has been appropriately validated psychometrically, they have been shown to be of value both as descriptors and prognosticators. Hence, they are in wide use today. However, they are not measures of quality of life since they lack items pertaining to psychological and social functioning. Therefore, valid measures of quality of life must include at least psychologic functioning and social functioning in addition to measures of physical functioning.

IV. WHO SHOULD MEASURE QUALITY OF LIFE?

In measuring quality of life, the measurer (whether patient or observer) is asked to make a comparison. As stated by Keyserlingk, this is "a comparison of the qualities *this* patient now has with the qualities deemed by *this* patient to be normative and desirable".[24] Who should make this comparison? The answer must take into account the words "normative" and "desirable". Normative relates to prescribing norms or standards. When measuring quality of life, what are desirable norms and who should prescribe them, i.e., who sets the normative standard? Is it society — or the health care provider — or the patient?

Since we are dealing with the *patient's* quality of life can there be doubt that it is the *patient's* right to set the normative standard? If the patient sets the standard then it follows that the patient should evaluate the extent to which his or her quality of life meets that standard. If an observer, no matter how observant or how well-informed, is asked to rate the quality of another's life, the observer will be influenced by his own perception of what the standard should be. Not only will the evaluation be inaccurate but the effects could be extremely dangerous. The evaluation will be inaccurate because the assessment will not reflect the patient's own view of what he feels *his* or *her* quality of life to be, and dangerous because the failure by a patient to meet some preconceived standard set by others can endanger the freedom of that patient's access to health care and, subsequently, the freedom to choose the possible alternatives available for care. Thus, there can really be only one answer to the question of who should set the normative standard, and that is — the patient.

All possible means must be used to find out what the patient's responses are to the questions posed and the only exception is those circumstances in which the patient is unable to give a response.

The results of research support the contention that we should seek answers directly from patients. In one study, when the rating of patients and health care providers were compared, an unacceptable variance was found.[25] In another, although the trend of observers' and patients' ratings were in the same direction, observers' ratings consistently tended to underrate quality of life as compared to the patient's own ratings.[26] These results are not surprising given that the assessment of psychosocial aspects of life is subjective and, therefore, difficult to ascertain by an observer.

Another reason for asking patients to rate their quality of life is that a patient's perception of what is an acceptable normative standard, i.e., "good" quality, may change with time. At the beginning of the illness, when a patient expects a cure, the patient's normative standard may be much higher than towards the end of the illness when the patient knows the illness is incurable, and the patient's primary concern may be comfort. This change in a patient's expectations must form a part of the considerations in the care of that patient.

V. HOW SHOULD IT BE MEASURED?

Even if there is agreement about which dimensions of life should be measured, another criticism leveled at measuring quality of life is that it can't be measured in quantitative terms since, ultimately, it is a subjective concept. This criticism is heard most frequently from clinicians (physicians and nurses), whose training is deficient in psychometric theory and investigation.[27] Psychometrics draws upon a vast body of experimentation in many fields (e.g., education, marketing) and is involved in the gathering of subjective information. This is often viewed as "soft" data as opposed to the "hard" data provided by biochemistry, hematology, etc. There are at least two ways in which "soft" data are made "hard" by appropriate attention to psychometrics. The first is that the measurement tools be rigorously constructed and tested for reliability, precision, responsiveness, and validity.[28-30] The second is that the numerical data resulting from tools that have been properly constructed be amenable to statistical analysis. The demonstration of the reproducibility of results[31] as well as the gathering of independent data for concurrent validity[32] are additional means of assuring clinical investigators of the validity of quality-of-life measures.

Since other chapters in this book deal in some detail with how to measure quality of life, only a brief statement about the general approach will be made here. If the exact purpose of measuring quality of life in a given situation is clearly known, an algorithm for proceeding to select the appropriate methods can serve as a guide.[18] If self-assessment instruments (questionnaires) seem most appropriate for the situation, close attention must be paid to their reliability, validity and responsiveness. If a new instrument needs to be developed, patients should be involved in providing the necessary information about their primary concerns so that the questions asked in the instrument can reflect these concerns. In addition, social scientists should be either consulted at the outset or directly involved in each study. Statisticians, preferably with some experience in dealing with quality-of-life data, should also be involved during the planning stages.

VI. OVERCOMING BARRIERS TO MEASURING QUALITY OF LIFE

Why are quality-of-life assessments not a routine part of clinical trials and clinical practice in oncology? The previous sections of this chapter have alluded indirectly to what might be called barriers to measuring quality of life. These barriers are the same as those encountered in any health status measurement, since measuring quality of life in patients with cancer is merely an example of measuring health status in a population defined by a group of diseases known as cancer. Deyo and Patrick state that the reasons for the lack of widespread use of health status measures include conceptual, methodologic, practical, and attitudinal barriers and that these barriers may be perceived in a different manner by researchers, clinicians, and policy-makers.[32] A similar taxonomy may be used for barriers to measuring quality of life.

A. ATTITUDINAL BARRIERS

There are a variety of attitudinal barriers to measuring quality of life, including negativism ("it's not worth doing" or "who cares?"), uninformed skepticism ("quality of life is subjective and can't be measured" or "what can measuring quality of life add to what is being done now?"), inertia ("too busy" or "it's too much trouble") and role rejection ("it's not my job") (Table 3). These attitudes among clinicians are understandable since clinicians generally have little knowledge about the body of work that already exists in this field.[27] They do not receive information relevant to measuring quality of life during their education in medical school or while specializing in oncology. Thus, they are largely uninformed of the methods used by psychologists and social scientists to carry out their research. As a result clinicians may feel either disinterest, lack of commitment, or a sense of uncertainty because of a lack of understanding of the reliability and relevance of quality-of-life data.

Quality-of-life assessments are of particular importance to clinical investigators who participate in clinical trials of new therapies in patients with cancer since the clinical trials setting allows for the systematic collection of all data that may be pertinent to the future use of a new treatment regimen. However, a major reason for the absence of quality-of-life measures in most current clinical trials settings appears to be a misconception about the scientific validity of quality-of-life data. Overcoming this barrier requires educational input directed at clinical-trials investigators by scheduling of symposia and by person-to-person contact. This approach has worked well in the Clinical Trials Group of the National Cancer Institute of Canada. As a result, this Group established a Quality of Life Committee in 1986 and has formulated a policy which requires that a statement be made in all phase III trials about whether or not quality-of-life measurement will be a part of the trial and, if so, how it will be measured. In addition, writing guidelines have been developed to assist protocol writers in the incorporation of quality-of-life measures into clinical trials protocols. Expert advice is also available from individual members of the Quality of Life Committee and from the statistical and data management personnel of the Clinical Trials Group central office.

Attitudinal barriers can be overcome by a variety of strategies directed at several levels. The most important goal is the acceptance by clinicians that the wishes of the patient in regard to quality of life are paramount in the construction of patient management plans. This goal can be achieved partly by instilling this attitude through appropriate education in medical school and in postgraduate training, but it is important, also, to begin earlier by selecting individuals with this attitude for entrance to medical schools. In medical schools and postgraduate training programs, information about the rigor and usefulness of quality-of-life measures should to be a part of the curricula of studies. It is important to demonstrate that psychometrically reliable measures, applied systematically, provide documentable and clinically meaningful information which is not otherwise obtainable. In trying to reach practicing clinicians and clinical investigators it is important for editors of journals and for directors of continuing medical education programs to be aware of the body of knowledge and research in this field. Because of the interdependence of medical teachers, administrators, practitioners, investigators, and students, and the multidisciplinary nature of quality-of-life assessment, strategies designed to increase awareness which, in turn, will influence attitudes requires a concerted effort at many levels by a variety of individuals.

TABLE 3
Barriers to Measuring Quality of Life

Attitudinal

Negativism
Inertia
Ignorance
Role uncertainty
Cynicism
Unreliability of subjective data

Conceptual and Methodological

Importance relative to biological/physiological outcomes
Reliability for screening purposes
Role in clinical decision making
Usefulness as utility measure
Definition of clinically significant outcomes
Ascertaining minimum clinically significant differences

Practical

Feasibility, i.e., time, manpower, organization, and cost
Raising unrealistic expectations
Choosing appropriate measures

B. CONCEPTUAL AND METHODOLOGICAL BARRIERS

Even when quality-of-life data are accepted as being relevant, there is remaining uncertainty about a number of key issues, such as whether the data should be collected by
observers or by self-assessment and which instruments to use. For example, some clinicians
regularly assess physical function or performance using well-known performance scales,
such as those described by Karnofsky[7] or Zubrod,[23] but are reluctant to incorporate any new
instruments into their assessment armamentarium, perhaps not realizing that newer instruments provide multidimensional information about dimensions other than physical activity
(for examples, see References 22, 26, and 33 through 43).

Another barrier to quality-of-life measurement is the lack of a clear concept of the
purpose of the measurement and its place in clinical care (Table 3). An essential difference
between quality-of-life outcomes and physiological outcomes is that the former may disclose
impairment in function not disclosed by the latter. In patients with cancer, an example of
a quality-of-life outcome not necessarily disclosed by a physiological measure is the fatigue
that may accompany therapy with radiation or antineoplastic drugs but not be associated
with any measurable physiological parameter (e.g., anemia or hypomagnesemia). A quality-
of-life measure may also disclose the extent to which the fatigue affects emotional well-
being in addition to impairment of physical activity. While these potential differences in
outcomes can readily be accepted in research on quality of life, how are they related to the
care of the patient? In particular, what level of importance should be assigned to functional
disabilities in the emotional or social dimensions of life in the management plan for the
patient? Should they be paramount considerations in the absence of documentable physiological impairment? Physicians may not wish to know about functional impairments that
they are unable to deal with effectively, or may they not know how much importance to
assign to them, particularly if it means interrupting potentially curative therapy. Thus, lack
of understanding of the purpose of measurement hampers the choice of an appropriate
measurement method. The purpose of obtaining quality-of-life data may be for screening
(or case-finding), for description, for clinical decision making or for assessment of patient

preferences.[18] (Another classification of the purpose for measuring quality of life is that the data can be used to discriminate among subjects at a single time, to measure change over time or to predict outcome.)[44] For most of these purposes, issues related to the sensitivity and specificity of most measurement instruments still needs further work. This is especially important if measuring quality of life is to be used for screening or clinical decision making where false positive and false negative results must be kept to a minimum. When patient preference is to be assessed, measures of utility need to be combined with measures of quality of life.

Overcoming these conceptual barriers requires careful thought about why quality of life is to be measured in a given situation. In the case of the clinical trials, a clear statement of the purpose of the trial will help the investigator to choose the most appropriate measure. In clinical practice, there needs to be an understanding that in order to give the best advice possible, a physician needs to have as much information as is reasonably possible. This attitude needs to be instilled at an early time in the physician's training.

When the choice is made to use previously developed self-assessment questionnaires, the investigators must be able to assess the reliability and validity of the existing instruments. Several recent reviews deal with the reliability and validity of questionnaires and provide a rating of existing questionnaires.[45-51] An algorithm for making choices in the process of measuring quality of life provides a step-by-step procedure which can assist relatively in-experienced investigators to reach a series of rational decisions.[18] However, seeking advice from investigators with experience in the field of health status measurement is the best way to learn the finer points of quality-of-life measurement. These advisors should include psychometricians, social scientists, statisticians, and clinicians.

One of the most difficult problems is the lack of a "gold standard" — a criterion which everyone accepts as being the best measure of quality of life either generally or in specific situations. The lack of criterion validity can be partly overcome by seeking concurrent validity.[32] This can be done by comparing the results of a particular quality-of-life assessment with the results other parallel measures, e.g., disease status or toxicity of therapy, etc. For example, if the results of a quality-of-life measure show a correlation between decreasing quality of life in at least some dimensions with increasing disease burden, then there is reason to believe that the measure of quality of life is probably valid. Another approach which provides some protection against the risk that a measure may not have validity is to assess convergent validity by comparing the results obtained by a new measure with the results obtained by previously accepted measures with known validity. For example, items purporting to measure anxiety/depression, which are embedded in a general quality-of-life measure, might be compared with either a simultaneously administered, widely accepted measure for anxiety/depression, or with the results of an in-depth interview before the new measure is accepted as being a valid measure of this construct. Thus, both concurrent validity and convergent validity can substitute, to some extent, for the lack of criterion validity.

Currently, there is probably no single questionnaire that will provide answers to all aspects of quality of life in all patients with cancer. However, choosing a generic or "core" questionnaire which can be given together with a specific questionnaire designed to address the constructs or details relevant to the particular research question, but which are not covered in the "core" questionnaire, is a reasonable approach to this issue.[39,42]

C. PRACTICAL BARRIERS

Several practical barriers relate to the feasibility of carrying out measurement (Table 3). Measuring quality of life requires sufficient financial support to provide an adequate in-frastructure, including appropriate personnel and materials to carry out the study and analyze the results. Quality-of-life research demands the same scientific rigor and attention to collecting data as does any other clinical investigation. This is time consuming and clinicians by themselves often are unable to give it the necessary attention. Therefore, an otherwise well-conducted study with adequate clinical and biological data (disease status, toxicity, and laboratory and diagnostic data) may still have inadequate quality-of-life data. Since contact with patients is required to collect quality-of-life data, studies should employ appropriately trained personnel to administer the measures, whether they be interviews or questionnaires. The feasibility of a study may be increased if the investigators can use self-administered questionnaires and these are reasonably short so that they may be administered repeatedly to ill as well as to relatively asymptomatic patients. However, it should be remembered that repeatedly administered questionnaires should be administered and completed under similar conditions on each occasion in a particular study, since varying the environment (e.g., the clinic on one occasion, the home on another, and by telephone on still another) introduces variability.

Approaching patients to repeatedly carry out quality-of-life measures raises another concern. The clinician's expression of caring about quality of life may create an atmosphere which raises patients' expectations unrealistically about what can be done to improve quality of life. However, it is more likely that the improved communication between the care giver and the patient resulting from an increased awareness of the patient's concerns will serve to dispel the risk of making promises that cannot be fulfilled. Indeed, dealing with patients in an atmosphere in which quality-of-life concerns are not in the forefront may result in patients feeling fear and disappointment or dissatisfaction with the care being provided.

VII. A GLOSSARY OF TERMS

The jargon of psychometrics can prove to be daunting to the uninitiated. The following glossary is intended as an aid to readers. The trained psychometrician and social scientist may wish to use different wording in the definitions below, but the wording is intended to be as understandable as possible to clinicians who are new to this field. Further details may be found in standard reference works.[52,53]

Category scale:	a series of descriptive phrases which either may be ordered in a particular sequence, e.g., from best to worst (Guttman scale) or may be answered by a "yes" or "no" response.
Convergent validity:	the extent to which two or more instruments purported to be testing the same construct agree with each other.
Content validity:	the extent to which the content of a questionnaire appears to logically examine the dimension or domain it is intended to examine.
Concurrent validity:	the independent corroboration, by other means, that an instrument is measuring what it is supposed to be measuring. An example would be decreasing physical activity as measured by a self-report questionnaire which is paralleled by other observable and/or documentable events such as reports by a family member, weight loss, hospitalization, etc.

Construct validity: the extent to which a questionnaire tests the hypotheses or ideas about the overall concepts it is supposedly measuring.

Criterion validity: the degree to which a questionnaire measures the true situation (referred to as the "gold standard").

Discriminant validity: the extent to which an instrument reflects differences in individuals, or populations of individuals, who would be expected to be different from each other at any given moment in time.

Dimension (domain):   a particular, definable aspect of life, e.g., physical activity, emotional state, social interaction, etc.

Factor analysis: a maneuver carried out to determine which items belong to the same dimension and the extent to which each item influences another dimension.

Face validity: the presentation or appearance of a questionnaire, e.g., is it easy to read, does it appear professionally prepared? (Sometimes equated erroneously with content validity.)

Instrument: a structured assessment tool, e.g., questionnaire, that can be submitted to formal statistical analysis. The application of a well-designed instrument will provide a quantitative result.

Internal consistency: the extent to which the questions relating to a particular dimension, e.g., physical activity, tap only this dimension and no other.

Inter-rater reliability: the extent to which two or more individuals agree, or the extent to which the results agree for similar populations in two or more institutions.

Item-total score correlations: the extent to which each item (question) within a particular dimension contributes to the total score for that dimension. If there is a strong correlation, this produces a high internal consistency as expressed numerically by, for example, Cronbach's alpha coefficient.

Likert scale: a rating system, subdivided numerically into a series of ordered responses e.g., from "never", through "sometimes" to "always". The responses may also be represented by a series of consecutive numbers, e.g., 1, 2, 3, 4, 5, which denote gradations in the possible range of responses.

Linear analog scale:
: a line or space of defined length, anchored at each end by a descriptive word or phrase each representing the extremes of a health state, e.g., "worst", "best". The subject places a mark on the line (or in the space) indicating the point at which his/her response best answers the question being asked.

Psychometric validation:
: the process by which an instrument is assessed for reliability and validity through a series of defined tests using actual subjects for whom the instrument is designed.

Reliability:
: a statistical description of the amount of random error associated with a measurement. There are certain parameters, such as test-retest stability, inter-rater reliability, internal consistency and situation-specificity, that need to be assessed before a measurement tool can be declared to have reliability.

Responsiveness (sensitivity to change):
: the extent to which an instrument actually reflects changes occurring in an individual or a population over a period of time.

Scaled:
: capable of being divided into dimensions each having a few or several items which, when summed, provide a single score for the dimension.

Test-retest stability:
: the extent to which an answer obtained initially is reproducible at a later time during a stable health state, using the same measurement instrument.

Time-framed:
: the time period which the question being asked refers to, e.g., "today", "this past week", etc.

Utility:
: a value, usually a number, which expresses a single person's preferences among available alternatives (e.g., health states).

Validity:
: an assessment of whether a measurement method measures what it is intended to measure. A valid instrument should have been assessed psychometrically for reliability and have content, construct and discriminant validity. It can only be said to have validity after it has been tested repeatedly in the populations for which it was designed.

REFERENCES

1. Shakespeare, W., *Hamlet*, Act IV, Scene 3.
2. National Cancer Institute of Canada, *Canadian Cancer Statistics 1990*, Toronto, 1990.
3. Sugarbaker, P. H., Barofsky, I., Rosenberg, S. A., and Gianola, F. J., Quality of life assessment of patients in extremity sarcoma trials, *Surgery*, 91, 17, 1982.
4. Till, J., Uses (and some possible abuses) of quality-of-life measures, in *Effect of Cancer on Quality of Life*, Osoba, D., Ed., CRC Press, Boca Raton, FL, 1991, chap. 11.
5. Coates, A., Gebski, V., Bishop, J. F., Jeal, P. N., Woods, R. L., Snyder, R., Tattersall, M. H. N., Byrne, M., Harvey, V., Grantley, G., Simpson, J., Drummond, R., Browne, J., van Cooten, R., and Forbes, J. F., Improving the quality of life during chemotherapy for advanced breast cancer. A comparison of intermittent and continuous treatment strategies, *N. Engl. J. Med.*, 317, 1490, 1987.
6. Roseman, J. and Choi, N. C., Improved quality of life of patients with small-cell carcinoma of the lung by elective irradiation of the brain, *Int. J. Radiat. Oncol. Biol. Phys.*, 8, 1041, 1982.
7. Karnofsky, D. A. and Burchenal, H. H., The clinical evaluation of chemotherapeutic agents in cancer, in *Evaluation of Chemotherapeutic Agents*, McLeod, C. M., Ed., Columbia University Press, New York, 1949, 191.
8. Ruckdeschel, J. C. and Piantadosi, S., Assessment of quality of life (QL) by the Functional Living Index — Cancer (FLIC) is superior to performance status for prediction of survival in patients with lung cancer, *Proc. Am. Soc. Clin. Oncol.*, 8, 311, 1989 (abstr. 1209).
9. von Neumann, J. and Morgenstern, O., *Theory of Games and Economic Behaviour*, 2nd ed., Princeton University Press, Princeton, NJ, 1947.
10. Torrance, G. W., Thomas, W. H., and Sackett, D. L., A Utility Maximization Model for evaluation of health care programs, *Health Serv. Res.*, 7, 118, 1972.
11. Sutherland, H. J., Llewellyn-Thomas, H., Boyd, N. F., and Till, J. E., Attitudes toward quality of survival: the concept of "maximal endurable time", *Med. Decision Making*, 2, 299, 1982.
12. Loomes, G. and McKenzie, L., The use of QALYs in health care decision making, *Soc. Sci. Med.*, 28, 299, 1989.
13. Goldhirsch, A., Gelber, R. D., Simes, R. J., Glasziou, P., and Coates, A. S., Costs and benefits of adjuvant therapy in breast cancer: a quality-adjusted survival analysis, *J. Clin. Oncol.*, 7, 36, 1989.
14. Drummond, M. F., Stoddart, G. L., and Torrance, G. W., *Methods for Economic Evaluation of Health Care Programmes*, Oxford Medical Publications, Oxford, 1987.
15. Feeny, D., Can we use quality-of-life measures for economic evaluations?, *Qual. Life Cardiovasc. Care*, 4, 185, 1988.
16. Jaeschke, R., Singer, J., and Guyatt, G. H., Measurement of health status. Ascertaining minimal clinically important difference, *Controlled Clin. Trials*, 10, 407, 1989.
17. Wilson, C. R. M., *Hospital-Wide Quality Assurance*, W. B. Saunders, Toronto, 1987.
18. Osoba, D., Aaronson, N. K., and Till, J. E., A practical guide for selecting quality-of-life measures in clinical trials and practice, in *The Effect of Cancer on Quality of Life*, Osoba, D., Ed., CRC Press, Boca Raton, FL, 1991, chap. 7.
19. Gerson, E. M., On the quality of life, *Am. Soc. Rev.*, 41, 793, 1976.
20. Calman, K. C., The quality of life in cancer patients — an hypothesis, *J. Med. Ethics*, 10, 124, 1984.
21. Till, J. E., McNeil, B. J., and Bush, R. S., Measurements of multiple components of quality of life, *Cancer Treat. Symp.*, 1, 177, 1984.
22. Aaronson, N. K., Bullinger, M., and Ahmedzai, S., A modular approach to quality-of-life assessment in cancer clinical trials, in *Cancer Clinical Trials: A Critical Appraisal*, Scheurlen, H., Kay, R., and Baum, M., Eds., Recent Results in Cancer Research, Vol. 111, Springer-Verlag, Berlin, 1988, 231.
23. Zubrod, C. G., Schneiderman, M., Frei, E., et al., Appraisal of methods for the study of chemotherapy of cancer in man: comparative therapeutic trial of nitrogen mustard and triethylene thiophosphoramide, *J. Chronic Dis.*, 11, 7, 1960.
24. Keyserlingk, E. W., *Sanctity of Life or Quality of Life*, Minister of Supply and Services Canada, Ottawa, 1979.
25. Presant, C. A., Quality of life in cancer patients, *Am. J. Clin. Oncol.*, 7, 571, 1984.
26. Wood-Dauphinee, S. and Williams, J. I., The Spitzer Quality of Life Index: its performance as a measure, in *Effect of Cancer on Quality of Life*, Osoba, D., Ed., CRC Press, Boca Raton, FL, 1991, chap. 13.
27. Petersdorf, R. G. and Feinstein, A. R., An informal appraisal of the current status of "medical sociology", in *The Relevance of Social Science for Medicine*, Eisenberg, L. and Kleinman, A., Eds., D. Reidel, Boston, MA, 1981, 27.
28. Guyatt, G., Bombardier, C., and Tugwell, P. X., Measuring disease-specific quality of life in clinical trials, *Can. Med. Assoc. J.*, 134, 889, 1986.

29. Deyo, R. A. and Cantor, R. M., Assessing the responsiveness of functional scales to clinical change: an analogy to diagnostic test performance, *J. Chronic Dis.*, 39, 897, 1986.

30. Guyatt, G., Walter, S., and Norman, G., Measuring change over time: assessing the usefulness of evaluative instruments, *J. Chronic Dis.*, 40, 171, 1987.

31. Feinstein, A. R., Clinical biostatistics. XLI. Hard science, soft data, and the challenges of choosing clinical variables in research, *Clin. Pharmacol. Ther.*, 22, 485, 1977.

32. Deyo, R. A. and Patrick, D. L., Barriers to the use of health status measures in clinical investigation, patient care, and policy research, *Med. Care*, 27, S254, 1989.

33. Priestman, T. S. and Baum, M., Evaluation of quality of life in patients receiving treatment for advanced breast cancer, *Lancet*, 1899, 1976.

34. Baum, M., Priestman, T., West, R. R., and Jones, E. M., A comparison of subjective responses in a trial comparing endocrine with cytotoxic treatment in advanced carcinoma of the breast, in *Breast Cancer: Experimental and Clinical Aspects*, Mouridsen, H. T. and Palshof, T., Eds., Proc. 2nd EORTC Breast Cancer Working Conf., Pergamon Press, Oxford, 1980, 223.

35. Spitzer, W. O., Dobson, A. J., Hall, J., Chesterman, E., Levi, J., Shepherd, R., Battista, R. N., and Catchlove, B. R., Measuring the quality of life of cancer patients. A concise QL-index for use by physicians, *J. Chronic Dis.*, 34, 585, 1981.

36. Padilla, G. V., Presant, C., Grant, M. M., Metter, G., Lipsett, J., and Heide, F., Quality of life index for patients with cancer, *Res. Nurs. Health*, 6, 117, 1983.

37. Schipper, H., Clinch, J., McMurray, A., and Levitt, M., Measuring the quality of life of cancer patients: The Functional Living Index-Cancer: development and validation, *J. Clin. Oncol.*, 2, 472, 1984.

38. Selby, P. J., Chapman, J.-A. W., Etazadi-Amoli, J., Dalley, D., and Boyd, N. F., The development of method for assessing the quality of life of cancer patients, *Br. J. Cancer*, 50, 13, 1984.

39. Aaronson, N. K., Bakker, W., Stewart, A. L., van Dam, F. S. A. M., van Zandwijk, N., Yarnold, J. R., and Kirkpatrick, A., Multidimensional approach to the measurement of quality of life in lung cancer clinical trials, in *The Quality of Life of Cancer Patients*, Aaronson, N. K. and Beckmann, J. H., Eds., Monogr. Ser. European Organization for Research and Treatment of Cancer, Raven Press, New York, 17, 63, 1987.

40. Boyd, N. F., Selby, P. J., Sutherland, H. J., and Hogg, S., Measurement of the clinical status of patients with breast cancer: evidence for the validity of self assessment with linear analogue scales, *J. Clin. Epidemiol.*, 41, 243, 1988.

41. Levine, M. N., Guyatt, G., Gent, M., De Pauw, S., Goodyear, M. D., Hryniuk, W., Arnold, A., Findlay, B., Skillings, J. R., Bramwell, V. H., Levin, L., Bush, H., Abu-Zarra, H., and Kotalik, J., Quality of Life in stage II breast cancer: an instrument for clinical trials, *J. Clin. Oncol.*, 6, 1798, 1988.

42. Aaronson, N. K., Ahmedzai, S., Bullinger, M., Crabeels, D., Estape, J., Filiberti, A., Flechtner, H., Frick, U., Hurny, C., Kaasa, S., Klee, M., Mastilica, M., Osoba, D., Pfausler, B., Razavi, D., Rofe, P. B. C., Schraub, S., Sullivan, M., and Takeda, F., The EORTC quality of life questionnaire: interim results of an international study, in *Effect of Cancer on Quality of Life*, Osoba, D., Ed., CRC Press, Boca Raton, FL, 1991, chap. 14.

43. Levine, M. N., Quality of life in breast cancer, in *Effect of Cancer on Quality of Life*, Osoba, D., Ed., CRC Press, Boca Raton, FL, 1991, chap. 15.

44. Kirschner, B. and Guyatt, G., A methodological framework for assessing health indices, *J. Chronic Dis.*, 38, 27, 1985.

45. van Knippenberg, F. C. E. and deHaes, J. C. J. M., Measuring the quality of life of cancer patients: psychometric properties of instruments, *J. Clin. Epidemiol.*, 1043, 1988.

46. Frank-Stromberg, M., Single instruments for measuring quality of life, in *Instruments for Clinical Nursing Research*, Frank-Stromberg, M., Ed., Appleton and Lange, Norwalk, CT, 1988, 79.

47. Dean, H., Multiple instruments for measuring quality of life, in *Instruments for Clinical Nursing Research*, Frank-Stromberg, M., Ed., Appleton and Lange, Norwalk, CT, 1988, 97.

48. Donovan, K., Sanson-Fisher, R. W., and Redman, S., Measuring quality of life in cancer patients, *J. Clin. Oncol.*, 7, 959, 1989.

49. Maguire, P. and Selby, P., Assessing quality of life in cancer patients, *Br. J. Cancer*, 60, 437, 1989.

50. Moinpour, C. M., Feigl, P., Metch, B., Hayden, K. A., Meyskens, F. L., Jr., and Crowley, J., Quality of life end points in cancer clinical trials: review and recommendations, *J. Natl. Cancer Inst.*, 81, 485, 1989.

51. Barofsky, I. and Sugarbaker, P. H., Cancer, in *Quality of Life Assessments in Clinical Trials*, Spilker, B., Ed., Raven Press, New York, 1990, 419.

52. Helmstadter, G. C., *Principles of Psychological Measurement*, Appleton-Century-Crofts, New York, 1964.

53. Nunally, J. C., *Psychometric Theory*, McGraw-Hill, New York, 1978.

Chapter 4

PREDICTION OF PSYCHOSOCIAL DISTRESS IN PATIENTS WITH CANCER

Neill Iscoe, J. Ivan Williams, John Paul Szalai, and David Osoba

TABLE OF CONTENTS

I. INTRODUCTION

Prediction of events, apart from being a popular human pastime, is a necessary human activity. Governments predict what their budgets will be for the next year, economists and analysts may focus on economic trends and stock activity, gamblers bet on the next card, sporting event, or lottery. In health or illness, patients wish to know what their individual prognosis is or if a given action or behavior predicts future health. With respect to the psychosocial issues in patients with cancer these concerns can be distilled into the following questions. Do particular psychosocial behaviors predict for the development of cancer? Is the psychosocial make-up of patients in itself a prognostic factor? Finally, following the diagnosis of cancer can we predict which patients will develop psychosocial distress? It is not our intention to address either of these first two questions. Evidence linking the development of cancer to particular psychosocial groups that is not mediated by known etiologic agents, such as tobacco, is inconclusive.[1] Initial observations[2] relating adjustment responses to prognosis have not been confirmed by other studies.[3]

In this chapter we will focus on the last question: can professionals predict which patient will have psychosocial distress following the diagnosis of cancer? As with quality of life the concept of psychosocial distress means different things to different people. We define it as the grief an individual experiences as a result of inadequate or inappropriate psychological or social function. The distinction here from grief posed by a poor quality of life is that the other major component, physical function, is ignored. Hence, though a person might have suboptimal quality of life due to paralysis, it would be possible to have no psychosocial distress by virtue of adequate social and psychological function.

Given that people view cancer as "sort of being like leprosy" and equate it with "pain and death",[4] it could well be asked — won't all patients with cancer need assistance in adjusting to their diagnosis? A cross-sectional study[5] suggests that patients with cancer have no more difficulty in terms of mental health problems than patients with other chronic medical illnesses. Even if one wanted to offer assistance to all patients with cancer there is the practical issue of inadequate resources to manage all patients when the disease affects up to one in three people during their lifetime and with one half of all cancers diagnosed in persons 65 years of age or older.

If medical professionals wish to treat people with a disease as opposed to a disease in people, it will be necessary to address the psychosocial and behavioral issues that surround patients with cancer. Prediction of future psychosocial distress is a desirable objective from two perspectives. First, it may permit the identification of the determinants of subsequent distress and by doing so, present logical opportunities for care that will prevent or modify this distress. Second, the professions will be able to focus on a group of patients in which therapy may prove to be useful and avoid interventions in patients who do not require this care.

As already stated, patients want physicians to predict their future. Studies to determine prognostic factors are best viewed within the framework of studies describing the clinical course of an illness,[6] in which a primary objective is to define the determinants of the outcome in question. The criteria may be loosely grouped into *patient-related factors:* inception cohort, description of referral pattern, and complete follow-up; and *measurement or analytic issues:* blinded assessment, objective outcome criteria, and adjustment for prognostic factors.

An inception cohort is a group of patients who are defined as having a particular condition being diagnosed within a specified time frame. This is routinely done in many clinical trials in which patients with some condition are treated with regimen A or B and then followed to compare the relative efficacy of treatment. However, even within clinical trials, an inception cohort may not be defined. For example, in the treatment of metastatic breast cancer, eligibility criteria do not generally include a statement defining the time from diagnosis of metastases. Would a patient with slowly progressive metastatic disease who has been asymptomatic for a year be expected to have a similar outcome to a symptomatic patient who was just discovered to have metastases? Surely the answer is no and is related to the length-time bias inherently present when patients are selected without considering the time from the event in question. Within the context of psychosocial distress in patients with cancer, numerous logical sets of inception cohorts can be constructed: e.g., newly diagnosed patients without evidence of disease after initial therapy, all newly diagnosed patients irrespective of the extent of disease, patients developing recurrent disease, patients commencing their first course of chemotherapy or radiotherapy, and patients at the time of admission to palliative care or hospice programs.

Striving to attain complete follow-up is an obvious goal in studies designed to relate present information to future events. "Losing" patients poses two problems: loss of information weakening the study and the consideration that those lost are systematically different than those remaining in the study. In studies of patients with malignancy, failure to return is always accompanied by the specter of death.

A description of the referral pattern permits the reader to decide if the patients being studied resemble those of his practice. Were the patients described in the context of a general practitioner's office or in a specialized treatment center? If the latter, how many layers of specialists or treatment centers did the patients pass through before being entered into the study. For example, cancer patients given palliative care in the community by a general practitioner may be very different than those cared for by oncologists in institutional settings.

Measurement issues related to psychosocial distress mirror those related to quality of life. Does the measurement reproducibly reflect the concept or concepts in question when often no universally accepted "gold standard" exists? Studies based on instruments for which no reliability or validity information exists should be viewed very critically. Furthermore, assessments should be made in a blinded manner so that any preconceived ideas of the assessor do not influence the outcome assessment.

In studies where prognostic factors or factors predictive of future states are unknown, a goal of the study would be to test which of various hypothesized predictors are truly related to the outcome or outcomes of interest. In the case of predicting future psychosocial distress, one could test the hypothesis that patients with poor prognosis at diagnosis will have more distress than patients with more favorable prognosis or that patients with a history of psychological difficulties will have greater difficulty adjusting to their diagnosis or treatment. Clearly other hypotheses can be developed based on theories present in the literature and personal beliefs. Moreover, the hypotheses need not be the same for different cohorts of patients, e.g., newly diagnosed, immediately following recurrence or pre-terminal patients. Beyond these general methodologic concerns there are issues related to the size of the target group and the accuracy of the prediction. Is the objective to predict which *groups* of patients are at risk for future psychosocial distress and might benefit by early intervention or is the goal to predict an *individual's* risk in which case less variability would be tolerated.

Finally, how accurate must the predictive model be and how was the analysis performed? Was the analysis based on binary outcomes, that is the presence or absence of psychosocial distress? This form of analysis lends itself to the definition of probabilities for the model. Whereas clinical judgment often declares a patient to be sick or not as opposed to very sick, marginally sick, or some gradation thereof; self report measures using scales generally result in scores that are treated as continuous variables analytically. These scales may permit comparison of one group to another but do not permit an *a priori* decision as to what score constitutes depression, anxiety, distress, etc. in any individual patient or group.

Given the prevalence of cancer, if psychosocial disability commonly accompanies the disease, successful management of this disability would have profound effects on the health of large numbers of people. To date, the large surveys that have been conducted have been cross-sectional in design and have compared 190 outpatients with cancer to other outpatient groups with chronic illnesses,[5] 245 patients with various malignancies at one of three centers in the eastern U.S.[7] or assessed 505 female outpatients with one of five different malignancies.[8]

The comparative study of Cassileth's[5] demonstrated that the anxiety, depression, and mental health index scores did not differ significantly among five chronic physical illnesses (one of which was cancer) when measured by the Rand Corporation Mental Health Index. Indeed, the mental health index scores of the 190 patients with cancer did not differ from the scores generated in the Rand survey of 5089 members of the general public. Unfortunately the meaning of a particular score in a given patient is unclear. Therefore, it is impossible to state with any certainty how many of the patients with cancer were depressed or anxious, though it seems sensible to believe that these disabilities are no more likely to be present in patients with cancer than patients with arthritis, diabetes, renal disease, or dermatologic conditions.

Lansky et al.[8] interviewed 505 women without clinical evidence of an organic brain syndrome to determine the prevalence of major depressive disorders. Seventy-six patients (15%) were hospitalized at the time of the interview. All patients were assessed for depression by the Hamilton rating scale and the Zung scale, as well as having their functional performance status and level of pain measured. Decision points for the determination of depression were similar to those used in other studies. Only 5.3% of the population were deemed depressed based upon scores that defined major depressive symptomatology. These patients had significantly poorer performance status, greater pain, lower socioeconomic status, and were more likely to have a past history of depression. In-patients, as expected, had greater pain and poorer levels of function and tended to have worse scores on the Zung and Hamilton depression scales.

The Psychology Oncology Group Study[7] assessed 215 patients in three large cancer centers in the eastern U.S. and determined the rates of psychiatric illness based on psychiatric interviews supplemented by self-report measures and clinical measures of function. All patients were new to the institutions but may not have represented newly diagnosed patients and, in contrast to the other studies, 61% were in-patients. Additionally, the patients had to have a Karnofsky performance status of 50 or greater, implying some minimal level of functioning. One hundred and one (47%) had a DSM-III psychiatric diagnosis with only 7 (3%) having a personality disorder. Six percent had a major affective disorder (akin to the 5.3% in the study by Lansky) but a further 32% had an adjustment disorder that was felt by the authors to be the type of disorder responsive to psychological interventions. An accompanying editorial[9] hastens to point out the prevalence of major affective disorders (6%) and anxiety disorders (2%) is similar to those seen in general population surveys.

What does all this mean? Do patients with cancer have morbidly ill psyches or do they have similar patterns of disability as the general population? We believe the truth is probably a rephrasing of the two observations. Major psychiatric illness is probably rare and no different than the general population. Minor psychiatric disturbance including the DSM-III adjustment disorders may well be common but may be no different than the minor affective disorders that often accompany physical complaints seen in the general practice setting and for which the prognosis is favorable.[10]

II. METHODS

We have performed a Medline English language literature computer search using the key words cancer and quality of life for the years 1985 through 1989. Further articles were obtained by examining the reference lists of the articles obtained and from our own files.

Of the 200 publications retrieved and reviewed, those included in this chapter were selected based on their purposes, e.g., identification of factors associated with the development of psychosocial distress and the design of trials with psychosocial outcomes, e.g., randomized prospective trials or cohort intervention studies. Cross-sectional studies, which cannot be predictive, were not included unless the information was deemed valuable due to the number of patients surveyed, the uniqueness of the information, or because the results were controversial.

Descriptive studies are useful for making observations and posing hypotheses to be tested. However, unless the observations are startling, it is not possible to establish with what degree of certainty an association exists. To do the latter, analytic methods are necessary and require counts or measurements with the problems attendant when measuring an attribute for which no "gold standard" exists.

This chapter, with rare exceptions, reflects what is known about adults with cancers, as very little information exists in the pediatric age group. The adult studies have been grouped according to the nature of the inception cohort: (a) patients at diagnosis, (b) patients receiving a specific intervention (c) patients receiving palliative or hospice-based care and in whom life expectancy is limited. We shall also present some data from a longitudinal study performed at this center.

In the review that follows a variety of research designs and an even greater variety of measurement techniques have been employed. We will comment on the research design only in so far as it affects the validity of the observation or affects the generalizability of the result. The tables do not make reference to the criteria of referral pattern or blinded outcome assessment as in only one report was either one of these criteria explicitly described. The nature of the practice can only be inferred from the institutional affiliation of the authors. No attempt has been made to review all the scales used but we attempt to provide our assessment of the merits of those scales listed in the tables. Interested readers are asked to review the appropriate references for further details.

III. CHILDHOOD CANCER

As the probability of childhood cancer is relatively rare, it was not until the recent, dramatic improvements in survival that follow-up studies of children have been possible. Depending on the diagnosis, up to 90% of children with cancer can expect to survive into adulthood with the prospect of living relatively normal lives.

Gotay[11] has reviewed the early studies on the quality of life among the survivors of childhood cancer, most of which were based on small numbers and lacked control or comparison groups. Physiological effects of the diseases and treatments were noted in all systems of the body; vision, hearing, dentition, and growth and developmental problems including stature and sexual maturation. Longer-term problems also include a 10- to 20-fold increased risk of developing subsequent cancers.

Global and specific cognitive defects were noted in a number of studies, particularly those focusing on children with brain tumors or lesions of the central nervous system. Gotay found it difficult to estimate the size of the effects because of the variability of the definitions and methods used to assess neuropsychological disabilities.

Gotay noted the studies were fraught with flaws in methods and designs. She called for improved staging efforts, more reliable instruments that are responsive to the effects to be assessed, better tracking systems to follow patients and their problems, and procedures for determining the specific problems survivors encounter in their schooling. She also discussed a number of strategies that could be used to minimize the difficulties survivors might encounter.

There are two studies that used siblings as controls, have high response rates, and relatively long follow-up periods. Teta et al.[12] identified 666 survivors of childhood and adolescent cancer cases in the Connecticut Tumor Registry who were diagnosed between 1945 and 1974, under 20 years of age at time of diagnosis, and survived 5 or more years. Five hundred and forty-two (81%) were interviewed. They provided 856 siblings (eligible controls) of whom 732 (86%) were interviewed. They excluded 149 proxy responses for siblings and were left with 450 survivors and 587 siblings. The psychosocial consequences studied included a standardized interview for depression, behavioral indicators of maladjustment, educational advancement, employment, and the ability to obtain life insurance.

There were no differences between survivors and controls with respect to depression, suicide, running away, or psychiatric hospitalization. Male survivors were less likely to gain entry into the military, college, and employment than their male sibs, but there were no differences for college and employment between the group of females. Survivors did encounter difficulties in obtaining life and health insurance. While the survivors were not at excess risk for depression, they did encounter difficulties in achieving major socioeconomic goals.

Byrne and colleagues[13] identified 2498 eligible survivors in five data registries who were diagnosed with cancer between 1945 and 1975, were under 20 years of age at the time, had survived for 5 years, and were at least 21 years of age by the end of 1979. They were able to interview 2283 (91%) of the survivors and 3270 (91%) of 3604 eligible, sibling controls. The outcomes of interest were marital histories, specifically marriage and divorce. Most of the differences observed applied to survivors of brain and central nervous system tumors. Compared to their sibling controls, CNS tumor survivors married later, were more likely to be divorced, and had first marriages that lasted a shorter time.

There is a disparity in findings between the latter two studies and earlier ones. As the earlier studies had small samples, lacked adequate controls and used questionable measures, the estimates of the long-term effects of cancer and treatment may have been grossly overestimated. Or, the adverse effects may have abated with time so that the differences would have been less pronounced if the children had been followed longer. In either set of studies, children who survive cancers of the brain or central nervous system are a greater risk of negative longer term outcomes than survivors of other childhood cancers.

IV. ADULT CANCER

A. WHEN CANCER IS DIAGNOSED

We have found seven published reports examining the psychosocial morbidity of patients with cancer as it relates to the diagnosis of the malignancy. The reports reviewed do not focus on any particular therapy or its impact and in only one report[14] is a single disease, lung cancer, examined. Four of the reports are longitudinal (Table 1) and had worrisome follow-up rates. A southern California cross-sectional study[15] observed a complex interaction between dimensions of social support and the extent of disease. Though the adequacy of attachment was important in the case of patients with localized disease, they observed the effects of both the adequacy of attachment and the availability of social integration were much more strongly (p <0.001) associated with nonlocalized disease. This suggests that patients in failing health are more profoundly affected by the ability to maintain (availability) meaningful social relationships (adequacy of attachment). In the context of this chapter this would suggest that more advanced or progressive disease predicts for poorer social function and heightened psychosocial distress. A Dutch cross-sectional study[16] observed patients who were undergoing treatment with chemotherapy or just after their initial surgery perceived more positive and less negative support (p <0.001) from those around them. These researchers noted patients perceived more support with increasing disability. These two cross-sectional studies illustrate the difference between social support and social function. A final

TABLE 1
Longitudinal Studies Following The Diagnosis of Cancer

Sample	Inception cohort	Follow-up	Outcome criteria	Prognostic factors	Ref.
221	Yes	73% at 1 year	POMS combined with Index of Vulnerability[b]	Multiple noted, including: more advanced disease or physical symptoms, high anxiety, low ego, psychiatric or alcohol abuse history, particular coping strategies, poor social support	18
31	Yes	70% at 6 to 12 months	Q-Sort index[a]	Severity of illness and prognosis	19
			Global Psychosocial Status[a]	Psychosocial stability, living arrangements	
60	Yes	73% at 3 months (11/14 unavailable due to death)	SCL 90-R,[c] Locke Wallace Marital Adjustment,[c] three others[a]	Marital adjustment, spousal support	14
369	Yes	68% at 9 to 12 months (15/114 lost died) 29% at 2+ years (29/260 lost died)	Rand MHI,[c] Role Limitation Measure,[c] Interview Scale for Social Interaction[b]	Initial MHI psychological status	20

Note: Outcome criteria assessment:

[a] Unique measure, no psychometric information available.
[b] Unique measure, some psychometric information available.
[c] Standard measure, psychometric information available.

cross-sectional study[17] reports on work disability in 247 patients selected from a tumor registry who had been working prior to their diagnosis. These patients were assessed within 1 year of diagnosis (86% by 6 months) and physical, emotional, and work characteristics were related to the patient's present work status. Failure to return to work was highly correlated with more advanced disease, greater physical dysfunction, and higher physical demands of the job.

The longitudinal studies offer the potential for assessing predictive factors. Table 1 summarizes the studies in chronological order of appearance according to the principles of a study of the clinical course of an illness already described. The report from Harvard[18] assembled a cohort of 221 patients with various malignancies within 10 days of diagnosis and intensively assessed them with a battery of self-report and interview-based measures. Outcome measures were based on the combination of the POMS (Profile of Mood States) with an interviewer rated Index of Vulnerability. Patients exceeding a preset standardized score were deemed to be distressed. No independent validation of this classification was offered. Dichotomizing the patients into sick and well permitted the development of a predictive or screening model that was 86% accurate with 7% false positives and 7% false negatives and that explained 56% of the outcome variance. At any given time the patients were assessed after study entry the medical factors of extent of disease, severity of symptoms, treatment, and health concerns, accounted for 40 to 60% of the explained variance with 25 to 38% of the remaining variance being explained by what is referred to as non-medical concerns, e.g., prior marital problems, life regrets, etc. Apart from the issue of whether these factors are indeed predictive of future psychosocial distress and the accuracy of the prediction are the issues of the validity of the outcome definition and the generalizability of this labor intensive process.

Mages et al.[19] interviewed 31 patients up to 4 months after initial therapy and reviewed 70% 6 and 12 months later. Psychosocial adaptation was judged by interviewers who used two rating schemes to assign people to adaptation groups. They noted that initial coping mechanisms persisted in all but two patients, even if the initial coping mechanisms were viewed as maladaptive. They also observed that higher psychosocial morbidity was strongly associated with increasing severity of illness ($p < 0.001$), poor prognosis ($p < 0.001$), living alone ($p < 0.01$) and decreased psychological stability as indicated by patients describing themselves in a manner that reflected feelings of unworthiness, victimization, embitterment, etc. ($p < 0.001$).

Quinn et al.[14] studied 60 men with lung cancer 1 month after diagnosis and reviewed the status of 44 4 months later (11 of 16 not in follow-up died). Patients completed scales designed to assess coping, marital adjustment, social support, anxiety, and depression at study entry and had coping, anxiety, and depression assessed 4 months later. Their wives were interviewed to assess the degree of marital intimacy and completed the marital adjustment, anxiety, and depression scales at study entry and the anxiety and depression scales at follow-up. Results from both the patients and the wives indicated a significant association between poor marital adjustment and future anxiety and depression. The authors also noted certain coping strategies such as "self-blaming denial" were more likely associated with subsequent anxiety and depression.

A second report of the southern California group[20] describes the longitudinal phase of the study referred to previously. Of 1732 patients reviewed, 797 were eligible and of these, 369 (46%) agreed to participate in this study designed to identify the determinants of subsequent mental health. Of the initial patients enrolled (77% were women) only 253 were assessed 9 to 12 months later and only 109 were assessed at a period of 24 months or more after entry into the study. Psychological status, determined by the Rand Corporation's Mental Health Index, was determined at study entry and at each follow-up visit. Factors recorded at study entry included sense of control, social relationship, socioeconomic status, and stage of disease. A number of important observations were made. First, if one divides the initial mental health scores into three groups: mean ± 0.5 SD, and groups above or below this level, regression towards the mean of subsequent mental health scores was noted. Notwithstanding this observation, initial mental health state was the most powerful predictor of the subsequent mental health state ($p < 0.001$) and explained approximately 50% of the variance. Other factors did not contribute significantly to the model. The follow-up rate was extremely poor (27%) with only 39 deaths out of the 260 failing to return at 24 months. The 221 lost to follow-up were similar to those who refused to participate in the study, in this case described as non-white male. Patients lost to follow up also tended to have greater role limitations, lower sense of control, lower social integration and lower mental health scores at study entry. These observations suggest a systematic loss and cast significant doubts on the generalizability of this and potentially any other study with a high initial refusal rate or a high drop out rate.

We have conducted a study at this Cancer Centre to determine if patients at high risk for psychosocial distress can be identified on the basis of factors collected at registration. The outline of this study is shown in Figure 1 and patient eligibility listed in Table 2. The independent variables of anxiety, depression, social support, future expectations, performance status, and history of alcohol abuse or psychologic counseling were determined at study entry and were correlated to the level of anxiety and depression as measured by the SCL-90 at 6 to 9 months following study entry or to the presence of clinically evident

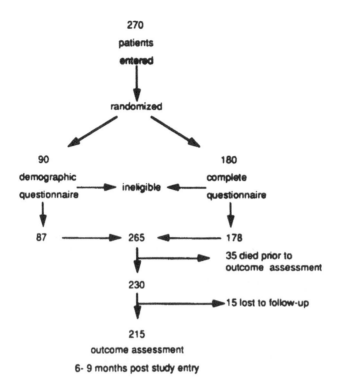

FIGURE 1. Prediction of psychosocial distress in patients with cancer.

TABLE 2
Eligibility Criteria

1. Pathologically confirmed diagnosis of cancer other than non-melanotic skin cancer
2. No prior history of cancer
3. Registration at the Toronto-Bayview Regional Cancer Centre within 3 months of the diagnosis of cancer
4. Ability to read and communicate in English
5. Available for follow-up
6. Ambulatory for at least part of the day
7. At least 18 years of age and able to give informed consent
8. No evidence of primary or secondary cerebral neoplasm

psychosocial distress as manifest by referral or recommended referral to a member of the Centre's psychosocial consultation team. A unique feature of this study was the randomization of the 270 patients following stratification by disease site to an experimental group (n = 180) receiving the full battery of psychosocial assessment and a control group (n = 90) receiving a demographic questionnaire. We felt it necessary to demonstrate the absence of heightened psychosocial awareness and potentially increased distress as a result of the assessment process.

The randomization produced two groups in which no significant differences were noted in the groups' male-female ratio, age or the clinical parameters of performance status at registration, performance status at follow-up, status at last follow-up, response to therapy or follow-up time. The size of the population studied and the actual values obtained demonstrated the age of the experimental group would be within 7% of the control group 95% of the time and that the ability to detect small to medium effects respectively in male-female ratio or the clinical parameters was very high (80 to 95% power). We also observed no statistically discernible difference in the rates of referral or observations of distress during follow-up and could have observed a small effect, had one existed, with 90% certainty. The self-report outcome assessments of anxiety and depression were not significantly different between the groups. However, the ability to state the results of the groups were equivalent was limited by the large standard deviations which equaled or exceeded the mean scores for anxiety and depression. Moreover, while the differences in the means of the outcome scores, 0.14 (0.42 vs. 0.28) for anxiety and 0.18 (0.68 vs. 0.50) for depression, approach statistical significance ($p = 0.09$ and $p = 0.08$, respectively), we do not feel these small differences are clinically meaningful. Hence, we were satisfied the assessment of the putative determinants of psychosocial distress did not affect the clinical course of disease.

Five patients were found to be ineligible. During the course of follow-up only 14 (5.2%) of the eligible patients were noted to have clinically overt psychosocial distress. This figure is remarkably similar to that noted by Lansky et al.[8] and to the frequency of major affective disorders seen in the Psychology Oncology Collaborative Research Group cross-sectional study.[7] Due to the rarity of patients noted to be overtly distressed it was not possible to assess the relationship of the independent variables to this clinical outcome. Possibly more important is the fact that we were unable to determine what level of SCL-90 anxiety or depression scores might serve as a useful decision point for defining clinical distress rather than the statistical or numerical decisions made in other studies.

The relationship of the independent variables to the outcome of anxiety or depression was assessed with stepwise multiple regression techniques. The R^2 value of 38.5% for the anxiety outcome was virtually all due to the initial measure of anxiety ($R^2 = 36\%$). The R^2 value of 43% for the depression outcome was related to the initial state measures of anxiety ($R^2 = 33\%$) and depression ($R^2 = 6\%$). One final note of caution is that during the development of our questionnaire we tested previously developed scales to measure recent life events and locus of control and could not reproduce the reliability estimates originally reported though acceptable values were obtained with the SCL-90.

Collectively these studies suffer from the variable quality of outcome assessment criteria, short follow-up and low follow-up rates. If common themes emerge, it appears that initial states of distress are the major determinants of subsequent distress in that Mages et al.[19] noted negligible change in patterns of coping and that both Ell et al.[20] and we have noted the major predictor of a future state is the initial measure of the same determinant. Less consistent observations suggest that more advanced disease, worse performance status, and poorer levels of social support are associated with more distress.

B. PSYCHOSOCIAL DISTRESS IN PATIENTS RECEIVING A SPECIFIC INTERVENTION

Of the 28 reports reviewed, 18 can be grouped according to the nature of the two most commonly investigated areas: primary treatment of breast cancer (6 reports — Table 3) and psychosocial interventions in the variety of diseases (12 reports — Table 4). The other reports will be discussed within this section and are not listed in the tables.

Two studies reported on the psychosocial outcomes of patients with soft tissue sarcomas of the extremities treated at the National Cancer Institute of the U.S. The first study[21] randomized eligible patients to extremity amputation or limb-sparing surgery and radiation with both groups receiving chemotherapy. Patients undergoing amputation reported better emotional outcomes as measured by the Sickness Impact Profile and less disturbed sexual functioning as measured by the Psychosocial Adjustment to Illness Scale. In a follow-up study of 88 patients undergoing limb-sparing surgery Chang et al.[22] noted poorer sexual function despite improved overall quality of life as measured by the Functional Living Index-Cancer. This seemingly contradictory result demonstrates the difficulties in adequately defining quality of life. Two randomized trials compared the effects of different chemotherapy regimens on the psychological response in patients with lung cancer[23] and overall quality

TABLE 3
Psychosocial Distress Associated with Mastectomy

Sample	Inception cohort	Study design	Follow-up	Outcome criteria	Prognostic factors	Ref.
40 breast cancer 25 surgery 25 healthy controls	Yes	Longitudinal cohort	50% used for analysis, 15 week follow-up	State-Trait Anxiety Inventory,[c] Wakefield Depression Inventory,[c] Rosenberg Self-Concept Scale[c]	Cancer and surgery group significantly more depressed than control group. Cancer group tended to be more anxious and have lower self esteem than control group	31
41 mastectomy or lumpectomy and radiation	Yes	Randomized trial	95% at 11 months, 82% at 18 months	Rotterdam Symptom[c] Checklist, body image,[b]	Significantly improved body image in lumpectomy group without heightened fear of recurrence	33
43 mastectomy or 36 lumpectomy or 44 lumpectomy and radiation	Yes	Cross-sectional survey within a randomized trial	100%	CES-D,[c] body image[b]	Radiation group more depressed than other groups. Body image of lumpectomy groups significantly superior to mastectomy group. Fear of recurrence similar in all groups.	34
83 mastectomy or lumpectomy +/- radiation	Yes	Randomized trial	3% studied area 6 months to 4 years after surgery	Brief Symptom Inventory[a]	Lumpectomy group had significantly better emotional and body image scores and lower fear of recurrence	35
98 (approx. 70% chose lumpectomy +/- radiation	Yes	Longitudinal cohort	100% at 3 months	POMS,[c] social support,[b] Karnofsky Performance Status[c]	Lumpectomy group were significantly more angry and depressed and described less support	36
78 mastectomy, 41 lumpectomy	Yes	Longitudinal cohort	82% followed "up to" 16 months post surgery	POMS,[c] PAIS,[c] Marital adjustment,[c] Sexual function[a]	Patients undergoing lumpectomy were significantly less angry and had better sexual function	32

Note: Outcome criteria assessment:

[a] Unique measure, no psychometric information available.
[b] Unique measure, some psychometric information available.
[c] Standard measure, psychometric information available.

TABLE 4

Studies of Interventions Reporting on Efforts to Reduce Psychosocial Distress in Patients with Cancer

Sample	Inception cohort	Study	Follow-up	Intervention	Outcome criteria	Comments	Ref.
56 patients, 41 controls	Yes, no	Nonrandomized cohort	25—70%, up to 12 months	Individual counseling	Self-rating scale,[c] Tennessee self-concept,[c] Sexual function,[a] POMS,[c] Employment[a]	Sexual activity greater in counseled group. No other difference seen in this small study	37
Control 1—83, intervention 157, control 2—68	Yes — breast, lung, melanoma	Nonrandomized cohorts with control groups before *and* after	64% at 6 months, 30 deaths overall	Individual counseling	Structured, interviewed,[a] MAACL,[c] Langner Psychiatric Scale,[c]	No adverse effect of intervention General decline in levels of difficulties noted in all groups. Intervention group scores tended to be better for patients with lung cancer. Scores very similar in other sites.	38
75 intervention, 77 controls	Yes, mastectomy patients	Randomized	100% (12—18 months)	Individual counseling and follow-up by a trained nurse	Interviewer[a]	12—18 months post surgery, psychiatric morbidity counseled 12%, control 39%. Counseling group had as many early problems but they were recognized and managed.	39

Sample	Cancer	Design	Follow-up	Intervention	Measure	Results	Ref
50 intervention, 36 controls	? Metastatic breast cancer	Randomized trial	Post-randomization exclusion of 32%, 34% completed study at 1 year	Support group	POMS,[c] denial,[a] maladaptive coping[a]	More favorable outcomes for those in support groups: total mood, anxiety, vigor, fatigue, confusion, coping, responses	40
26 intervention, 26 controls	No	Randomized trial	84% at 4 weeks	Group education program	State-Trait Anxiety,[c] purpose in life[b]	Lower anxiety for patients in intervention group p <.0001	41
62 intervention, 58 controls	? Advanced cancer in men	Randomized trial	Assessed at 1, 3, 6, 9, and 12 months, 20% alive at 12 months	Counseling	POMS,[c] Self-esteem,[c] life satisfaction,[c] alienation[c]	Significantly more favorable outcomes in experimental group	42
105 patients in two studies Intervention, control	No	Randomized trial	77% at 12 weeks	Education Support group	Cancer Patient Behaviour Scale[a]	Anxiety reduced with education Activity reduced with support	43
75 intervention, 77 controls	Yes, mastectomy patients	Randomized	100% (12—18 months)	Individual nurse counseling	Interviewer based[a]	More favorable social adjustment	44
59 randomized to one of two interventions	Yes, identified as high risk by screening	Randomized trial of interventions compared to historical no treatment control	100% at week 24	Psychotherapy, cognitive skills training	POMS combined with Index of Vulnerability[b]	No differences in effectiveness of interventions, less compared to control though, 7/21 baseline comparisons statistically different	45
48 intervention 52 controls	? Before radiotherapy	Nonrandomized cohort study	100% at 12 weeks	Individual psychotherapy for 10 weeks	Modified Schedule of Affective Disorders and Schizophrenia[a]	Favorable effect of psychotherapy (p <0.05) at end of radiotherapy and 8 weeks later	46

TABLE 4 (continued)
Studies of Interventions Reporting on Efforts to Reduce Psychosocial Distress in Patients with Cancer

Sample	Inception cohort	Study	Follow-up	Intervention	Outcome criteria	Comments	Ref.
13 coping 14 support 14 controls	No, distressed patients as determined by structured interview	Randomized trial	100% at 6 weeks	Group coping skills, Support group therapy, No intervention	POMS, [c] CPIS, [c]	Both intervention group had much better outcome on POMS than control group	47
12 compliant 10 non-compliant	?	Retrospective allocation by medication compliance	100% (post-hoc analysis)	Antidepressant medication (imipramine)	Hamilton Rating Scale, [c] PAIS, [c] clinical judgment[a]	More favorable outcome in those with major depressive symptoms who took medication	48

Note: Outcome criteria assessment:

[a] Unique measure, no psychometric information available.
[b] Unique measure, some psychometric information available.
[c] Standard measure, psychometric information available.

of life in patients with advanced colorectal cancer.[24] In both instances a difference was noted favoring a particular regimen. In patients with inoperable lung cancer randomized to radiotherapy or chemotherapy Norwegian investigators noted lesser psychosocial distress in patients receiving radiotherapy[25] and observed psychosocial function was not related to the side effects induced by a particular treatment but to the physical function ($p < 0.01$) of the patient.[26]

The impact of chemotherapy on quality of life was assessed in a randomized trial in the adjuvant treatment of breast cancer and in randomized trials in advanced breast cancer. In the adjuvant setting, chemotherapy was associated with higher overall psychiatric morbidity as measured by the General Health Questionnaire when compared to a concurrent group randomized to receive radiation.[27] The higher levels of anxiety tended to persist following the discontinuation of chemotherapy, a finding supported by observations of Meyerowitz et al.[28] The reports[29,30] in advanced disease support the notion that aggressive therapy, though more physiologically toxic, was associated with better psychosocial outcomes when compared to groups randomized to a less intensive regimen.

The psychosocial sequelae of breast cancer surgery has been a common focus of interest. Surgery itself does not appear to be an event that precipitates distress as patients with breast cancer were observed to feel more helpless and tended to be more anxious or more distressed on multiple psychological measures, irrespective of the extent of surgery, when compared to a control group having surgery for benign conditions.[31,32]

Other studies were designed to assess the impact of more radical to less radical breast surgery within or outside the setting of a randomized trial. The observation of more favorable body image without increased fear of recurrence in the three randomized trials[33-35] is supported by improved sexual function in the cohort study of Wolberg et al.[32] However, the Pittsburgh group[36] noted patients choosing a more conservative operation were more confused, angry, depressed, and had less support when compared to the mastectomy group. The authors suggest these unanticipated observations may be related to the timing of the Profile of Mood States assessment at the end of radiation treatment. This suggestion is supported by Lasry's finding of increased depressive symptoms associated with radiation treatment following lumpectomy.[34] Other possibilities offered to explain the Pittsburgh results include the suggestion that patients may not be comfortable making a choice for themselves, particularly when choosing a practice that had just become accepted as appropriate medical care.

The 12 reports[37-48] of various psychosocial maneuvers include 6 randomized controlled trials, a randomized trial in which patients were randomized to one of two interventions and compared to a historical control, three studies in which patients were compared to a nonrandomized contemporary control group and one drug study in which the comparison was between compliant and noncompliant patients. In all instances, including the six randomized trials, intervention was associated with improved psychosocial outcomes whether measured as social functioning[44] or psychologic functioning.[39,40,42,43,47] The two small randomized studies of Jacobs et al.[43] did demonstrate greater negative effects associated with the peer support group on activity and with both education or the peer support group on self competency when compared to standard care. Whether a particular intervention is superior to another is unclear as contradictory results favoring a particular method are advocated by Telch[47] but not by Worden.[46] The one drug study reported demonstrates that of 13 people with major depression, those who complied with treatment recommendations improved and that those who did not comply, did not improve.[48] While the improvement cannot clearly be ascribed to the medication, the effects of following medical advice or some combination thereof, it should be noted compliance with medical advice did not seem to affect the outcome in the few patients with lesser degrees of depression.

Flaws in these studies mirror those noted in the previous section: variable quality in the outcome assessment criteria, short follow-up and often very poor follow-up rates. Notwithstanding these obvious deficiencies it appears the development of psychosocial distress seems to be associated with the type of therapy received. Furthermore, it appears this distress can be ameliorated with therapy in advance of discernible pathology. Beyond these generalities no specific statements are possible as the permutations and combinations of therapies and circumstances make any generalizations impossible. For example, though some studies demonstrate chemotherapy is associated with more distress than radiation therapy, the generalizability of that observation to all chemotherapy regimens is not possible as different regimens are associated with different disabilities.[23]

C. PALLIATIVE CARE

In this section we review the information related to predicting psychosocial distress in patients and families who are deemed to be in the terminal stages of their illness or at the time of admission to a palliative care or hospice program. To our knowledge patients have to consent to be managed in a palliative care or hospice program. The very idea of palliative or hospice care is viewed as accepting defeat by some patients and rejected. Hence, we believe these studies are not generalizable to all patients entering the terminal stages of their illness.

All four reports arise from the National Hospice Study which compared the effects of hospice care to conventional care and the quality of life of patients and their families. Nonrandom cohorts of 833 hospital hospice (HH) patients, 624 home care (HC) hospice patients and 297 conventional cared for (CC) patients were assessed at 14-day intervals until the patient's death. As well, bereavement follow-up assessed outcomes in primary care providers at 90 to 120 days after death. Outcomes measures included a modified form of the Spitzer index for overall quality of life, social quality of life, measures related to the satisfaction of care and the emotional state of the caregiver before and after death. The analyses adjusted for differences in the baseline characteristics of the study populations.

As might be expected those in conventional care had higher utilization rates of laboratory tests or radiologic examinations. There was no difference detectable in caregiver satisfaction in the three settings, despite the fact that home based hospice patients were heavily dependent on their caregivers for assistance. There were marked differences in the site of death for the patient; deaths in the home occurred in 62% in HC, 27% in HH, and 13% in CC. The hospice group caregivers were more satisfied with where the patient died than those involved in conventional care and higher satisfaction with care in institutionalized patients was reported by hospice caregivers. In follow-up the HC hospice caregivers had levels of emotional distress slightly higher than CC caregivers but significantly higher than HH caregivers. This was the only finding that suggested an adverse effect of the increased caregiver's burden imposed by home based care.[49] For the patients themselves the major predictor of deteriorating quality of life is the proximity to death with changes evident in the period three weeks prior to death,[50] findings replicated in a series of cancer patients cared for in nursing homes and in the community.[51] Finally using a subset of patients from the NHS, Wallston et al.[52] reported that, in the caregiver's opinion, patients achieved their "ideal" death more often in a hospice setting when compared to those who died in conventional care settings.

In summary it appears the major predictor of psychosocial distress in patients in the palliative care setting is proximity to death and that clients who select the hospice mode of care are happier than those who could not or did not choose this type of care.

V. SUMMARY AND CONCLUSIONS

Severe clinical psychosocial distress is an uncommon occurrence following the diagnosis of cancer. The frequency of meaningful psychosocial distress is undoubtedly much greater and may occur in more than 40% of patients during the course of their illness. The search for the determinants of psychosocial distress has been plagued by multiple problems: an acceptable conceptual definition of the outcome, an agreed upon way to measure the outcome, short term studies, low follow-up rates and the generalizability of the investigative methods. Measures that do not easily and accurately define a group at increased risk for psychosocial distress and are not easily used in the clinical setting will not result in altered clinical practice. Despite these concerns some general observations can be made. Psychosocial distress consistently is more evident in those with poor functional states and advanced disease, varies with the type of therapy, is reduced by strong support systems and seems to be highly correlated with any initial state measures of distress or maladaptation. Perhaps the most encouraging observation is that various therapeutic maneuvers designed to reduce psychosocial morbidity appear to have the desired effect. This observation and those confirming the benefits of lesser breast surgery and highlighting unanticipated problems in the case of limb-sparing sarcoma surgery demonstrate the worth of pursuing these studies and improving upon the foundation they have established.

ACKNOWLEDGMENTS

We wish to thank Natasha Slinko for her secretarial assistance and Marco Katic for performing the analysis related to our study. Part of this work was supported by a grant from the Sunnybrook Trust for Medical Research.

REFERENCES

1. Hurny, C., Psyche and cancer, *Ann. Oncol.*, 1, 6, 1990.
2. Greer, S., Morris, T., and Pettingale, K. W., Psychological response to breast cancer: effect on outcome, *Lancet*, ii, 785, 1979.
3. Cassileth, B. R., Walsh, W. P., and Lusk, E. J., Psychosocial correlates of cancer survival: a subsequent report 3 to 8 years after cancer diagnosis, *J. Clin. Oncol.*, 6, 1753, 1988.
4. Cassileth, P. and Cassileth, B. R., Learning to care for cancer patients, the students' dilemma, in *The Cancer Patient, Social and Medical Aspects of Care*, Cassileth, B. R., Ed., Lea & Febiger, Philadelphia, 1979, 304.
5. Cassileth, B. R., Lusk, E. J., Strouse, T. B., Miller, D. S., Brown, L. L., Cross, P. A., and Tenaglia, A. N., Psychosocial status in chronic illness: a comparative analysis of six diagnostic groups, *N. Engl. J. Med.*, 311, 506, 1984.
6. Department of Clinical Epidemiology and Biostatistics, How to read clinical journals. III. To learn the clinical course and prognosis of disease, *Can. Med. Assoc. J.*, 124, 869, 1981.
7. Derogatis, L. R., Morrow, G. R., Fetting, J., Penman, D., Piasetsky, S., Schmale, A. M., Henrichs, M., and Carnicke, C. L. M., The prevalence of psychiatric disorders among cancer patients, *JAMA*, 249, 751, 1983.
8. Lansky, S. B., List, M. A., Herrmann, C. A., Ets-Hokin, E. G., DasGupta, T. K., Wilbanks, G. D., and Hendrickson, F. R., Absence of major depressive disorder in female cancer patients, *J. Clin. Oncol.*, 3, 1553, 1985.
9. Glass, R. M., Psychiatric disorders among cancer patients, *JAMA*, 249, 782, 1983.
10. Goldberg, D. P. and Blackwell, B., Psychiatric illness in general practice. A detailed study using a new method of case identification, *Br. Med. J.*, 2, 439, 1970.
11. Gotay, C. C., Quality of life among survivors of childhood cancer: a critical review and implication for intervention, *J. Psychosoc. Oncol.*, 5(4), 5, 1988.
12. Teta, M. J., Del Po, M. C., Kasl, S. V., Meigs, J. W., Myers, M. H., and Mulvihill, J. J., Psychosocial consequences of childhood and adolescent cancer survival, *J. Chronic Dis.*, 39(9), 751, 1986.
13. Byrne, J., Fears, T. R., Steinhorn, S. C., Mulvihill, J. J., Connelley, R. R., Austin, D. F., Holmes, G. F., Holmes, F. F., Latourette, H. B., Teta, M. J., Strong, L. C., and Myers, M. H., Marriage and divorce after childhood and adolescent cancer, *JAMA*, 262(19), 2693, 1989.
14. Quinn, M. E., Fontana, A. F., and Reznikoff, M., Psychological distress in reaction to lung cancer as a function of spousal support and coping strategy, *J. Psychosoc. Oncol.*, 4, 79, 1986.

15. Ell, K. O., Mantell, J. E., Hamovitch, M. B., and Nishimoto, R. H., Social support, sense of control and coping among patients with breast, lung, or colorectal cancer, *J. Psychosoc. Oncol.*, 7, 63, 1989.

16. Tempelaar, R., De Haes, J. C. J. M., De Ruiter, J. H., Bakker, D., Van Den Heuvel, W. J. A., and Van Nieuwenhuijzen, M. G., The social experiences of cancer patients under treatment: a comparative study, *Soc. Sci. Med.*, 29, 635, 1989.

17. Greenwald, H. P., Dirks, S. J., Borgatta, E. F., McCorkle, R., Nevitt, M. C., and Yelin, E. H., Work disability among cancer patients, *Soc. Sci. Med.*, 29, 1253, 1989.

18. Weissman, A. D. and Worden, J. W., Coping and vulnerability in cancer patients, *Monogr. of Harvard Medical School and the Massachusetts General Hospital*, 1976.

19. Mages, N. L., Castro, J. R., Fobair, P., Hall, J., Harrison, I., Mendelsohn, G., and Wolfson, A., Patterns of psychosocial response to cancer: can effective adaptation be predicted?, *Int. J. Radiat. Oncol. Biol. Phys.*, 7, 385, 1980.

20. Ell, K., Nishimoto, R., Morvay, T., Mantell, J., and Hamovitch, M., A longitudinal analysis of psychological adaptation among survivors of cancer, *Cancer*, 63, 406, 1989.

21. Sugarbaker, P. H., Barofsky, I., Rosenberg, S. A., and Gianola, F. J., Quality of life assessment of patients in extremity sarcoma clinical trials, *Surgery*, 9, 17, 1982.

22. Chang, A. E., Steinberg, S. M., Culnane, M., Lampert, M. H., Reggia, A. J., Simpson, C. G., Hicks, J. E., White, D. E., Yang, J. J., Glatstein, E., and Rosenberg, S. A., Functional and psychosocial effects of multimodality limb-sparing therapy in patients with soft tissue sarcomas, *J. Clin. Oncol.*, 7, 1217, 1989.

23. Silberfarb, P. M., Holland, J. C. B., Anbar, D., Bahna, G., Maurer, L. H., Chahinian, A. P., and Comis, R., Psychological response of patients receiving two drug regimens for lung carcinoma, *Am. J. Psychiatry*, 140, 110, 1983.

24. Glimelius, B., Hoffman, K., Olafsdottir, M., Pahlman, L., Sjoden, P. O., and Wennberg, A., Quality of life during cytostatic therapy for advanced symptomatic colorectal carcinoma: a randomized comparison of two regimens, *Int. J. Cancer Clin. Oncol.*, 25, 829, 1989.

25. Kaasa, S., Mastekaasa, A., and Naess, S., Quality of life of lung cancer patients in a randomized clinical trial evaluated by a psychosocial well-being questionnaire, *Acta Oncol.*, 27, 335, 1988.

26. Kaasa, S. and Mastekaasa, A., Psychosocial well-being of patients with inoperable non-small cell lung cancer, *Acta Oncol.*, 27, 829, 1988.

27. McArdle, C. S., Calman, K. C., Cooper, A. F., Hughson, A. V. M., Russell, A. R., and Smith, D. C., The social, emotional and financial implications of adjuvant chemotherapy in breast cancer, *Br. J. Surg.*, 68, 261, 1981.

28. Meyerowitz, B. E., Watkins, I. K., and Sparks, F. C., Psychosocial implications of adjuvant chemotherapy: a two-year follow-up, *Cancer*, 52, 1541, 1983.

29. Coates, A., Gebski, V., Stat, M., Bishop, J. F., Jeal, P. N., Woods, R. L., Snyder, R., Med, M., Tattersall, M. H. N., Byrne, M., Harvey, V., Gill, G., Simpson, J., Drummond, R., Browne, J., Van Cooten, R., and Forbes, J. F., Improving the quality of life during chemotherapy for advanced breast cancer: a comparison of intermittent and continuous treatment strategies, *N. Engl. J. Med.*, 317, 1490, 1987.

30. Tannock, I. A., Boyd, N. F., DeBoer, G., Erlichman, C., Fine, S., Larocque, G., Mayers, C., Perrault, D., and Sutherland, H., A randomized trial of two dose levels of cyclophosphamide, methotrexate, and fluorouracil chemotherapy for patients with metastatic breast cancer, *J. Clin. Oncol.*, 6, 1377, 1988.

31. Gottesman, S. and Lewis, M. S., Differences in crisis reactions among cancer and surgery patients, *J. Consult. Clin. Psychol.*, 50, 381, 1982.

32. Wolberg, W. H., Romsaas, E. P., Tanner, M. A., and Malec, J. F., Psychosexual adaptation to breast cancer surgery, *Cancer*, 63, 1645, 1989.

33. deHaes, J. C. J. M., van Oostrom, M. A., and Welvaart, K., The effect of radical and conserving surgery on the quality of life of early breast cancer patients, *Eur. J. Surg. Oncol.*, 12, 337, 1986.

34. Lasry, J. M., Margolese, R. G., Poisson, R., Shibata, H., Fleischer, D., Lafleur, D., Legault, S., and Taillefer, S., Depression and body image following mastectomy and lumpectomy, *J. Chronic Dis.*, 40, 529, 1987.

35. Kemeny, M. M., Wellisch, D. K., and Schain, W. S., Psychosocial outcome in a randomized surgical trial for treatment of primary breast cancer, *Cancer*, 62, 1231, 1988.

36. Levy, S. M., Herberman, R. B., Lee, J. K., Lippman, M. E., and d'Angelo, T., Breast conservation versus mastectomy: distress sequelae as a function of choice, *J. Clin. Oncol.*, 7, 367, 1989.

37. Capone, M. A., Good, R. S., Westie, K. S., and Jacobson, A. F., Psychosocial rehabilitation of gynecologic oncology patients, *Arch. Phys. Med. Rehabil.*, 61, 1980.

38. Gordon, W. A., Freidenbergs, I., Diller, L., Hibbard, M., Wolf, C., Levine, L., Lipkins, R., Ezrachi, O., and Lucido, D., Efficacy of psychosocial intervention with cancer patients, *J. Consult. Clin. Psychol.*, 48, 743, 1980.

39. **Maguire, P., Tait, A., Brooke, M., Thomas, C., and Sellwood, R.,** Effect of counselling on the psychiatric morbidity associated with mastectomy, *Br. Med. J.,* 281, 1454, 1980.

40. **Spiegel, D., Bloom, J. R., and Yalom, I.,** Group support for patients with metastatic cancer, *Arch. Gen. Psychiatry,* 38, 527, 1981.

41. **Johnson, J.,** The effects of a patient education course on persons with chronic illness, *Cancer Nurs.,* April, 117, 1982.

42. **Linn, M. W., Linn, B. S., and Harris, R.,** Effects of counseling for late stage cancer patients, *Cancer,* 49, 1048, 1982.

43. **Jacobs, C., Ross, R. D., Walker, I. M., and Stockdale, F. E.,** Behavior of cancer patients: a randomized study of the effects of education and peer support groups, *Am. J. Clin. Oncol.,* 6, 347, 1983.

44. **Maguire, P., Brooke, M., Tait, A., Thomas, C., and Sellwood, R.,** The effect of counselling on physical disability and social recovery after mastectomy, *Clin. Oncol.,* 9, 319, 1983.

45. **Worden, J. W. and Weisman, A. D.,** Preventive psychosocial intervention with newly diagnosed cancer patients, *Gen. Hosp. Psychiatry,* 6, 243, 1984.

46. **Forester, B., Kornfeld, D. S., and Fleiss, J. L.,** Psychotherapy during radiotherapy: effects of emotional and physical distress, *Am. J. Psychiatry,* 142, 22, 1985.

47. **Telch, C. F. and Telch, M. J.,** Group coping skills instruction and supportive group therapy for cancer patients: a comparison of strategies, *J. Consult. Clin. Psychol.,* 54, 802, 1986.

48. **Evans, D. L., McCartney, C. F., Haggerty, J. J., Nemeroff, C. B., Golden, R. N., Simon, J. B., Quade, D., Holmes, V., Droba, M., Mason, G. A., Fowler, W. C., and Raft, D.,** Treatment of depression in cancer patients is associated with better life adaptation: a pilot study, *Psychosom. Med.,* 50, 72, 1988.

49. **Greer, D. S., Mor, V., Morris, J. N., Sherwood, S., Kidder, D., and Birnbaum, H.,** An alternative in terminal care: results of the national hospice study, *J. Chronic Dis.,* 39, 9, 1986.

50. **Morris, J. N., Suissa, S., Sherwood, S. Wright, S. M., and Greer, D.,** Last days: a study of the quality of life of terminally ill cancer patients, *J. Chronic Dis.,* 39, 47, 1986.

51. **Morris, J. N. and Sherwood, S.,** Quality of life of cancer patients at different stages in the disease trajectory, *J. Chronic Dis.,* 40, 545, 1987.

52. **Wallston, K. A., Burger, C., Smith, R. A., and Baugher, R. J.,** Comparing the quality of death for hospice and non-hospice cancer patients, *Med. Care,* 26, 177, 1988.

Chapter 5

N OF 1 RANDOMIZED CONTROLLED TRIALS FOR INVESTIGATION OF QUALITY OF LIFE IN CANCER

Roman Jaeschke and Gordon H. Guyatt

TABLE OF CONTENTS

I. INTRODUCTION

The efficacy of cancer treatment may be assessed using numerous outcome measures. Traditionally, important questions which are considered by patients and clinicians caring for them are: Does treatment have the potential to eradicate the disease?; What is the probability of prolonging the life of the patient?; What is the chance of delaying the progression of a disease? These aspects of management problems are commonly studied in clinical trials.

During the last several years another aspect of assessing a therapeutic regimen's usefulness in dealing with cancer patients, labeled as Health Related Quality of Life (HRQL), gained recognition. It has become clear that the subjective aspects of the disease and of the treatment process (e.g., pain, nausea, anxiety, depression, distress in the family, etc.) should be taken into the account when management decisions are made. That the clinicians' role does not end on the attempts to prolong life or delay cancer-related symptoms has also become more and more recognized: optimizing the care of terminally ill, suffering or even dying patients is acknowledged as an equally important part of clinicians' role.

Use of HRQL measures in the setting of clinical trials of cancer patients is already accepted,[1] but creates a number of formidable challenges to the clinicians — how to choose a reliable, valid, and responsive instrument; how to interpret changes in the instrument score; to what degree can the results of a given trial be applied to the care of an individual patient. In this chapter we will concentrate on the attempts to overcome some of these difficulties using the methodology of N of 1 Randomized Controlled Trials (N of 1 RCTs).[2] Remembering that different aspects of quality of life could be investigated using this approach our discussion will be based on a specific example — exploring the possibility that a specific analgesic A (drug A) works better than drug B in patients experiencing pain caused by bone metastases.

When deciding which therapy is more beneficial for a given patient, clinicians often cannot rely on the results of randomized control trials (RCTs). One possibility is that the relevant trial comparing drug A with other forms of therapy may never have been done. Second, even if a well designed and executed trial has been performed and drug A was shown to control pain better than drug B in the population of patients, this result may not be applicable to the patient at hand — the patient may not meet criteria of the study, or may represent the minority of patients who do not conform to the overall trial result. Under these circumstances, clinicians typically conduct the time-honored "trial of therapy" in which the patient is given a treatment and the subsequent clinical course determines whether the treatment is judged effective and continued.

Many factors may mislead physicians conducting conventional therapeutic trials. They include the placebo effect, the natural history of the illness, the expectations that the clinician and patient have about the treatment effect, and the desire of the patient and the clinician not to disappoint one another.

To avoid these pitfalls, trials of therapy would have to be conducted with safeguards that would keep both patients and their clinicians "blind" to the kind of treatment being administered. Such safeguards are routine in large-scale RCTs involving dozens or hundreds of patients. Use of an N of 1 RCT design allows similar safeguards in defining beneficial (or better) therapy in single subject.

II. N OF 1 RCT — THE GENERAL CASE

Experimental studies of single subjects have long been an important part of psychological research.[3-5] The methodology is known as "single case" or "single subject" research, N = 1, or, as we call it, N of 1 randomized controlled trials (N of 1 RCTs). We have previously described how N of 1 RCTs may be used in medical practice to determine the optimum treatment of an individual patient and described an "N of 1 service" designed to assist

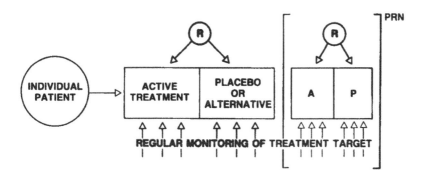

FIGURE 1. N of 1 study design.

clinicians who wish to conduct such a trial. More recently, we have provided detailed guidelines for clinicians interested in conducting their own N of 1 RCTs and reviewed our own 3 years experience in conducting such studies.[6,7]

In general terms the N of 1 RCT design is based on pairs of active/placebo, high dose/ low dose or first drug/alternate drug combinations, the order of administration within each pair determined by random allocation (Figure 1). Treatment targets (directed specifically at patient's complaints) are monitored in a double-blind fashion on a regular, predetermined schedule throughout the trial. The trial continues as long as the clinician and patient agree that they need more information to get a definite answer regarding the efficacy or superiority of the treatment, or until the patient or clinician decides for any other reason to end the trial. The main attractiveness of N of 1 trials is that results pertaining directly to the patient involved are immediately available after the patient has completed the trial.

Several criteria have to be satisfied before N of 1 RCT is attempted. In short, in addition to the effectiveness (or superiority) of treatment being in doubt, the disorder should be relatively chronic and stable. The treatment, if effective, should be continued relatively long term, and the patient should be eager to collaborate in designing and carrying out an N of 1 RCT. In addition, the treatment(s) must have a rapid onset and termination of action, and an optimal treatment duration should be known and practical. Last but not least, the co-operation of a pharmacy prepared to cooperate in the conduct of N of 1 RCT (for example, in the preparation of blinded medication) has to be secured.[6]

III. N OF 1 RCT — EVALUATION OF THE HRQL IN INDIVIDUAL CANCER PATIENT

Solving difficult management dilemmas while caring for cancer patients provides a unique opportunity for the use of N of 1 RCT. Let's assume that the problem the clinician is faced with is pain associated with the metastases to bones. Such a situation fulfills all the requirement necessary to conduct N of 1 RCT — the discomfort is long lasting, most analgesics have a rapid onset and termination of action, the medication, if effective, will be continued relatively long term. The treatment targets most important for the patients may be established prior to the trial and tailored to the individual case. Potential examples include severity of pain, frequency of medication administration, discomfort due to nausea and vomiting while in pain, psychological distress due to pain-related inability to care for dependents, discomfort due to other people noticing discomfort, inability to get a good night's sleep, family discomfort due to patient's heavy sedation, etc. The simplest outcome measure could be just preference of one medication over the other. If one would like to quantify the degree of symptoms and explore the reasons behind preference, the response options depend on the nature of the treatment target. We have found the seven-point Likert-type scale an optimal method for recording the severity of symptoms.[8] For example one may ask:

Please indicate how much discomfort you have been experiencing due to back pain during the last 12 h by choosing one of the options from the scale below:

1.   Extreme discomfort
2.   Severe discomfort
3.   Quite of lot of discomfort
4.   Moderate discomfort
5.   Mild discomfort
6.   A little discomfort
7.   No discomfort at all

Experience drawn from conducting numerous N of 1 RCTs indicates, that in a usual case one should aim for at least three treatment pairs (in our hypothetical case each consisting, for example, of two 24-h treatment periods, with outcome measures taken every 12 h). With relatively short duration of treatment periods the number of pairs could obviously be greater.

IV. N OF 1 RCT — STATISTICAL INTERPRETATION OF THE RESULTS

Upon conclusion of the study the results may be analyzed in a number of ways. The advantages and disadvantages of different methods presented below are discussed elsewhere.[9]

The simplest way of evaluating the data is visual inspection. Such inspection can be made rigorous by systematic consideration of the appropriate graphing of the data, the variability within and between periods, the degree of overlap between periods on different drugs, and the consistency of the difference between periods. If there are apparent differences between treatment periods, their magnitude in relation to the variability seen within periods can be examined. Finally, if there is an apparent effect of treatment, its consistency over pairs of treatment periods can be examined. A deduction that the treatment is effective is supported to the extent that there is a minimal variability within periods, that the difference between drug A and drug B periods is large in relation to the within period variability that is seen, and to the extent that the magnitude of the difference between treatment periods is consistent. Using the visual inspection of data one tries therefore to draw conclusions about direction, magnitude, and consistency of difference between drugs in an intuitive way. The main advantage of this approach is that visual inspection makes intuitive sense to both patient and clinician.

An alternative approach to analysis of data from N of 1 RCTs is to utilize a statistical test of significance. The *p* value associated with the test provides a more formal quantification of the strength of evidence for a treatment effect, and the confidence interval establishes a range of likely treatment effects.

A number of tests are possible candidates in the N of 1 situation. These tests fall into two main classes: nonparametric tests (also called randomization tests), and parametric tests. In its simplest form a randomization test would be based on the direction (i.e., sign) of the observed treatment difference in each pair. Suppose we have conducted an N of 1 RCT of two analgesics for the patients with bone metastases with five treatment pairs. If the two treatments do not differ, any pair is as likely to favor one drug as the other. Under this hypothesis, the chance that patient favors any treatment in a given pair is therefore 1/2; the chance that the patient will prefer analgesic A over B in each of the five pairs is 1/32 or 0.0313, indicating that the result is unlikely to be due to chance alone. This type of nonparametric test is called the sign test since it considers only the sign (and not the magnitude) of the difference in score for each treatment pair. Other nonparametric tests, which do incorporate the size of the outcome score differences are available (the Wilcoxon Signed

Rank test or a "pure" quantitative randomization test).[10,11] The main problem with the use of nonparametric tests is their limited power — for example, with three treatment pairs the probability that patient prefers drug A in each pair (by chance alone) is $1/2 \times 1/2 \times 1/2 = 1/8$ (or $p = 0.125$), still above conventional level of statistical significance.

The main way in which we have been conducting statistical analysis of N of 1 RCTs completed to date was with the use of a parametric test — the Student's paired t test. Mean values for all symptom scores for each treatment period, the mean differences between treatment periods' scores, the 90% confidence interval around the differences, and the probability of differences seen being due to chance are to be calculated. The most important advantage of parametric tests is the increased ability to detect difference between treatments (if such difference exist) — in our experience in about one third of N of 1 RCT with three pairs of treatment the conventional level of statistical significance was reached.[7] The paired t has a number of advantages over nonparametric tests in addition to increased range of possible p values: it is very commonly used and is familiar to most readers of the scientific literature. In addition it is frequently the analytic approach of the cross-over trial, the multisubject equivalent of the N of 1.

V. N OF 1 RCT — CLINICAL INTERPRETATION OF THE RESULTS

One of the biggest problems facing an investigator wanting to include HRQL measures in assessing the effectiveness of any therapeutic intervention is how to interpret the results and communicate them in a meaningful fashion to other clinicians.

The effect of any treatment should be expressed in terms of both statistical significance and clinical relevance. Meeting criteria of statistical significance carries no guarantee that the differences observed are large enough to mandate treatment or that the outcomes which result are particularly satisfying. When discrete events are the measures of outcome (mortality or disease recurrence), the effect of an intervention may be translated into number of lives saved, number of disease-free years, cost of hospitalization saved, etc. In these circumstances the significance of the treatment effects is likely intuitively apparent to the physicians, patients, patients' families, and society.

For most HRQL measures the interpretation is much more difficult. Measuring HRQL involves analysis of patients' subjective assessment of their level of physical dysfunction or psychological discomfort. If one finds a mean change of 0.4 cm on a 10 cm visual analog scale measuring pain, does this constitute a large difference, or a clinically trivial difference? Is a difference of 0.4 point per question on a five-point Likert-type scale measuring the severity of nausea worth continuation of treatment?

Translating changes in a HQRL instrument score into clinically meaningful terms is clearly crucial in the interpretation of study results. This is true for quantifying both the minimal important difference as well as larger effect sizes. The minimal important difference (MID) can be defined as the smallest difference in score in the domain of interest which patients perceive as a change and which would mandate, in the absence of troublesome side effects and excessive cost, modification in the patient's management. While the clinician would participate in the decision regarding modification of management, the definition otherwise focuses on the patient's experience. This follows from a conceptual or philosophical perspective which sees quality of life, including HRQL, as part of an individual's subjective experience.

Conducting N of 1 RCTs provides an opportunity to define the size of the MID and other effect sizes. The strategy which we have used in the N of 1 RCTs performed to date could be summarized as follows.[12]

All N of 1 RCTs were designed to examine the efficacy of specific interventions in ameliorating symptoms due to a variety of conditions. Although in no case have we dealt with cancer patients, some cancer treatments, especially these influencing HRQL, are potentially well suited for N of 1 RCTs. The primary outcome measure in each N of 1 RCT was a HRQL questionnaire measuring the severity of symptoms identified by patients as related to their disease and important in their day-to-day life. The operational definition of the MID which we have used was the smallest difference which was important enough that patients would choose to continue indefinitely with intervention.

Each trial was conducted according to the principles outlined in the previous sections. To assess drug efficacy (or one drug's superiority over the other) in the N of 1 RCT an individualized questionnaire examining the severity of symptoms identified by patients as part of their disease and as being important in their day-to-day life was constructed. The specific symptoms to be measured were obtained from detailed interviews with patients in which information regarding patients' experience of the illness, and what bothered them most, were elicited. The questionnaire that was developed on the basis of the interview consisted of four to seven items (symptoms) with severity of symptoms measured on a seven-point Likert-type scale (see response option example in Section III). The difference in the mean score per question between treatment periods for each treatment pair was established.

To directly assess the patient's perception of drug's benefit (or superiority) we asked the following questions after each pair of treatment periods:

Overall in which of the two periods did you feel better?

1. First period
2. Second period
3. No difference

If patient expressed a preference on the above question we then asked:

Would you continue drug A indefinitely if it was actually drug A that made you feel better?

1. Yes
2. No

When the patient answered YES to the above questions we asked him/her to provide us with the magnitude of the drug effect by asking the following question (Global Rating):

If it turns out that you felt better during the period in which you were on drug A, we would like you to rate how important the difference between the two periods is to you:

1. Not important
2. Slight importance
3. Some importance, consistent benefit
4. Moderate importance, consistent benefit
5. Much importance, good deal of benefit
6. Very important
7. Great importance

A Global Rating score of 0 was assigned if the patient indicated that there was no difference between periods, or if the observed difference was not sufficient to make him or her take the drug indefinitely.

We subsequently examined the relation between patient's subjective assessment of drug efficacy (Global Rating) and differences in the quality-of-life questionnaire score in every pair of every N of 1 RCTs in which data were available. As different questionnaires included from four to seven questions, the difference in the quality-of-life questionnaire score was expressed as total difference in score divided by the number of questions in a particular questionnaire. The MID was defined as difference in the questionnaire score corresponding to a small degree of importance (answers 1 to 3 on the Global Rating); moderate benefit as differences corresponding to answers 4 or 5, and large benefit as differences corresponding to answers 6 or 7.

For individual patients the clinical interpretation of the observed symptom questionnaire score difference was self-evident after each trial was completed. To generalize observations from different patients, we presented our results as mean differences on the HRQL questionnaire score corresponding to small, moderate, and large degree of importance expressed by patients across all trials. The differences on the quality-of-life questionnaire score increase through the range of the differences on Global Rating of the Drug Guess. A mean difference of 0.29 points per question in HRQL questionnaire score correspond to the MID. Differences of approximately 0.66 points per question corresponded to the moderate difference as ranked by the Global Rating; differences of about 1.09 points per question represented a marked difference.[12]

While analyzing the size of MID in the setting of N of 1 RCTs we observed large between-patient variability in the changes in symptom questionnaire score corresponding to varying estimates of drug efficacy. Some portion of this variability is certainly due to the less than perfect validity of the independent standard (in this case, the Global Rating of drug efficacy). However, it is likely that patients have different standards about the changes in symptoms that they view as important or trivial. Such variability in the clinical significance of a particular change in score or outcome is seen in physiological as well as subjective measures. On the other hand, establishing the range of changes in score that correspond to small, medium, and large effects across a group of patients undergoing N of 1 RCTs and confirming that these changes conform to the previous estimates[13] provided us with information allowing meaningful interpretation of study results and were useful in the planning of future studies.

VI. N OF 1 RCTS — INVESTIGATING NEW DRUGS

In the preceding sections we have described application of N of 1 RCTs in deciding about optimal therapy in individual patients. The concept of N of 1 RCT, however, could also be used to draw more general conclusions regarding drug efficacy. The main role of this methodology is likely in the early stages of drug development.[14]

Let's assume again, that a new medication potentially acting on the discomfort due to bone metastases is developed, and that investigators wish to compare it with currently used modes of therapy. In large-sample parallel-group trials patients are assigned at random to one of the treatments under study, for example drug A and drug B. The different treatment groups are followed for the response variable of interest. These trials are the standard approach to establishing drug efficacy, and to persuading regulatory agencies that a new medication should be placed on the market. There are three major hurdles that need to be taken before such large-sample parallel-group studies of the efficacy and safety of a new drug can be undertaken. First, it must be determined whether the new drug shows sufficient promise to justify the initiation of a large clinical research program. Second, the patient population to be studied must be defined. Third, the dose regimen to be used in the major trials must be established.

These decisions are generally based on findings from early clinical safety, tolerance, pharmacology and drug disposition studies in healthy volunteers and patients, augmented by ideas gained from initial small-scale efficacy studies. These efficacy studies are often open, and use baseline status or a historical reference group as a control. Such studies tend to yield anecdotal information of questionable validity. Classical double-blind randomized parallel-groups studies may be used in the early exploration of drug properties, but their small sample size results in findings which leave considerable uncertainty about the three key questions described above.

Thus, when designing the first large-sample efficacy study, investigators are faced with difficult decisions concerning both dose regimen and sample selection. They may gamble on a single dose, or take a safer approach which includes two or more different regimens for comparison. At the same time, they may hazard a guess at a suitable homogeneous target population of patients, or take a more conservative approach which includes a heterogeneous (possibly stratified) population.

If the investigators decide to gamble or guess and turn out to be wrong, the large-sample efficacy study misfires. Nevertheless, the choice for gambling and guessing is frequently made. The reason is that even with a well-defined, homogeneous patient population, a parallel-groups study of a single dose of new drug often requires large numbers of patients for adequate statistical power. The extra numbers required for a heterogeneous patient population and/or several different dosage regimens may well be considered prohibitive.

Even if, through good luck or sound judgment, the first large-sample efficacy study is successful and the study population is clearly shown to benefit from the selected dosage of the new drug, important questions are likely to remain. Would as marked benefit have been obtained at lower doses, or would there be additional benefit with higher doses? Are there subgroups of patients who are particularly responsive or resistant to the new drug?

Several successive rounds of large-sample parallel groups studies may well fail to provide clear cut answers. One reason is that in such studies, there is usually much uncontrolled variation between patients. The result of this variation is that the determination of the profiles of responsive and drug resistant sub-populations of patients is hindered and at times rendered impossible.

In this context N of 1 trials share many features in common with traditional cross-over trials. The fundamental difference between the N of 1 approach and traditional cross-over trials is their primary purpose: N of 1 trials attempt to establish effects in an individual, cross-over trials attempt to establish effects in a group. As a secondary goal, one may use a cross-over trial to examine individual responses. By the same token, one may analyze a series of N of 1 trials with a similar design as a multiple cross-over trial. However, the N of 1 trial will be designed so that individual effects can be reliably detected; the cross-over trial will be designed so that individual estimates of response are imprecisely estimated but the magnitude of the average group effect can be efficiently determined.

In some therapeutic indications (including our hypothetical example), the problems faced by investigators involved in drug development may be overcome by including in the program a short series of carefully designed N of 1 RCTS. These studies will permit the reliable identification of responders and nonresponders, and an estimate of the proportion of patients in each category. They may also make it possible to determine the optimal dosage regimen for individual patients. The availability of this type of information makes the design of large-scale parallel groups studies less problematic.

In relating the foregoing example to the general use of N of 1 RCTs in drug development we will deal in turn with the following six issues: the role of open run-in period, determining the rapidity of onset of drug action, optimising dose, measuring outcome, assessing potential drug impact, and predicting response (Table 1).

A.   THE ROLE OF OPEN RUN-IN PERIOD

To increase the efficiency of generating data in early drug development one could argue for conducting formal N of 1 RCTs only among patients who showed an apparent benefit

TABLE 1
Using N of 1 Trials in Drug Development — Issues and Opportunities

1. The role of open trials of medication
   Does a negative open trial exclude benefit?
2. Determining the rapidity of onset of drug action
   How quickly does the drug begin to act, and cease acting?
3. Optimizing dose
   What is the "best" dose? Does it differ between patients?
4. Measurement of outcome
   What outcomes are most influenced by the new drug?
5. Assessing potential drug impact
   Will the drug have a significant impact on the disease?
6. Predicting response
   Are there features that discriminate between responders and nonresponders?

related to a new drug during an open run-in period. In open therapeutic trials potential biases, including patient and physician expectations and the placebo effect generally favor a conclusion that the new treatment is beneficial. Thus, a false positive conclusion (concluding the drug works better when it doesn't), is far more likely than a false negative (concluding the drug does not work when in fact it does). Accordingly, it would be reasonable to conduct formal N of 1 studies only on patients with apparent benefit of a new drug in open trials. Obviously, any estimates of the degree to which patients prefer drug A over drug B have to take into account that only potential respondents were included in formal evaluation.

B. DETERMINING THE RAPIDITY OF ONSET AND TERMINATION OF ACTION

Conducting visual and statistical analyses of the data generated while obtaining numerous measurements during each treatment period may help in determining the rapidity of the onset and termination of treatment effect. Subsequent N of 1 RCTs may thus be modified to incorporate this knowledge. Precise information about the rapidity of action may also add to the understanding of the drug mechanism of action — a drug exerting its action within minutes of administration and another drug acting first after days of use are likely to have different biological modes of action.

C. OPTIMIZING DOSE

When the optimal dose of the drug is not known, one option is to allow open, unblinded dose titration aiming at a response in the individual patient. One of many alternative approaches would be to begin an N of 1 trial with the lowest acceptable (from the patient's comfort point of view) dose of a new drug. If the first pair showed superiority of drug B (accepted method of treatment), a higher dose of drug A could be used in the next pair. The process could continue until side effects appeared, the highest acceptable dose of drug A was reached, or a difference between drug A and drug B favors the new medication. This last observation could be confirmed by conducting additional pairs of treatment on the apparently favorable dose of drug A. This approach would not only help determine the optimal dose, but would reveal whether this optimal does differed in different patients, an issue that would be very difficult to elucidate by parallel group studies. In addition, it would be possible to modify the doses used after only a few trials, if a high incidence of toxicity (use lower doses), or a low incidence of response (use higher doses) were found.

D. MEASUREMENT OF OUTCOME

In the initial study of a new drug, investigators may be uncertain about the outcomes on which to focus. This is particularly true if the primary outcomes relate to patients' symptoms, and if the condition being treated results in a spectrum of problems. For example, an analgesic for cancer patient with bone metastases may have differential impact on the pain, cognitive functions, or the associated symptoms of nausea and vomiting. These differences may become apparent in initial positive N of 1 RCTs, giving the investigator an opportunity to shift the focus of outcome measurement to the areas most likely to benefit.

E. ASSESSING POTENTIAL DRUG IMPACT

When a number of N of 1 trials have been conducted, one is in a position to evaluate the potential impact of the new medication. Assume that approximately one quarter of the investigated patients responded favorably to drug A. In a condition of major importance to a relatively large population of patients, when the drug (at the doses used) is inexpensive and nontoxic, a 25% response rate suggests an important role for the medication. If only one out of 20 patients has a positive (for drug A) N of 1 RCT, a drug may not be worth further development; if 15 out of 20 patients favor a new analgesic, one clearly has an important new treatment. Between such extremes, the decision concerning further study will depend on factors such as the prevalence of the condition being treated, its associated morbidity, the expense and toxicity of the treatment, and the availability of other effective treatments. We should note that in a condition which results in severe morbidity and for which there is no other treatment, an inexpensive and nontoxic drug might be worth developing and using even if only a small proportion of patients gained a clinically important benefit.

If N of 1 RCTs suggest further study is warranted, the results can help in planning subsequent investigations. For example, sample size for a parallel groups study can be informed by prior N of 1 RCTs which provide accurate information concerning both within-person variability over time and heterogeneity of treatment response. The lower the response rate in preceding N of 1 RCTs, the larger the sample size required in subsequent parallel group designs.

F. PREDICTING RESPONSE

N of 1 RCTs can also help determine eligibility criteria for subsequent studies. The precise identification of responders and nonresponders allows powerful examination of predictors of response. If there is very little overlap between responders and nonresponders (for example, if virtually all people over 50 years of age or with vertebral column metastases respond, and all those under 50 and with rib cage do not) a small number of N of 1 RCTs will allow identification of variables associated with response. If a larger number of N of 1 RCTs have been completed, weaker predictors may also be identified. If the number of trials is large enough, one can use logistic regression methods to determine the independent contribution of a set of variables in differentiating responders from nonresponders.

Identifying variables associated with response is important for clinicians in deciding when to use a drug. In addition, the ability of N of 1 RCTs to precisely define responders may provide a solution to one of the major dilemmas facing those investigating a new drug: choosing the population for the first large-sample parallel groups RCT.

In summary, N of 1 RCTs have an important potential role to play in the development of new drugs influencing quality of life of cancer patients. Information regarding rapidity of onset and termination of drug action, the optimal dose, the outcomes on which to focus, and predictors of response may be obtained most efficiently using N of 1 RCTs. The ultimate impact of a new medication can be assessed early on in the process of clinical testing.

The arguments presented here are theoretical; N of 1 RCTs have not as yet played a major role in the development of a new drug. As a result, the best ways of conducting N of 1 RCTs in this setting remain to be established. Questions include the necessity for double-blind N of 1 RCTs when a preliminary open trial in the same patient is negative, the size of each trial (e.g., the optimal number of pairs of treatment periods), the choice of design, and the relative merits of fixed vs. variable period length and parametric vs. nonparametric analysis. However, the method has sufficient promise that these questions should be addressed through use of N of 1 RCTs as an important part of the strategy for testing of new drugs.

REFERENCES

1. **Coates, A., Gebski, V., Bishop, J. F., et al.,** Improving the quality of life during chemotherapy for advanced breast cancer: a comparison of intermittent and continuous treatment strategies, *N. Engl. J. Med.,* 317, 1490, 1987.
2. **Guyatt, G. H., Sackett, D., Taylor, D. W., Chong, J., Roberts, R., and Pugsley, S.,** Determining optimal therapy — randomized trials in individual patients, *N. Engl. J. Med.,* 314, 889, 1986.
3. **Kratchwill, T. R.,** *Single Subject Research: Strategies for Evaluating Change,* Academic Press, Orlando, FL, 1978.
4. **Barlow, D. H. and Hersen, M.,** *Single Case Experimental Designs: Strategies for Studying Behaviour Change,* 2nd ed., Pergamon Press, New York, 1984.
5. **Kazdin, A. E.,** *Single-Case Research Designs: Methods for Clinical and Applied Settings,* Oxford University Press, New York, 1982.
6. **Guyatt, G. H., Sackett, D. L., Adachi, J. D., et al.,** A Clinician's guide for conducting randomized trials in individual patients, *Can. Med. Assoc. J.,* 139, 497, 1988.
7. **Guyatt, G. H., Keller, J. L., Jaeschke, R., Rosenbloom, R., Adachi, J. D., and Newhouse, M. T.,** Clinical usefulness of the N of 1 randomized control trials: three year experience, *Ann. Intern. Med.,* 112, 293, 1990.
8. **Jaeschke, R., Singer, J., and Guyatt, G. H.,** A comparison of 7 point and visual analogue scales: data from a randomized trial, *Controlled Clin. Trials,* 11, 43, 1990.
9. **Roberts, R. S., Jaeschke, R., Keller, J., and Guyatt, G. H.,** Design and analysis of N of 1 randomized trials: the options, submitted.
10. **Conover, W. J.,** *Practical Nonparametric Statistics,* John Wiley & Sons, New York, 1971.
11. **Edgington, E. S.,** *Randomization Tests,* 2nd ed., Marcel Dekker, New York, 1987.
12. **Jaeschke, R., Guyatt, G. H., Keller, J., and Singer, J.,** Ascertaining the meaning of a change in quality-of-life questionnaire score: data from N of 1 randomized control trials, *Controlled Clin. Trials,* in press.
13. **Jaeschke, R., Singer, J., and Guyatt, G.,** Measurement of health status: ascertaining the minimal clinically important difference, *Controlled Clin. Trials,* 10, 407, 1989.
14. **Guyatt, G. H., Heyting, A., Jaeschke, R., Keller, J., Adachi, J. D., and Roberts, R. S.,** N of 1 randomized trials for investigating new drugs, *Controlled Clin. Trials,* 11, 88, 1990.

Chapter 6

QUALITY OF LIFE OF THE TREATMENT PROCESS IN PEDIATRIC ONCOLOGY: AN APPROACH TO MEASUREMENT

David Feeny, Ronald D. Barr, William Furlong, George W. Torrance, and Sheila Weitzman

TABLE OF CONTENTS

I. INTRODUCTION

Success in achieving remission and disease-free survival for many types of childhood cancer has increasingly focused attention on two important issues: long-term sequelae and the morbidity experienced during the process of treatment. The latter is the focus of the paper.

For childhood cancers with very high survival rates, such as Wilms tumor (Stages 2 to 3, approximately 90% 5-year survival rate; Stages 4 to 5, approximately 75% survival rate), the outcome appears to justify the morbidity burdens of the surgery, radiotherapy, and chemotherapy needed to achieve survival. Thus attention is focused on achieving survival success while reducing the incidence of long term sequelae and the morbidity burden of the treatment process.

Other childhood cancers have remained resistant to treatment. For instance, the 5-year survival rate for inoperable Stage 3 and Stage 4 neuroblastoma is approximately 10%. With such a low rate of success it is important to ask whether aggressive therapy aimed at cure does more harm than good. An alternative would be to consider palliative care.

In order to evaluate new therapies aimed at reducing the morbidity of treatment, it is essential that a measure of the quality of life of the treatment process be developed. As part of a larger evaluation of treatments for three major childhood cancers (Wilms tumor Stages 2 to 5; high risk acute lymphoblastic leukemia (ALL); neuroblastoma, inoperable Stage 3 and Stage 4), quality of life measures both for treatment process and for outcome have been developed. The former will be described here. The primary purpose of the paper is to describe an approach to quantifying the quality-of-life burden of treatment and illustrate its application in pediatric oncology.

The quality of life effects of cancer and its treatment have received increased attention in the last decade.[1-6] Although quality of life issues have not received the same attention in pediatric oncology as they have for adult oncology, the literature has begun to grow rapidly.[7-21]

To date the focus in the literature, on the quality of life of the treatment process in pediatric oncology, has been on organ toxicity, pain, nausea, vomiting and the consequences of bone marrow suppression, with increasing attention being given to psychological adjustment.[10,13,22] There have been relatively few attempts to assess comprehensively the quality of life burden of treatment. Our goal was to develop a framework within which to provide such an assessment.

II. UTILITY APPROACH TO MEASURING HEALTH-RELATED QUALITY OF LIFE

There are a variety of generic and specific approaches to measuring health-related quality of life.[23] In this case the utility approach was chosen for several reasons. Before elaborating on those reasons, a brief description of the approach is necessary.

The utility approach is a generic method for measuring health-related quality of life. It is derived from economic and decision theory and based on a well developed set of axioms for decision making under uncertainty.[24-34] The utility approach has been applied to a variety of diseases and health-care problems. One of its advantages is that it allows for broad comparisons.

By convention utility is measured on a dead (0.0) to perfect health (1.0) scale. It provides a single global score of health-related quality of life. Thus utility scores summarize both the positive and negative (i.e., adverse) effects of treatment. This summarization is both a blessing and a curse. The single score provides a valuable measure of the net effect on quality of life; the single score does not, however, reveal to the investigator the aspects of quality of life which have been influential in generating that score. For this reason, utility measures are sometimes administered in conjuction with less aggregated types of measures from which such detail is available.

The utility approach was chosen for this application in part because it permits the analyst to combine measures of the quality of life of the treatment process with the quality of life of the outcome. In addition to measuring the quality of life of the treatment process, a multi-attribute health status classification system was developed to characterize the quality of life for survivors of childhood cancer. The system is comprised of seven attributes: audio-visual function, physical mobility, emotional function, cognitive function, self-care, pain, and fertility. Three to five levels of function are defined for each attribute (ranging from very poor to normal function). A multi-attribute utility function was estimated to provide utility scores for the outcome health states experienced by patients cured of cancer. The multi-attribute system is designed to describe health states associated with combinations of sequelae from the disease and its treatment. Thus it goes beyond the standard reports in the late effects literature which enumerate the sequelae suffered by survivors and provide separate estimates of the number of patients who experience each sequela. The multi-attribute approach provides an overall assessment of the quality of life of the patient.

To supplement these measures of the quality of life of the outcome of treatment, it was necessary to obtain measures of the quality of life experienced during the treatment process itself. Taking into account both the frequency and duration of each health state, these two types of utility measurements may be aggregated to characterize the combined impact on quality of life of treatment and outcome.

III. MEASURING QUALITY OF LIFE DURING TREATMENT

The quality-of-life measurements reported here were not conducted within a prospective study. Prospective assessment would allow the investigator to measure the quality of life of the health state while the subject is experiencing it. Because that was not possible in this study, it was necessary to obtain quality-of-life measurements for a set of hypothetical health states which are thought to be representative of the experience of patients undergoing treatment for childhood cancer. The set of hypothetical states was chosen so that the states would be mutually exclusive and exhaustive.

There are well defined phases in the treatments for Wilms tumor, ALL, and neuroblastoma. For Wilms tumor, surgery (nephrectomy) and chemotherapy are followed by radiotherapy (in some patients) and additional chemotherapy. Palliative care is a relevant phase for only a small minority of Wilms patients. Similarly, initial chemotherapy for ALL attempts to induce remission of the systemic disease. This phase is followed by cranial irradiation (in some patients) and intrathecal chemotherapy, and then continuing systemic administration of drugs. Other possibilities include subsequent attempts to induce remission (following relapse), further intensive chemotherapy, bone marrow transplantation, and palliative care. The phases for neuroblastoma include surgery, radiotherapy (in some patients), chemotherapy, bone marrow transplantation, and palliative care.

Health-state scenario descriptions were developed to describe each of the health states associated with the separate phases of therapy for the three reference diseases. These descriptions were based on the treatment protocols used at the Children's Hospital at Chedoke-McMaster (Hamilton) and the Hospital for Sick Children (HSC, Toronto). These protocols include the National Wilms' Tumor Study protocols,[35] the SIOP protocol,[36] the Dana-Farber Cancer Institute protocols,[37-38] the BFM protocol,[39] the MADDOC protocol,[40] and the St. Jude's protocol.[41]

The content of the descriptions was designed to provide information, when relevant, for each of the first six attributes (excluding fertility) of the multi-attribute health-status clas-

TABLE 1
Example of Health-State Description for Initial Treatment of Neuroblastoma

1. You will live in hospital for 1 month and receive drugs, or blood transfusions. On a few occasions you will need to visit another hospital and lie frustratingly still for radiation treatments or X-rays.
2. In the first week an operation will be performed to insert a plastic tube through the skin of your chest and along a vein to your heart.
3. During the fourth week you will have another major operation to remove tumors from your abdomen and chest.
4. On one occasion during this month a needle will be inserted into your pelvic bone to obtain a bone marrow sample.
5. For the first and fourth weeks of this month you will have to remain in bed and be helped to wash, dress, and use the toilet. During the second and third weeks you will gradually be able to walk and play.
6. You will have a slightly sore mouth, skin rash, and a few stomach aches. You can also expect to vomit occasionally, and lose some of your hair.
7. The disease, needles, strange surroundings and unknown people will make you feel afraid. You will be angry, or passive and withdrawn. This will be a fairly stressful time for your family.

Note: This state corresponds to state 19, T1N-PH in Table 3.

TABLE 2
Example of Health-State Description for Maintenance Phase of Treatment for ALL

1. You will live at home for 2 years except for one occasion, lasting 2 weeks, when you will be admitted to hospital for treatment of an infection. While living at home you will visit the hospital once per week to have drugs injected through your chest tube.
2.
3.
4. On 24 occasions during the course of these 2 years you will receive a needle into a muscle and on 8 other occasions a needle into your spine. You will need to take tablets by mouth every day.
5. For most of these 2 years you will be able to play and go to school.
6. You will have an occasional sore mouth but generally feel well.
7. You will be irritated by the need to visit the hospital for treatments which disrupt your social activities. You will be hopeful of being cured but realize there is a chance the disease may return.

Note: This state corresponds to state 5, T3A-EH/PH in Table 3. Information normally contained in paragraphs 2 and 3 are not applicable for this health state and therefore left blank.

sification system mentioned above. In addition, other aspects of treatment which were felt to be important to patients were included. The format of these descriptions and order of presentation of each type of information were standardized. Each description consists of seven paragraphs that provide details about the duration of the state, where the patient resides during that phase of treatment (in-patient or ambulatory care), major surgical procedures (such as the insertion of a right atrial catheter or excision of a tumor), the administration of other forms of therapy (such as number and mode of administration of injections), self-care function, adverse effects (such as nausea, vomiting, hair loss, facial swelling), and emotional state (such as anger and fear of unknown surroundings). Examples are presented in Tables 1 and 2. The standardized format and order of presentation were designed to facilitate the comparisons among states. The scope of the health-state descriptions is broader and more comprehensive than the coverage of other measures described in the literature, such as the performance measure devised by Lansky et al.[10]

In order to standardize time for the utility measurements, the treatment states were divided into two sets: a set of 1 month and a set of 2-year states. The former was designed to represent the duration of initial intensive phases of therapy and other acute periods. The 2-year period was designed to reflect the later phases of treatment such as continuing ''maintenance'') chemotherapy, not the chronic outcomes that are the health states experi-

TABLE 3
Summary of Health States Associated with the Treatment Process of Childhood Cancers

State #	Label	Description	Duration
1	T1A-PH	ALL: initial induction of remission	1 month
2	T1A-PL	ALL: initial induction of remission	1 month
3[a]	T2A-PH	ALL: intensive treatment	1 month
4	T2A-PL	ALL: intensive treatment	1 month
5	T3A-EH/PH	ALL: less intensive treatment	2 years
6	T3A-EH/PL	ALL: less intensive treatment	2 years
7[a]	T3A-EL/PH	ALL: less intensive treatment	2 years
8	T3A-EL/PL	ALL: less intensive treatment	2 years
9	T4A-PH	ALL: further intensive treatment	1 month
10[a]	T4A-PL	ALL: further intensive treatment	1 month
11	T5A	ALL: bone marrow transplantation	1 month
12	T6A	ALL: second induction of remission	1 month
13	T1W-PH	Wilms: surgery and chemotherapy	1 month
14	T1W-PL	Wilms: surgery and chemotherapy	1 month
15[a]	T2W-PH	Wilms: radiotherapy and chemotherapy	1 month
16	T2W-PL	Wilms: radiotherapy and chemotherapy	1 month
17[a]	T3W-PH	Wilms: chemotherapy	2 years
18	T3W-PL	Wilms: chemotherapy	2 years
19[a]	T1N-PH	Neuroblastoma: surgery and initial treatment	1 month
20	T1N-PL	Neuroblastoma: surgery and initial treatment	1 month
21[a]	T2N-PH	Neuroblastoma: chemotherapy and second phase	2 years
22	T2N-PL	Neuroblastoma: chemotherapy and second phase	2 years
23[a]	T3N	Neuroblastoma: bone marrow transplantation	1 month
24	T1PS	Palliative care: initial short phase	1 month
25[a]	T1PE	Palliative care: initial extended phase	2 years
26	T2P	Palliative care: end-stage short phase	1 month

Note: A = ALL, PH = Physical High, PL = Physical Low, EH = Emotional High, EL = Emotional Low, W = Wilms tumor, N = neuroblastoma, P = palliative, T = temporary, S = short, and E = extended.

[a] Denotes that the state was assessed on the chance board and rating scale.

enced by patients after the cessation of therapy. For some diseases, such as ALL, children are sometimes on "maintenance" chemotherapy for more than 2 years.

Draft health-state descriptions were reviewed by pediatric oncology specialists including physicians, nurses, and child-life workers. They were asked to classify patients currently on therapy at the Children's Hospital of Chedoke-McMaster (Hamilton) according to the health-state descriptions given. In order to represent the full range of experience during the phases of treatment, it was necessary to create a number of variations on the descriptions which had been developed according to the clinically defined phases of treatment. In particular, the feedback from the pediatric oncology specialists indicated that there were various combinations of physical high or low, and emotional high or low functioning that different patients experienced during the same phases of treatment. On the basis of frequently observed combinations of physical and emotional coping, a number of new health-state descriptions were created. The aim was to create a reasonably compact set of mutually exclusive and exhaustive health states, the combinations of which would describe the full treatment experience for any patient.

The full set of 26 states is presented in Table 3. States 1 and 2 both refer to the initial remission induction phase for ALL. State 1 describes induction which is well tolerated (physical high). State 2 is a variation representing poorly tolerated induction (physical low).

Similarly there are two variations on intensive treatment for ALL (states 3 and 4), four variations on less intensive treatment for ALL (states 5 through 8), and two variations on further intensive treatment (states 9 and 10). Similar variations were identified for treatments for Wilms tumor and neuroblastoma.

IV. ASSESSORS FOR MEASURING HEALTH-RELATED QUALITY OF LIFE

This evaluation of the quality of life of the treatment process was conducted in the context of a larger study evaluating economic and quality-of-life effects of treatments for childhood cancer. On-going prospective measurement of the quality of life of actual patients during the phases of treatment would be the method of choice. In this study that was not possible for several reasons.

Methods for measuring quality of life in pediatric populations are less well developed than for adult populations.[42] Furthermore, given the wide range of ages in those afflicted with childhood cancer, much of the patient population is too young to give meaningful answers with standard instruments. In addition, the effects of the disease and treatment incpacitate some subjects to the point that they are unable to provide meaningful scores. Finally, the small number of patients available at two major tertiary care centers limits the generalizability of results that could be obtained from direct quality-of-life measurements.

These general concerns are intensified because the utility approach for measuring health-related quality of life is cognitively demanding. Therefore, it was decided that proxy respondents would be used.

The evidence on the validity of proxy respondents for collecting data on health-related quality of life is mixed.[43-46] Pain, emotional states, and other not directly observable dimensions of health status are generally less adequately measured through proxy respondents than dimensions which are directly observable.[44] In some studies of adults, proxies underrate the patient's physical health and the ability to perform a number of activities of daily living.[45] In other studies of adult populations, female proxy respondents consistently underreported health problems compared with self-report for male respondents.[43,46] The degree of underreporting varied with symptom or problem. Underreporting decreased, however, with the persistence of the health problem.

The evidence on the use of proxies in pediatric populations is also mixed.[8,18,44] Proxy responses by adults in behalf of teenage subjects may be especially problematic. For concrete, serious, or obvious events or problems, Herjanic and Reich[44] found high levels of agreement on symptom reporting by children (ages 6 to 16) and their mothers. However, levels of agreement were lower for behaviors and subjective feelings. Children reported more subjective symptoms than mothers. For family coping, Kupst et al.[8-9] found reasonably high correlations between ratings by family members and mental health professionals but only moderate agreement between the ratings of mothers and fathers. O'Malley et al.[18] found moderate correlation between psychiatric evaluations and self assessments. Lansky et al.[10] found reasonable agreement among assessments of play performance of pediatric oncology patients made by mothers of patients, fathers of patients, pediatric oncology nurses, and research interviewers. In sum, proxy respondents are likely to be reliable for readily observable, or relatively serious conditions or events but less reliable for subjective phenomena. On the basis of the published evidence, it was concluded that, although the use of proxy respondents was not ideal, it was nonetheless a practical and useful way to obtain at least some information on the quality of life of the treatment process in pediatric oncology.

Parents were chosen as the natural proxy respondents. Two samples of parents were selected. The first set was a random sample of parents in the general public, more precisely a random sample of parents of children enrolled in junior kindergarten through grade 5 of

TABLE 4
Demographic Characteristics of Parent Samples

Characteristic	General public/A	General public/B	Parent of patient/A and B
Total number	109	109	50
Number male	51	50	15
Number female	58	59	35
Exclusions[a]	8	14	5
Number available for analysis	101	95	45
Number male	48	44	13
Number female	53	51	32
Mean Age	37.1	37.6	34.2
(SD)	(5.5)	(5.5)	(5.8)
Minimum	28	23	24
Maximum	61	55	53
Mean number of children	2.6	2.5	2.4
(SD)	(0.8)	(0.9)	(1.0)
Minimum	1	1	1
Maximum	5	5	6

Note: The health states included in Schedule A describe treatments for ALL; health states in Schedule B describe treatments for Wilms tumor and neuroblastoma.

[a] The reasons for the exclusions are discussed in the text.

the Hamilton Board of Education and Hamilton-Wentworth Roman Catholic Separate School Board in Hamilton, Ontario. Two hundred ninety-three parents from this sample participated in interviews concerning the quality of life of treatment outcomes and provided data for the estimation of the multi-attribute utility function. Two hundred eighteen parents, a subsample of the 293 parents, participated in the second interview devoted to an assessment of the quality of life of the treatment process. One hundred nine parents evaluated the states associated with the treatment of ALL (labeled as Schedule A); 109 evaluated states associated with Wilms tumor and neuroblastoma (Schedule B). General public parents were randomized to receive Schedule A or B. Seven states were contained in both sets of interviews.

The second set of parents was a sample of convenience selected from the roster of parents of patients actually undergoing therapy in the Children's Hospital at Chedoke-McMaster Hospitals (Hamilton) or the Hospital for Sick Children (Toronto). It was felt that parents who had observed their child's experience with the treatment of childhood cancer would provide most knowledgeable assessments of the hypothetical health states. A total of 59 parents participated in the first interview on treatment outcomes; 50 parents were available for the second interview on treatment process. Forty parents of patients with ALL evaluated those states (Schedule A); ten parents of patients with Wilms tumor or neuroblastoma evaluated the second set of states (Schedule B). The parents of patients were assigned to the Schedule that contained the health states associated with the treatment protocols which their child was receiving.

A summary of demographic characteristics of the two sets of parents appears in Table 4. For the subset of demographic variables displayed there, it can be seen that the two groups were, in general, quite similar. The major exception is the gender mix. The parent-of-patient sample frame was one of convenience. Whichever parent was available was interviewed, usually the mother. In the general public sample, efforts were made to obtain equal numbers of male and female respondents. The groups were also similar on the basis of other information collected including marital status, education, religion, and income.

V. METHODS FOR MEASURING UTILITY SCORES

Utility scores were obtained in carefully designed interviews conducted by trained professional interviewers. All interviews were tape recorded as a routine component of quality assurance. The mean duration of the interviews for the temporary health states associated with treatment was 70.5 min (SD = 14.73); the minimum duration was 30 min and the maximum was 130 min. Most interviews were conducted in the respondent's home; some of the parent-of-patient interviews were conducted privately at the clinic. The interviews of parents in the general public sample were conducted between November 1987 and April 1988; parent-of-patient interviews were conducted between January 1988 and July 1988.

Interview subjects were asked to imagine that they were a child undergoing treatment for a serious disease. (The disease label, cancer, was not mentioned to general public parents in order to avoid a labeling effect; see Reference 47.) They were asked to imagine themselves in each situation described and to respond on the basis of the quality-of-life burden they thought that they would experience. Subjects were informed that prognosis was unaffected by the nature of the health state being experienced. This was an attempt to obtain an evaluation of the quality of life of the particular treatment phase independent of the outcome to which it might lead.

Interview subjects were first asked to rank health states (of the same duration) on a visual analog scale referred to as the feeling thermometer. The scale varies from 0 (the least desirable state) to 100 (perfect health). In the first portion of the interview the subjects evaluated the 11 1-month states associated with ALL (or 10 1-month states associated with Wilms tumor and neuroblastoma). After ranking these states, subjects then further evaluated three of the states with the chance board (see Figure 1).

The chance board is a device that corresponds to the theory which underlies utility measurement. The theory prescribes the standard gamble approach as the method for measuring utility. A standard gamble question is illustrated in Figure 2. In the standard gamble the subject is presented with two alternatives: 1 or 2. In alternative 2 the subject would be certain to get the health state described as state i (previously ranked as intermediate between states presented in alternative 1). In alternative 1 the subject is offered a lottery with a probability p of obtaining the more desirable outcome (healthy in this example) and a probability $1-p$ of obtaining the less desirable outcome (dead in Figure 2). The probability is varied until the subject is indifferent between alternatives 1 and 2. The probability indifference value occurs when the expected utilities for alternatives 1 and 2 are equal. The chance board (Figure 1) provides subjects who are less familiar or comfortable with probabilities with a means of expressing their preferences in probability terms. The measurement scores obtained from the chance board and its underlying standard gamble approach provide cardinal (interval scale) utility scores.

After obtaining rankings for all of the states of 1 month duration and chance board scores for a subset of them, the subjects are then asked to rank the five 2-year states associated with ALL (or six 2-year states associated with Wilms tumor and neuroblastoma). Three of these are evaluated on the chance board.

The quality-of-life assessment interviews included interview evaluations of the quality of the interview process. Interviewers were asked to provide information on the degree of cooperation of the subject (three-point scale), thoughtfulness of the subject (three-point scale), understanding (three-point scale), and overall impression (five-point scale). It was decided in advance, before examining the utility scores, to exclude from the analysis any data from subjects who were rated in any one of the lowest categories for each of the above mentioned criteria. Our assumption was that utility scores provided by subjects who were not thoughtful, or who did not understand the tasks were unlikely to be accurate representations of their preferences. Given the relatively small number of exclusions, it is unlikely

CHOICE "A"

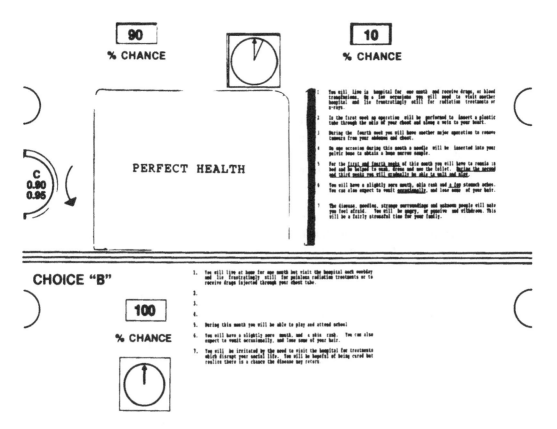

CHOICE "B"

FIGURE 1.   Chance board.

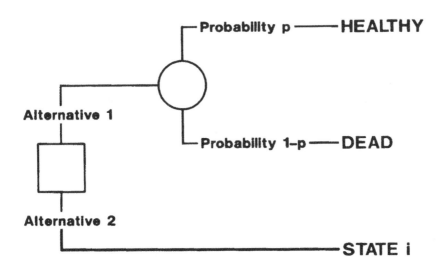

FIGURE 2.   Standard gamble.

that the exclusions affect the results. (Interviews for which there was missing data were also excluded). For the general public/schedule A group this resulted in 8 of the 109 being excluded, leaving 101 subjects available for analysis. For the general public/schedule B group there were 14 exclusions, leaving 95 usable subjects. For the parent-of-patient groups, 5 of the 50 were excluded, leaving 45 available for analysis (35 for schedule A; 10 for schedule B).

VI. METHODS FOR THE ANALYSIS OF UTILITY SCORES

Two sets of scores are available for the nine states assessed on both the feeling thermometer and chance board. For the remaining 17 states, only feeling thermometer scores are available. Technically scores from the visual analog scale (feeling thermometer) are value scores while scores from the standard gamble (chance board) are utility scores.[48] A key distinction (in decision science) between the concepts of value and utility is that the risk preferences of the subject are represented in the latter but not in the former. In order to assess the quality of life of the treatment process and to be able to integrate that analysis with the quality of life of the treatment outcome, it is necessary to transform the value scores into utility scores. In general, these scores can be related to each other through a power function.[49-50]

The case here is slightly more complicated. The value scale used on the feeling thermometer was defined by the interval having a minimum value assigned to the lowest ranked health state (usually 0) and a maximum value assigned to perfect health (usually 100). The scale used on the chance board, however, was defined as having a minimum utility of death (0.0) and a maximum utility of perfect health (1.0). Therefore, the transformation of individual value scores into utility scores needs to allow for the general power function relationship, for the value scale defined by the respondent, and for an adjustment to align the value scale to the conventional 0.0 to 1.0, dead to healthy, utility scale.

For convenience the power function was estimated for disutility scores as a function of disvalue scores. Disvalue scores are equal to 1 minus the value; disutility scores are 1 minus the utility. Thus perfect health has a disvalue and a disutility of 0. Death has a disutility of 1.0.

The power function took the following form: $u = 1 - k(1 - v)^a$ where v is the measured value of a particular health state, k and a are parameters of the conversion function, and u is the calculated utility of the health sate. A power function of this form was estimated for each subject. The individual's power function was then used to determine utility scores for health states for which only feeling thermometer measurements were available. (If the calculated score was less than zero, worse than death, it was assigned a value of zero.) In this fashion utility scores for all 26 states were calculated on the basis of the directly measured value scores and the estimated relationship between utility and value scores for each individual. Both value and utility scores were measured directly for a collection of nine states.

VII. RESULTS

The summary statistics for utility scores of health states evaluated on the Chance Board are given in Table 5. Utility scores for the full set of health states based on the fitting process described in Section VI are given in Table 6.

Several sets of comparisons are meaningful. First, for the general public sample, scores for states 17, 19, and 25 (the states assessed on the chance board in both Schedules A and B) obtained from parents who were given interview schedule A are in close, but not perfect agreement with scores obtained from parents who were given schedule B. Given that parents were randomized between the two interview schedules one would expect that the scores

TABLE 5
Summary of Descriptive Health Statistics for Measured
Temporary "A" and "B" Health-State Utility Scores

State #	Health states description		General public parents, A (n = 101) B (n = 95)				Parent-of-Patients, A (n = 35) B (n = 10)			
	Label	Duration	Mean	SD	Min	Max	Mean	SD	Min	Max
3	T2A-PH	1 month	0.85	0.211	0.00	1.00	0.91	0.110	0.45	1.00
7	T3A-EL/PH	2 years	0.82	0.157	0.15	1.00	0.84	0.138	0.51	1.00
10	T4A-PL	1 month	0.76	0.247	0.00	1.00	0.81	0.175	0.35	1.00
15*	T2W-PH	1 month	0.91	0.126	0.31	1.00	0.96	0.047	0.86	1.00
17	T3W-PH	2 years	0.87	0.158	0.19	1.00	0.91	0.076	0.73	1.00
17*	T3W-PH	2 years	0.86	0.165	0.25	1.00	0.92	0.081	0.73	1.00
19	T1N-PH	1 month	0.72	0.244	0.00	1.00	0.78	0.168	0.35	1.00
19*	T1N-PH	1 month	0.80	0.209	0.05	1.00	0.89	0.101	0.74	1.00
21*	T2N-PH	2 years	0.72	0.247	0.00	1.00	0.72	0.197	0.35	0.97
23*	T3N	1 month	0.63	0.248	0.00	1.00	0.67	0.303	0.00	0.95
25	T1PE	2 years	0.59	0.266	0.00	0.98	0.59	0.243	0.15	0.95
25*	T1PE	2 years	0.64	0.264	0.00	1.00	0.63	0.184	0.35	0.95

Note: * denotes state measured on Temporary Schedule B. States 17, 19, and 25 were included on both interview schedules.

would be nearly the same. Using a t-test to test for differences between the scores for these three states, the hypothesis is confirmed for States 17 and 25 but not for state 19 (for which the difference is significant, $p < 0.025$). Parents of patients were not randomized between the two interview schedules. Nonetheless, scores for those given Schedule A and Schedule B for states 17 and 25 are in close agreement and the difference between scores is not statistically significant. The difference for state 19 is, however, statistically significant ($p < 0.05$).

Second, it appears that the parents of patients generally rate the health states as slightly better than parents from the general public sample. This result, that persons with experience tend to rate a state somewhat better than those for whom it is strictly hypothetical, is consistent with previous findings.[47] However, when the apparent trend for parents of patients to report higher utility scores than general public parents is tested, again using states 17, 19, and 25 for which the sample sizes are largest, the difference is only significant for state 17 ($p < 0.025$).

In addition to statistical test results, it is also important to consider the magnitude of the differences. The minimum important difference in utility scores has received relatively little attention in the utility measurement literature. Nonetheless a working definition of the minimally important difference is 0.10 (on the 0.0 to 1.0 scale). By this standard, only one of the three statistically significant differences (parent-of-patient A vs. parent-of-patient B for state 19) is large enough to be considered important. The other two differences, 0.05 (difference between general public and parent-of-patient patents for state 17) and 0.08 (difference between general public parents schedule A and general public parents schedule B for state 19), fall below the threshold. Thus overall it would appear that ratings by parents of patients and by general public parents are approximately equal and there are few important differences in scores provided by different assessors.

There are, however, differences in ratings among health states. Parents report differences in quality of life (utility) among health states associated with treatment for childhood cancer. States such as number 15 are viewed as involving a mild burden of morbidity. In contrast, states such as numbers 23 or 25 are viewed as involving a heavy burden.

TABLE 6
Descriptive Statistics of "Fitted" Utility Scores For All Temporary "A" and "B" Health States

	Health states description		General public parents, A (n = 101) B (n = 95)				Parent-of-patients A (n = 35) B (n = 10)			
State #	Label	Duration	Mean	SD	Min	Max	Mean	SD	Min	Max
1	T1A-PH	1 month	0.72	0.272	0.00	1.00	0.82	0.209	0.00	1.00
1*	T1A-PH	1 month	0.80	0.203	0.00	0.99	0.85	0.206	0.29	0.99
2	T1A-PL	1 month	0.62	0.319	0.00	1.00	0.75	0.264	0.00	1.00
3	T2A-PH	1 month	0.85	0.210	0.00	0.99	0.90	0.114	0.42	0.99
4	T2A-PL	1 month	0.81	0.229	0.00	0.99	0.87	0.135	0.45	1.00
5	T3A-EH/PH	2 years	0.85	0.320	0.00	1.00	0.84	0.135	0.49	1.00
5*	T3A-EH/PH	2 years	0.81	0.225	0.00	1.00	0.64	0.299	0.00	0.97
6	T3A-EH/PL	2 years	0.83	0.340	0.00	1.00	0.78	0.181	0.31	1.00
7	T3A-EL/PH	2 years	0.84	0.324	0.00	1.00	0.83	0.141	0.52	0.99
8	T3A-EL/PL	2 years	0.84	0.331	0.00	1.00	0.79	0.190	0.22	0.99
9	T4A-PH	1 month	0.86	0.193	0.00	1.00	0.90	0.112	0.59	1.00
10	T4A-PL	1 month	0.77	0.236	0.00	0.99	0.82	0.160	0.46	0.99
11	T5A	1 month	0.45	0.371	0.00	0.97	0.58	0.351	0.00	0.99
12	T6A	1 month	0.57	0.341	0.00	1.00	0.70	0.288	0.00	1.00
13*	T1W-PH	1 month	0.84	0.185	0.09	1.00	0.89	0.120	0.67	1.00
14*	T1W-PL	1 month	0.79	0.221	0.00	1.00	0.88	0.147	0.49	0.99
15*	T2W-PH	1 month	0.91	0.126	0.31	0.99	0.96	0.047	0.85	0.99
16*	T2W-PL	1 month	0.84	0.196	0.00	1.00	0.93	0.075	0.79	0.99
17	T3W-PH	2 years	0.88	0.276	0.00	1.00	0.90	0.080	0.73	0.99
17*	T3W-PH	2 years	0.85	0.168	0.24	0.99	0.92	0.081	0.73	0.99
18*	T3W-PL	2 years	0.76	0.237	0.00	1.00	0.78	0.199	0.41	0.98
19	T1N-PH	1 month	0.73	0.240	0.00	0.99	0.78	0.168	0.41	0.99
19*	T1N-PH	1 month	0.79	0.215	0.00	0.99	0.87	0.106	0.69	0.98
20*	T1N-PL	1 month	0.71	0.253	0.00	0.98	0.72	0.320	0.00	0.98
21*	T2N-PH	2 years	0.72	0.234	0.00	0.99	0.74	0.164	0.49	0.97
22*	T2N-PL	2 years	0.46	0.337	0.00	1.00	0.26	0.340	0.00	0.93
23*	T3N	1 month	0.67	0.242	0.00	0.99	0.70	0.322	0.00	0.97
24	T1PS	1 month	0.63	0.348	0.00	1.00	0.72	0.322	0.00	1.00
24*	T1PS	1 month	0.75	0.235	0.00	1.00	0.70	0.366	0.00	0.98
25	T1PE	2 years	0.81	0.356	0.00	1.00	0.64	0.228	0.24	0.97
25*	T1PE	2 years	0.66	0.255	0.00	0.99	0.61	0.195	0.37	0.95
26	T2P	1 month	0.66	0.323	0.00	1.00	0.69	0.346	0.00	0.99
26*	T2P	1 month	0.75	0.270	0.00	1.00	0.73	0.316	0.00	0.99

Note: * denotes state measured on Temporary Schedule B. For description of fitting process see text.

VIII. SIMULATIONS OF QUALITY-OF-LIFE BURDEN OF COMBINED PHASES OF TREATMENT

In order to obtain a picture of the quality-of-life burden of the full course of therapy, nine case scenarios of patient experience during therapy were developed (Table 7). Case A represents a child with ALL who spends 1 month in state 1, 1 month in state 3, and then 2 years in state 5. Case A represents the least morbidity and the lower bound estimate of the quality-of-life burden associated with the treatment of ALL. The burden may be summarized using an index of health-related quality of life, the quality-adjusted life year, QALY (described in References 32 to 34). In this approach spending the 2.17 years (2 years and 2 months of treatment) in perfect health would represent 2.17 QALYs — 2.17 years times a utility of 1.0 (perfect health). Using the utility scores reported by parents of patients for

TABLE 7

Quality-of-Life Experience During Treatment Process

Case	1-month states	2-year states	Duration in years	QALYs[a]	Quality-of-life burden[b] (%)
A	1, 3	5	2.17	1.82	16
B	2, 3	6	2.17	1.70	22
C	1, 3, 12, 26	7, 25[c]	2.83	2.24	21
D	13[d], 15	17[e]	1.63	1.50	8
E	14[d], 16	17[e]	1.63	1.49	8
F	14[d], 16, 24, 26, death		0.29	0.23	20
G	20	21[f]	1.08	0.80	26
H	19, 23	21[e]	0.67	0.50	25
I	20, 24, 26	22[c], death	0.75	0.31	59

[a] Using parent-of-patient utility scores from Table 6. For the ALL scenarios (A through C), the scores are the means for parents of ALL patients (those who completed Schedule A of the interview); for the Wilms and neuroblastoma scenarios (D through I), scores are the means for parents of patients who completed Schedule B interviews.

[b] The quality-of-life burden is defined as the number of QALYs that would have been obtained if the period had been spent in perfect health, 2.17 in Case A, minus the QALYs experienced during treatment, 1.82 in Case A, divided by the QALYs under perfect health, expressed as a percent.

[c] Health state is experienced for 6 months.

[d] Health state is experienced for 2 weeks.

[e] Health state is experienced for 18 months.

[f] Health state is experienced for 1 year.

states 1, 3, and 5 (see Table 6), and weighting the scores for states 1 and 3 by 0.08 years (1 month each) and the score for state 5 by 2.0 years, Case A represents 1.82 QALYs, a quality-of-life burden of 16% (Table 7). In other words, the difference between the quality of life experienced by a child undergoing the course of therapy described in Case A and the quality of life of that child in perfect health for the same period of time represents 16% of the maximum potential quality of life. (Using the general public utility scores from Table 6, Case A represents 1.83 QALYs, also a burden of 16%). QALYs and measures of morbidity, using parent-of-patient utility scores, for nine case scenarios are presented in Table 7.

Case A represents the most favorable treatment experience for high-risk ALL. Case B represents a treatment scenario in which some problems are encountered during therapy but there is no relapse. Case C is a scenario for a case involving relapse, failure to obtain a second remission, and palliative care followed by death.

Wilms tumor scenarios are described in Cases D through F. Case D represents the most common scenario, Case E is reasonably common, and Case F is very unusual.

Neuroblastoma scenarios are described in Cases G through I. Case G represents a realistic "best-case" scenario. Case H depends upon the availability of a bone marrow donor. Case I is the most common scenario.

Several generalizations emerge from an examination of the simulation results in Table 7. First, treatment, even in the most favorable cases, involves an important burden of morbidity. Second, there is a substantial variance in that burden of morbidity. Third, typical scenarios for ALL and neuroblastoma patients seem to involve a heavier burden of morbidity, as well as less favorable survival, when compared to the experience for Wilms tumor.

IX. CONCLUSIONS

The utility approach to measuring health-related quality of life offers an advantage in that it can be used to quantify the quality-of-life burden of the treatment process. Estimates of that burden, such as the ones presented here, may be integrated with estimates of the quality of life of the treatment outcomes to provide a comprehensive assessment of the quality-of-life effects of treatments for childhood cancer. Although the validity of these particular results may have been affected by the use of proxy respondents for the quality-of-life measurement, in general these methods can be used to assess the quality-of-life effects of alternative courses of therapy and may contribute to the development of improved patient management.

ACKNOWLEDGMENTS

The authors acknowledge the contributions of Robin Roberts, Dr. Peter Rosenbaum, John Horsman, Yueming Zhang, Dr. Alvin Zipursky, the interviewers and staff of Social Data Research Ltd., Lori Scapinello, and Carol Siksay to the research project. The authors also acknowledge the contributions of the team of pediatric oncology specialists in Hamilton who assisted in the development of the health-state descriptions. The team includes Dr. Maureen Andrew, Dr. Mohan Pai, Susan Dawson, Ruth Snider, and Sharon Smith. The cooperation of the Hamilton Board of Education of Hamilton-Wentworth Roman Catholic Separate School Board are also acknowledged. Dr. David Osoba and Dr. J. E. Till provided helpful comments on a draft of the paper. The financial support of the Ontario Ministry of Health Grant 01386 and Merck Foundation are also gratefully acknowledged. The usual disclaimer applies.

REFERENCES

1. Stjernsward, J. and Teoh, N., Chapter 1, this volume.
2. Osoba, D., Chapter 3, this volume.
3. Donovan, K., Sanson-Fisher, R. W., and Redman, S., Measuring quality of life in cancer patients, *J. Clin. Oncol.*, 7, 959, 1989.
4. Fayers, P. M. and Jones, D. R., Measuring and analyzing quality of life in cancer clinical trials: a review, *Stat. Med.*, 2, 429, 1983.
5. Mor, V. and Guadagnoli, E., Quality of life measurement: a psychometric tower of Babel, *J. Clin. Epidemiol.*, 41, 1055, 1988.
6. van Knippenberg, F. C. E. and de Haes, J. C. J. M., Measuring the quality of life of cancer patients: psychometric properties of instruments, *J. Clin. Epidemiol.*, 41, 1043, 1988.
7. Bloom, H. J. G., Wallace, E. N. K., and Henk, J. M., The treatment and prognosis of medullablastoma in children: a study of 82 verified cases, *Am. J. Roentgenol.*, 105, 43, 1969.
8. Kupst, M. J., Schulman, J. L., Maurer, H., et al., Coping with pediatric leukemia: a two-year follow-up, *J. Pediatr. Psychol.*, 9, 149, 1984.
9. Kupst, M. J. and Schulman, J. L., Long-term coping with pediatric leukemia — a 6-year follow-up study, *J. Pediatr. Psychol.*, 13, 7, 1988.
10. Lansky, S. B., List, M. A., Lansky, L. L., et al., The measurement of performance in childhood cancer patients, *Cancer*, 60, 1651, 1987.
11. Levine, A. S. and Hersh, S. P., The psychological concomitants of cancer in young patients, in *Cancer in the Young*, Levine, A. S., Ed., Masson, New York, 1982, 367.
12. Links, P. S. and Stockwell, M. L., Obstacles in the prevention of psychological sequelae in survivors of childhood cancer, *Am. J. Pediatr. Hematol. Oncol.*, 7, 132, 1985.
13. Maguire, G. P., The psychological sequelae of childhood leukemia, *Rec. Results Cancer Res.*, 88, 48, 1983.
14. Meadows, A. T., Gordon, J., and Massari, D. J., et al., Dysfunction in children with acute lymphocytic leukemia treated with cranial irradiation, *Lancet*, 2, 1015, 1981.
15. Meadows, A. T., Krejmas, N. L., and Belasco, J. B., The medical cost of cure: sequelae in survivors of childhood cancer, in *Status of the Curability of Childhood Cancers*, van Eys, J. and Sullivan, M. P., Eds., Raven Press, New York, 1980, 263.

16. Nesbit, M. E. et al., A follow-up report of long-term survivors of childhood acute lymphoblastic or undifferentiated leukemia, *J. Pediatr.*, 95, 727, 1979.

17. Monaco, G. P., Socioeconomic considerations in childhood cancer survival, *Am. J. Pediatr. Hematol. Oncol.*, 9, 92, 1987.

18. O'Malley, J. E., Koocher, G., Foster, D., et al., Psychiatric sequelae of surviving childhood cancer, *Am. J. Orthop.*, 49, 608, 1979.

19. Pastore, G., Zurlo, M. G., Acquaviva, A., et al., Health status of young children with cancer following dicontinuation of therapy, *Med. Pediatr. Oncol.*, 15, 1, 1987.

20. Wheeler, K., Leiper, A. D., Jannoun, L., et al., Medical cost of curing childhood acute lymphoblastic leukemia, *Br. Med. J.*, 296, 162, 1988.

21. Whitt, J. K., Wells, R. J., Lauria, M. M., et al., Cranial radiation in childhood acute lymphoblastic leukemia. Neuropsychologic sequelae, *Am. J. Dis. Child.*, 138, 730, 1984.

22. Pizzo, P. A. and Poplack, D. G., *Management of Problems Arising at Diagnosis and During Treatment*, J. B. Lippincott, Philadelphia, 1989.

23. Guyatt, G. H., van Zanten, S. J. O. V., Feeny, D. H., et al., Measuring quality of life in clinical trials: a taxonomy and review, *Can. Med. Assoc. J.*, 140, 1441, 1989.

24. Goodwin, P., Chapter 10, this volume.

25. Till, J. E., Chapter 11, this volume.

26. Feeny, D. and Torrance, G. W., Incorporating utility-based quality-of-life assessment measures in clinical trials: two examples, *Med. Care*, 27, S190, 1989.

27. Feeny, D., Labelle, R., and Torrance, G. W., Integrating economic evaluations and quality-of-life assessments, in *Quality of Life Assessments in Clinical Trials*, Spilker, B., Ed., Raven Press, New York, 1990, 71.

28. Froberg, D. G. and Kane, R. L., Methodology for measuring health-state preferences. I. Measurement strategies, *J. Clin. Epidemiol.*, 42, 345, 1989.

29. Froberg, D. G. and Kane, R. L., Methodology for measuring health-state preferences. II. Scaling methods, *J. Clin. Epidemiol.*, 42, 459, 1989.

30. Froberg, D. G. and Kane, R. L., Methodology for measuring health-state preferences. III. Population and context effects, *J. Clin. Epidemiol.*, 42, 585, 1989.

31. Froberg, D. G. and Kane, R. L., Methodology for measuring health-state preferences. IV. Progress and a research agenda, *J. Clin. Epidemiol.*, 42, 675, 1989.

32. Torrance, G. W., Measurement of health state utilities for economic appraisal: a review article, *J. Health Econ.*, 5, 1, 1986.

33. Torrance, G. W., Utility approach to measuring health-related quality of life, *J. Chronic Dis.*, 40, 593, 1987.

34. Torrance, G. W. and Feeny, D., Utilities and quality-adjusted life years, *Int. J. Technol. Assess. Health Care*, 5, 559, 1989.

35. D'Angio, G. J., Breslow, N., Beckwith, B., et al., Treatment of Wilms' tumour: results of Third National Wilms' Tumour Study, *Cancer*, 64, 1989, 349.

36. de Kraken, J., Voute, P. A., and Lemerle, J., for the SIOP trial committee, Preoperative chemotherapy in Wilms' tumour: results of clinical trials and studies on nephroblastoma conducted by the International Society of Pediatric Oncology in *Renal Tumors: Proceedings of the First International Symposium*, Alan R. Liss, New York, 1982, 131.

37. Clavell, L. A., Gelber, R. D., Cohen, H. J., et al., Four agent induction and intensive asparaginase therapy for treatment of childhood acute lymphoblastic leukemia, *N. Engl. J. Med.*, 315, 657, 1986.

38. Desai, S. J., Barr, R. D., Andrew, M., et al., Management of Ontario children with acute lymphoblastic leukemia by the Dana-Farber Cancer Institute protocols, *Can. Med. Assoc. J.*, 141, 693, 1989.

39. Henze, G., Langermann, H. J., et al., Acute lymphoblastic leukemia therapy study BFM 79/81 in children and adolescents: intensified reinduction therapy for patients with different risk of relapse, *Kl. Paediatr.*, 194, 195, 1982.

40. Frantz, C. N., Gelber, R. D., Belli, J. A., et al., Aggressive treatment of neuroblastoma, in *Pediatric Oncology, Proc. 13th Int. Meet. Soc. Pediatric Oncol.*, Excerpta Medica, Amsterdam, 1982, 175.

41. Green, A. A., Hayes, F. A., and Rao, B., Disease control and toxicity of aggressive 4 drug therapy for children with disseminated neuroblastoma, *Proc. Am. Clin. Oncol.*, 5, 210, 1986.

42. Rosenbaum, P., Cadman, D., and Kirpalani, H., Pediatrics: assessing quality of life, in *Quality of Life Assessments in Clinical Trials*, Spilker, B., Ed., Raven Press, New York, 1990, 205.

43. Cartwright, A., The effect of obtaining information from different informants on a family morbidity inquiry, *Appl. Stat.*, 6, 18, 1957.

44. Herjanic, B. and Reich, W., Development of a structured psychiatric interview for children: agreement between child and parent on individual symptoms, *J. Abnorm. Child Psychol.*, 10, 307, 1982.

45. Magaziner, J., Simonsick, E. M., Kashner, T. M., et al., Patient-proxy response comparability on measures of patient health status and functional status, *J. Clin. Epidemiol.*, 41, 1065, 1988.

46. **Clarridge, B. R. and Massagli, M. P.**, The use of female spouse proxies in common symptom reporting, *Med. Care*, 27, 352, 1989.
47. **Sackett, D. L. and Torrance, G. W.**, The utility of different health states as perceived by the general public, *J. Chronic Dis.*, 31, 697, 1978.
48. **Keeney, R. L. and Raiffa, H.**, *Decisions with Multiple Objectives: Preferences and Value Tradeoffs*, John Wiley & Sons, New York, 1976.
49. **Torrance, G. W.**, Social preferences for health states: an empirical evaluation of three measurement techniques, *Soc. Econ., Planning Sci.*, 10, 129, 1976.
50. **Torrance, G. W., Boyle, M. H., and Horwood, S. P.**, Application of multi-attribute utility theory to measure social preferences for health states, *Oper. Res.*, 30, 1043, 1982.

Chapter 7

A PRACTICAL GUIDE FOR SELECTING QUALITY-OF-LIFE MEASURES IN CLINICAL TRIALS AND PRACTICE

David Osoba, Neil K. Aaronson, and James E. Till

TABLE OF CONTENTS

I. INTRODUCTION

Once the decision has been made by a clinical investigator or practitioner to measure quality of life, the next question is *how* to do it. This involves a consideration of many factors, including the purpose of the measurement, whether patients, families, and/or health care workers should be interviewed or asked to fill out self-assessment questionnaires, which questions should be asked, who will ask them, the psychometric properties of the items in questionnaires or structured interviews, whose normative standard should be used, whose answers will be compared to the normative standard, where the questions will be asked, how feasible it is to carry out the assessment, and how the results will be analyzed.

Some of these questions are addressed in recent reviews and editorials.[1-17] While some authors have recommended particular measures,[12,14,15] others have simply catalogued the properties of available self-assessment questionnaires.[7,9-11,16] These are all very useful sources of information, but they have not provided novice investigators with a set of easy-to-follow steps for reaching a rational, "tailored" decision, i.e., one which is best suited for the particular situation the investigator has in mind. The use of an assessment method or instrument "off the shelf", without a careful examination of whether that method or instrument is logical for the particular situation at hand, increases the risk that a suboptimal method or instrument may be applied and that the results will be invalid.

In this chapter, we provide a simple algorithm, or decision tree, as a step-by-step approach that can serve as a guide for the selection of appropriate methods and instruments. Also, we provide a checklist of properties or criteria that need to be considered when examining questionnaires to be completed either by health care professionals or as self-assessment instruments. Examples of particular instruments will be given to illustrate the criteria that we think should be considered.

II. AN ALGORITHM FOR SELECTING QUALITY-OF-LIFE MEASURES

An algorithm is a step-by-step set of guidelines for solving a complex problem by setting down individual steps and showing how each step follows the preceding one. When presented in graphic form as a tree with branches representing alternative decisions, it is known as a decision tree (see Figures 1 and 2). Algorithms are useful for solving various health care problems, by presenting for consideration alternative strategies which, if followed, result in varying probabilities of a clinically desirable outcome. Here we use an algorithm as an aid to answer the question of how to select the most appropriate measure for assessing quality of life in a variety of possible clinical situations, whether as a part of a clinical trial, or in day-to-day clinical practice. The importance of choosing the appropriate measure for a given problem cannot be overstated. The use of unsuitable measures will provide questionable data and these may lead to ineffective interventions. In addition, the use of inappropriate measures is a waste of human and material resources.

In this section we pose several questions that can be helpful in the selection of quality-of-life assessments. These are basic questions that should be answered before initiating the actual measurement, but in some situations there will be additional questions that need to be answered. Also, there is room for debate as to the exact chronological order in which these questions should be posed. The order given here seems reasonable, but conceivably may be altered for certain situations. In other words, while the algorithm we suggest will likely be applicable to most situations, exceptions will undoubtedly arise and these should be dealt with in a common-sense manner.

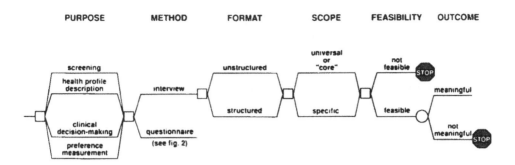

FIGURE 1.   An algorithm for selecting quality-of-life measures. This portion of the algorithm shows the initial steps, which are to determine the purpose of the measurement and to decide whether to use interviews or questionnaires, followed by the subsequent steps for the interview method. The subsequent steps for the questionnaire method are shown in Figure 2.

A. WHAT IS THE PURPOSE OF MEASURING QUALITY OF LIFE?

The algorithm for answering the general question "*how* should quality of life be measured in this situation?" begins with the specific question "for what *purpose* will the results of the measures be used?" Although many specific purposes could be listed, they can be reduced to four main ones: screening (or case finding), description of health profiles, preference measurement, and clinical decision making (Figure 1). This taxonomy is somewhat different than that proposed by Guyatt et al., but could be included within either health profiles or utility measures, the two broad categories that they suggest.[18]

1. Will the Measure be Used for Screening (or Case-Finding)?

Screening is the systematic examination of a large group of individuals in order to identify those displaying certain characteristics (in this context, quality-of-life characteristics). Typically, it is undertaken to identify "high risk" individuals for purposes of classification, for determining incidence, or for subsequent study and appropriate intervention. If a measure of quality of life is to be used for screening then a major consideration is the need to apply the measure routinely to a large sample of the population as compared to assessing a smaller sample when measuring quality of life for other purposes. Another important difference is that the amount of detail desired for screening may be much less than for the other purposes. Thus, for screening, lengthy multidimensional questionnaires may contain too much detail; a single global score or an aggregated score may be sufficient to allow identification of the parameter of interest. Noninformative detail adds to the work involved in data collection and analysis and should be avoided.

In addition to brevity, screening instruments should exhibit very high levels of reliability with, for example, a higher level of internal consistency (Cronbach's alpha >0.9) than that which is commonly accepted (>0.6) for measures intended to detect group differences in a particular quality-of-life dimension.[19] Furthermore, if screening measures are not to "label" individuals incorrectly, they should have high levels of sensitivity (true positive rate) and specificity (true negative rate). This is particularly important if screening is being carried out to identify individuals for subsequent intervention. Unfortunately, little precise information is available on the sensitivity and specificity of current quality-of-life measures. For example, to our knowledge, Receiver Operating Characteristic curves have not been published for any quality-of-life measure. Nevertheless, the brevity of certain instruments (see Section III) makes them possible candidates to consider as screening measures.

2. Will the Measure be Used for Obtaining Quality-of-Life Health Profiles?

When the purpose of the assessment is to obtain a quality-of-life profile, three subsidiary questions need to be asked.

1. Is the profile intended for descriptive purposes only? If so, the implication is that the data are intended to describe the current state of quality of life of a cohort (or an individual) as a single description to be collected at one time only.
2. Is the quality-of-life profile to be used for purposes of comparison? Two kinds of comparison are possible: (i) intergroup comparisons, such as a comparison of two or more groups of individuals after each has been subjected to differing interventions in a randomized clinical trial, and (ii) intragroup comparisons, such as comparison of the quality of life of a single cohort over time (e.g., pretreatment vs. post-treatment).
3. Is the reason for obtaining a quality-of-life profile to describe a cohort, before an intended intervention, for the purpose of stratification? An example would be the allocation of an individual to an appropriate stratum according to some quality-of-life parameter(s) (e.g., physical functioning, emotional well-being, etc.).

In all of these examples, the main purpose is to develop a profile of a state (or series of states) of quality of life. In each case much more detail is desirable than is required for screening. A detailed unidimensional measure may be appropriate if information is desired only for a single dimension of quality of life (e.g., emotional state). However, for most purposes, multidimensional measures will be more appropriate in that they will provide detailed information about different aspects of quality of life. Such detailed data may make it possible to distinguish between the effects of the disease and the effects of treatment on physical, emotional, and social functioning for individuals or for groups of individuals.

When using a quality-of-life measure before an intervention in order to stratify individuals into subgroups, one should have evidence that the measure has prognostic value. The Karnofsky and Eastern Cooperative Oncology Group (ECOG) performance status indices, or other similar measures of physical performance status are often used in this way.[20] While none of these can be considered as a valid measure of quality of life, since they deal only with physical functioning, their widespread use for purposes of stratification suggests that more broadly based quality-of-life measures may have a similar use. Indeed, an early report of the results of the Functional Living Index-Cancer (FLIC) in a study of patients with lung cancer suggests that it may have prognostic value in addition to that provided by histology and extent of disease.[21]

3. Will the Measure be Used for the Assessment of Preferences?

In preference assessment, patients are asked to express their preference for a particular health state. One widely used approach to the assessment of preferences is utility measurement, a process derived from economic and decision theories,[22,23] and intended to reflect the preferences of patients for different quality-of-life states as affected by their illness or its treatment. Utility measurement was developed as an aid for decision making under conditions of uncertainty. The utility score for a particular state of quality of life is expressed as a single number along a continuum extending from death or worst quality (0.0) to perfect health or highest quality (1.0). This procedure provides an assessment of quality of life according to the patients' subjective perceptions. Thus, stated in another way, it is the expression of patients' preferences for their present state of health, relative to specified lowest and highest extremes, on the basis of each patient's own normative standard. Since the result is usually expressed as a single number between zero and one, the responses must be quantifiable. (Further details on utility measurement applied to cancer care are found in other chapters of this book).[24-26]

If the only purpose is to assess preference, then a detailed measurement (with, for example, each dimension represented on a scale from 0.0 to 1.0) would be needed to evaluate the relative importance placed by individuals or groups on physical functioning vs. emotional or social functioning. However, when preference assessments (such as utility measurements) are to be combined with other measures, such as cost (e.g., in a cost-utility analysis), a single global score for evaluating quality of life may suffice.

4. Will the Measure be Used in Clinical Decision Making?

Our use of the term "clinical decision making" is reserved primarily for decision making in clinical practice, although it may be desirable to include interim analyses of quality-of-life data in clinical trials to decide whether or not a trial should continue or to modify or interrupt a particular intervention for a group of patients in the trial. Presumably, in such a situation, the quality-of-life data would closely parallel toxicity data, but this need not be the case if the toxicity data is expressed only in biological terms.

The most likely setting for including a quality-of-life measure for the purpose of clinical decision making would be in day-to-day clinical practice, where a physician or other health care practitioner is involved in decisions about the appropriate interventions for a particular patient as a result of changing circumstances or characteristics of quality of life. In this situation, the measure would be used repeatedly with the results of each assessment being compared with previous or baseline results.

It is likely that multidimensional measures would be preferable to unidimensional measures in clinical decision making, since such measures provide a broad profile of information on which to base a decision. However, if only a particular dimension of life is of interest, a unidimensional measure would be appropriate providing it gives sufficient detail to be clinically useful.

Ideally, if measures are to be used for clinical decision making for individual patients, they should have high levels of sensitivity and specificity, and Receiver Operating Characteristics curves[27] should be developed.

B. WHICH METHOD OF MEASUREMENT IS MOST APPROPRIATE FOR THE PURPOSE?

There are two main methods for assessing quality of life: by *interviews* (ranging from unstructured to structured) and by *questionnaires* (either self-assessment or observer assessment) (Figure 1). Each may be used to obtain responses from either patients or family members, health care personnel or from combinations of these.

In general, an unstructured interview is most suitable for exploratory studies, where the exact items (questions) have not been delineated, and it is desirable to obtain subject input into the kinds of questions that could be most revealing or informative. This approach is particularly suitable with small samples because of the extensive work involved in interpreting and coding individual responses. A fully structured interview, composed entirely of set questions and fixed response categories, is very similar to a self-assessment questionnaire, the difference being that an interviewer poses the questions. Semistructured interviews combine open- and closed-ended questions. They provide a greater degree of standardization than do unstructured interviews, while remaining flexible enough to allow the collection of some qualitative information.

Self-assessment questionnaires are more easily applicable to larger populations of subjects than are interviews, the exact numbers being dependent only marginally on the complexity of the questionnaire. They may be given to subjects directly, mailed to them, or form part of a telephone or face-to-face interview (in which case they are really indistinguishable from a fully structured interview). In certain clinical settings, questionnaires intended for self-completion can be presented in interview form (e.g., for patients with sight impairment).

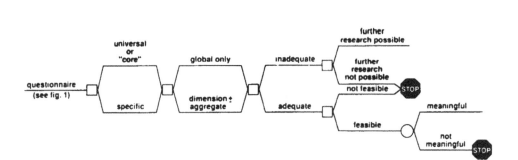

FIGURE 2.   An algorithm for selecting quality-of-life measures. This portion is a continuation of Figure 1 and suggests the steps to be followed when the questionnaire method has been chosen as the means of measurement.

If a quality-of-life measure is intended to measure a *patient's* quality of life, then the patient's own subjective normative standard is the "gold standard". For this reason self-assessment is always preferable to the opinions of observers, such as health care personnel. Nevertheless, in some situations, a "second-best" approach may be preferable to no assessment at all. Examples include assessment of quality of life in young children, in the mentally impaired or in those with certain physical handicaps, since these subjects may not be amenable to either direct interviewing or to self-assessment.

In some situations, it may be desirable to employ both patient self-assessment and observer rating (e.g., family member, health care worker, etc.). For example, one may be interested in studying the degree of concordance between patients' and partners' perceptions of the effect of the disease or its treatment on the patients' quality of life.

C. WHAT IS THE SCOPE OF THE ASSESSMENT?

Regardless of whether the interview or the questionnaire method of assessment has been chosen, the next step is to determine whether the *scope* of the assessment is to be general or specific (Figures 1 and 2). By a general assessment is meant an inquiry into several dimensions of quality of life, e.g., at least the physical, emotional, and social dimensions, whereas a specific assessment would focus on either a single dimension (e.g., psychological functioning) or be restricted even further to deal with some facet of one dimension (e.g., depression). A general assessment is likely to be applicable to most patients with cancer since it deals with issues common to all or most patients.

When the questionnaire method (observer-assessment or self-assessment) is to be used, and a general assessment is desired, a "core" (generic) questionnaire is most appropriate. A core questionnaire is broad in scope in that it contains items directed towards each of several dimensions of quality of life. Each dimension may be summarized by a single score, and these may be combined in some way to give an aggregate score. If the scope is narrow, and only a particular quality-of-life dimension is to be assessed, then a specific questionnaire restricted to items designed to explore only that domain will be appropriate.

D. ARE RELIABLE, VALID QUESTIONNAIRES AVAILABLE?

When either a self-assessment or an observer-assessment questionnaire has been selected, the next step is a critical appraisal of its reliability and validity (psychometric properties) (Figure 2). Although reliability and validity are also relevant for interviews, we will focus primarily on the appraisal of these properties in self-assessment questionnaires in a separate section (see Section III).

If the appraisal reveals that none of the available questionnaires has acceptable psychometric properties, then the investigator needs to decide whether or not to pursue the extensive research and development required to design and validate a new questionnaire. If further research is not feasible, an alternative to be considered is whether or not the original purpose of measuring quality of life in a given set of circumstances can be reframed in a way that allows a reiteration of the algorithm.

E. IS THE INTENDED ASSESSMENT FEASIBLE?

The next step is to determine the feasibility of carrying out the intended assessment. How frequently will the measure be applied? Is it intended to be used only once (e.g., for stratifying patients into subgroups) or will it be used daily to monitor closely the effects of therapy (e.g., the side effects of chemotherapy)? Are the human and material resources available? Does an infrastructure exist which will allow the assessment to proceed to completion? In other words, is there appropriate funding for trained personnel to administer, follow-up, monitor, and analyze the results of either interviews or questionnaires according to the planned objectives? What will be done to ensure quality control? All of these items should be carefully thought out and resolved before the study begins. An otherwise excellent plan will fail if there is poor compliance, i.e., missing data, inaccurate data, or inadequate analysis, due to lack of personnel or resources.

F. ARE THE RESULTS (OUTCOMES) MEANINGFUL?

Up to this point, all of the decisions in the algorithm can be made on the basis of available information. If the investigation proves to be feasible and proceeds according to plan, it will presumably yield information relevant to the quality-of-life research question that has been posed. The next critical step in the process involves the interpretation of the study results. Central to this interpretive step is to determine what can be considered as "meaningful" results.[28-30]

In this context, the term "meaningful" can be defined in two ways. It can be used to indicate that the study results can be interpreted with a certain degree of statistical certainty (i.e., statistically significant) or that the results are of clinical relevance. These two definitions of "meaningful" are not always synonymous. For example, if a quality-of-life assessment was carried out for purposes of screening a population of individuals for possible psychosocial intervention, the statistical value of the screening assessment can be determined by examining its sensitivity and specificity in relation to a presumably valid criterion measure (e.g., a psychiatric interview). Yet, in most situations, a balance needs to be struck between instrument sensitivity and specificity. The costs of failing to detect a psychosocial "case" (a question of sensitivity) needs to be weighed against the costs associated with the risk of misclassifying certain individuals as "cases" (a question of specificity). The acceptable degree of trade-off between sensitivity and specificity of a screening instrument can only be determined on the basis of clinical and related considerations (e.g., the relative costs of generating false positives vs. false negatives both in terms of health risk and health care financing).

If the original purpose of the quality of life investigation was to generate a quality of life "health profile", then statistical meaningfulness can be defined in terms of convergent validity (e.g., the degree to which different methods, e.g., a self-assessment questionnaire vs. a clinical interview yield similar results). Yet, such statistical evidence does not address directly the issue of clinical relevance. For example, given a sufficiently large sample size in a randomized clinical trial, very small group differences in the quality-of-life outcome may reach standard levels of statistical significance, but may be of only limited clinical interest. Recently, Jaeschke et al. have attempted to elucidate the minimal degree of change that can be reliably interpreted as being clinically meaningful.[30] It is likely that there are no general criteria for a minimal clinically important difference that can be applied to all studies and specific criteria may need to be developed for the particular situation in which quality-of-life measures are being used.

Regardless of the type of quality-of-life study to be conducted, the decision regarding what kind of quality-of-life outcome will be considered to be clinically meaningful should preferably be specified at the beginning of a study, rather than during the data analysis and interpretation stage. In this way, one can enhance the efficiency of the study (i.e., by setting appropriate sample size requirements) and can minimize the risk associated with attempting to capitalize on chance findings. At the same time, one should be open to the possibility of counterintuitive findings. Some recent quality-of-life studies in osteogenic sarcoma[31] and advanced breast cancer[32] have yielded results that ran contrary to *a priori* expectations. Such counterintuitive results, while deserving of very critical scrutiny, must be taken seriously and be submitted to replication. Nevertheless, if the tools and data collection are reliable, studies yielding counterintuitive results must be accepted. In this way old paradigms die and new ones are born!

If meaningful outcomes have been obtained, new or further research questions may now be addressed and a reiteration of the algorithm will be helpful in approaching the task.

III. CRITERIA FOR ASSESSING SUITABILITY OF QUESTIONNAIRES

In this section we give special attention to questionnaires. Although the interview method is useful in certain circumstances (see Section II.B), the most appealing characteristic of questionnaires is that the results are quantifiable, i.e., the results can be expressed numerically. Thus, comparisons between individuals or groups of individuals at one or more points in time may be expressed in statistical terms. Furthermore, during the development of a questionnaire, its psychometric properties can be quantified and analyzed. It is this property that defines reliability as a statistical description of the amount of random error associated with a questionnaire. The reliability of a measure is essential information when choosing a questionnaire that will be appropriate to the task. Another reason for the wide appeal of questionnaires is that their administration is usually less time-consuming and labor-intensive than are interviews, and the training required for personnel administering questionnaires is relatively simple.

There are multiple criteria for deciding which questionnaire(s) is most suitable for assessing the quality of life of patients. The remainder of this paper will focus on a list of questions which should be asked about questionnaires when using the algorithm presented in Section II (Figure 2). In addition, 11 selected questionnaires have been scrutinized by the suggested approach and the criteria fulfilled by each have been summarized (Table 1). These questionnaires are not intended to be an inventory of all the questionnaires that have been developed for use with cancer patients; they are presented for illustrative purposes only. Furthermore, the data presented for each questionnaire (compiled by David Osoba) are based on the information generated in field trials during its development and not during its subsequent performance when used to assess quality of life in various clinical situations. Some of the instruments have been used extensively since their initial development and the results are presented in more detail elsewhere in this book.[33,34]

A. WHO DEVELOPED THE QUESTIONNAIRE?

If a questionnaire is to reflect the concerns of most importance to patients, then its development should involve a cooperative effort by both health care workers *and* patients. Questionnaires not developed with input from patients may, nevertheless, be relevant and should not be discounted for this reason alone if they fulfill other relevant criteria.

B. WHAT IS THE QUESTIONNAIRE'S SCOPE?

Is the questionnaire meant to be used for patients with cancer at any site or is it meant to be restricted to patients with cancer at only a certain site? Is it meant to assess primarily the effects of the disease, or the effects of treatment, or of both disease and treatment on quality of life? Questionnaires intended for a broad assessment of quality of life in virtually all patients, regardless of the site of the tumor, have been termed "generic", "core", or "universal" questionnaires. When the intension is to determine the quality of life of patients having a particular form of cancer (e.g., lung cancer) or a particular form of treatment, the questionnaires are known as "specific" or "restricted" questionnaires. Since a core questionnaire may not provide sufficient detail about the effects of quality of life resulting from a specific form of cancer or treatment, it is recommended that a modular approach be used whereby a specific or restricted module (or modules) is added to a core or universal questionnaire. In this way one or more modules, each designated for a specific purpose, can be added to a single core questionnaire, depending upon the research question being asked.

C. WHO WILL CARRY OUT THE ASSESSMENT?

Is the questionnaire intended for self-assessment or is it intended for completion by a health care worker? If it is intended to assess the patients' quality of life, self-assessment is preferable to assessment by an observer because self-assessment will provide responses based upon the patients' own normative standard rather than the observers' standard or some abstract "societal" standard.

Brief questionnaires, taking less than 10 or 15 min to answer, are preferable to long questionnaires, particularly if they are to be administered repeatedly or to very ill patients. The questionnaire should be in the language best understood by the intended respondent and should be simple enough to be understood by all the respondents. While this seems logical, publications describing questionnaire development seldom indicate the level of education required for respondents to be able to answer the questions.

D. WHAT IS THE QUESTION TIME FRAME AND RESPONSE STRUCTURE?

The time frame of the questions should always be clear, since this will have an effect on whether the responses reflect random events, true events or personality traits influencing quality of life. In one study, it was found that short time frames (1 day) were associated with increased randomness in the responses, whereas long time frames (longer than 1 week) appeared to be associated with the personality trait of the respondent rather than with the actual symptom state being experienced.[35] Time frames of between 3 and 7 days are probably best.

Whether the response structure is in the form of a categorical scale (Likert scale) or a linear (visual) analog scale seems to depend upon the individual preferences of investigators. Categorical scales are easier for patients to understand than are visual analog scales, but the latter allow greater precision of measurement. An important issue is whether or not these methods differ in sensitivity to change (responsiveness), i.e., in their ability to detect minimal clinically important changes. Jaeschke et al. have reported that these two methods of presenting response options show similar responsiveness, and recommended the use of seven-point Likert scales because of their ease of administration, analysis, and interpretation.[36]

E. WHAT ARE THE DIMENSIONS TAPPED BY THE QUESTIONNAIRE?

Some questionnaires are designed to tap multiple, separate dimensions; others are unidimensional. The desirable number of dimensions that should be assessed by a questionnaire will depend upon the research question being asked, i.e., the purpose of the assessment. In general, measures for description of quality-of-life profiles and for decision-making purposes should be more detailed than measures for screening and for preference ratings, but even

TABLE 1

Summary of Criteria Fulfilled by Selected Quality of Life Measures Developed for Cancer Patients

	Authors										
Criterion	Priestman et al.[38,39]	Padilla et al.[40]	Schipper et al.[41]	Selby et al.[42,43]	Fayers and Jones[2]	Aaronson et al.[44,46]	Karnofsky and Burchenal[47]	Zubrod et al.[48]	Spitzer et al.[49] (QL-Index)	Spitzer et al.[49] (Uniscale)	Levine et al.[50]
Developed by											
Physicians/nurses	+	+	+	+	+	+	+	+	+	+	+
Allied workers	–	–	+	+	–	+	–	–	+	+	–
Patients/relatives	–	–	+	–	–	–	–	–	+	+	+
Intended scope											
All patients ("core")	–	+	+	–	+	+	+	+	+	+	–
Specific (restricted)	+	–	–	+	–	–	–	–	–	–	+
Assessment by											
Self assessment	+	+	+	+	+	+	–	–	+*	+*	–
Observer assessment	–	–	–	–	–	–	+	+	+*	+*	+
Response design											
Linear analog	+	+	±	+	–	–	–	–	–	+	–
Categorical	–	–	+	–	+	+	+	+	+	–	+
Time-framed	–	+	±	+	+	+	+	+	+	+	+
Dimensions tapped											
Physical	+	+	+	+	±	+	+	+	±	–	±
Emotional	+	±	+	+	±	+	–	–	±	–	+
Social	+	+	+	+	–	+	–	±	±	–	–
Pain	+	+	+	+	±	+	–	–	–	–	±
Other	–	+	+	+	+	+	–	–	–	+	+
Global	–	–	–	–	–	+	–	–	–	+	–
Reliability											
Internal consistency	–	–	–	+	–	+	–	–	–	–	+
Test-retest stability	+	+	–	+	+	+	+	+	+	+	+
Inter-rater/institutional	–	–	+	–	–	+	+	+	+	+	–

Validity										
Extensive testing	±	±	+	+	±	+	+	+	+	±
Content	+	+	+	+	+	+	+	+	+	+
Sensitivity to change	±	−	±	+	+	−	+	−	−	+
Situation-responsive	±	+	+	+	+	+	+	+	+	+
Cross-cultural testing	−	−	−	−	−	+	−	−	+	−
Aggregation/disaggregation										
Quantifiable data	+	+	+	+	+	+	+	+	+	+
Aggregate score	+	+	+	−	+	+	+	−	+	+
Item scores	+	±	+	−	+	−	−	−	−	−
Dimension scores	−	−	−	+	−	−	−	+	−	−
Global score	−	−	−	−	+	−	−	+	−	−

Note: The description of the instruments included in this table is based primarily upon initial published data during early development of each questionnaire. It has been compiled by one of the authors (D. Osoba). A "+" symbol is meant to indicate that a particular criterion has been fulfilled. Conversely, a "−" symbol indicates that the criterion was not fulfilled. A "±" symbol means that there is only partial fulfillment of that criterion. NK = not known.

a These instruments originally were developed for observer-assessment, but now are available for either observer-assessment or self-assessment.

b This is an interviewer guided self-assessment procedure in which the patient responds to questions by choosing answers from options listed on a card. It has recently also been converted to self-assessment.

the latter may cover the three basic dimensions (physical, emotional, and social) if they are suitably brief (see Sections II.A and C).

Questionnaires should have been subjected to factor analysis during development to determine how many factors (or dimensions) are being assessed. This provides a way for each of the dimensions tapped by the questionnaire to be identified and related to more than a single item. Such an analysis, along with item-total score correlations will reveal whether or not the items in a questionnaire can be grouped into separate subscales so that each subscale can be expressed by a single number.

Factor analysis may also provide some insight into the validity of the questionnaire, if the factors revealed by the analysis are interpretable in relation to the dimensions that the questionnaire is *intended* to measure.

F. WHAT IS THE RELIABILITY OF THE QUESTIONNAIRE?

The reliability of an instrument (i.e., the extent to which it is free of random error) is an important, basic consideration in choosing among available measures. Most often, reliability is defined in terms of "internal consistency". In nontechnical terms, this refers to the degree of correlation between items making up a scale. For a measure to be internally consistent, the individual items should exhibit a relatively high correlation with one another, as well as with the overall scale score. The most common statistical test for internal consistency is Chronbach's alpha coefficient.[37]

Reliability can also be defined in terms of test-retest stability. The period of time over which responses should remain stable will vary with the population being studied. Quality-of-life measures employed in patients with a rapidly changing course of illness or undergoing treatment might only be expected to remain stable over a short period of time (hours or days). Conversely, among patients whose illness is unchanging and who are not receiving treatment, the quality-of-life assessments should remain relatively stable over long periods of time (e.g., several weeks).

Finally, if observers (doctors, nurses, family members) are being used to rate the quality of life of patients, then data should be available regarding the inter-rater reliability of these assessments. It should be mentioned that a number of different statistics are available to assess inter-rater reliability with some providing a more stringent test than others. In comparing the inter-rater reliability of different candidate measures, one should take into consideration the type of statistic that has been applied (e.g., whether the statistic has corrected for chance agreement between raters).

G. ARE THE RESULTS LIKELY TO BE VALID?

The validity of a tool, such as a questionnaire, is always in doubt until the tool's usefulness has been proven in extensive clinical trials and in a variety of clinical situations. Therefore, in choosing a questionnaire for a particular purpose in a given situation, attention should be paid not only to the content of the questionnaire, but to whether it has been tested repeatedly in the same or similar groups of patients and has been shown to be responsive to changes in quality of life expected to occur longitudinally with time, (e.g., changes associated with improving or worsening disease status). In addition to being responsive to differing situations in the same individual, it should be able to detect differences between groups of patients in differing situations (e.g., one would expect, intuitively, that quality of life in patients whose disease is in complete remission and who are living at home would be higher than in hospitalized patients with advanced disease). Another example of situation-responsiveness is the ability of a questionnaire to reflect the acute changes in quality of life associated with a therapy that is likely to produce obvious short-term side effects and to distinguish these from the underlying quality of life attributable to the effects of the disease for which the treatment has been given.

Other aspects of validity include an examination of whether the item is logical for the situation in which the questionnaire will be used. For example, for the study of patients with cancer, it makes sense to use questionnaires that have been developed with this patient population in mind or, at the very least, that have been developed for patients with chronic illnesses. It would not be useful to employ questionnaires developed for other populations, (e.g., patients with a psychiatric illness).

There are a number of formal strategies available for examining the statistical validity of an instrument. The two most common strategies are criterion validity (whereby the instrument of interest is tested against a criterion with which it is known or expected to co-vary) and convergent validity (whereby the correlation between the instrument of interest and other instruments designed to measure similar and/or dissimilar quality of life domains are examined). A detailed discussion of these procedures is beyond the scope of this paper, but we recommend that when choosing among candidate quality-of-life measures, a psychometrician and/or statistician be consulted on these issues.

A special characteristic, of importance in multicultural communities or in multinational studies where respondents speak more than one language, is to determine whether appropriate cross-cultural testing has been carried out. A simple translation of the questions into the desired language is not sufficient to ensure a reliable translation of exact meaning, e.g., a literal translation of the English "Have you been feeling blue?" (a common item used in most depression scales), would be meaningless in most European languages. Therefore, a careful process of repeated translation back and forth between the original and desired languages is necessary to preserved the intended meaning.

H. WHAT KINDS OF LEVEL OF AGGREGATION/DISAGGREGATION WILL ANALYSIS PROVIDE?

A major advantage of questionnaires, as compared to unstructured interviews, is that questionnaires provide quantifiable data which may be expressed in several ways. These may be a single score resulting from a summation of all the items *(aggregate score)* or a set of separate scores for each of the dimensions represented *(dimension scores)* which then may be summed into an aggregate score. If none of these is desirable then each item may be represented by a separate score *(item score)*. A global question asking a single question such as "How is your quality of life?" is a method of generating a *global score*. Other than for screening or for preference measurement, a global score has the disadvantage that it does not discriminate between dimensions; identical scores for two patients may be derived from very different states of quality of life in different dimensions. At the other extreme, a separate score for each item produces a large amount of data for analysis, especially if the questionnaire is administered repeatedly. Thus, a multidimensional questionnaire producing separate dimension scores, which also may be summed to produce an aggregate score is desirable. Some questionnaires combine more than one approach by asking a global question about the subject's overall perception of quality of life, as well as having a broad multidimensional approach leading to dimension scores and an aggregate score.

IV. SUMMARY AND CONCLUSIONS

This practical, "consumers" guide is intended to help potential users of quality-of-life measures by providing a rational approach to selecting appropriate measures. The selection process is presented as an algorithm combined with a series of questions that may be used as a checklist. The algorithm begins with asking the user to make a decision about the purpose of measuring quality of life and then continues in a stepwise fashion through the selection of the method, scope, reliability and validity, feasibility and the meaningfulness of the outcomes of the assessment. The checklist provides a standard set of criteria against which the attributes of questionnaires may be compared. Eleven currently available questionnaires are used as examples of how the checklist may be used to provide information on the attributes of each questionnaire.

The algorithm presented in this chapter, by necessity, lays out the steps involved in selecting quality-of-life measures in a linear fashion. In practice, many of the considerations that we have outlined may occur in a somewhat different order, or may even occur simultaneously. For example, issues of feasibility may precede those of the validity and reliability of available candidate measures, e.g., one might first decide that, given the constraints operating in a given clinical setting, the only possibility would be to employ a short, self-administered questionnaire. One would then restrict the search for psychometrically robust instruments to just such brief questionnaires, and would not be interested in a lengthy interview, regardless of its psychometric properties.

Many of the steps described in this decision-tree are of a technical nature. Nevertheless, we would like to end this discussion where we began, by emphasizing the central place of the research question itself in this whole process. Ultimately, the value of quality-of-life investigations will rest on the relevance of the research questions that we pose. Methodological considerations should not influence the substantive direction of our research. To the contrary, our theoretical and clinical concerns should guide us in choosing appropriate methodologies.

REFERENCES

1. **Najman, J. M. and Levine, S.**, Evaluating the impact of medical care and technologies on the quality of life: a review and critique, *Soc. Sci. Med.*, 15, 107, 1981.
2. **Fayers, P. M. and Jones, D. R.**, Measuring and analyzing quality of life in cancer clinical trials: a review, *Stat. Med.*, 429, 1983.
3. **van Dam, F. S. A. M.**, Assessment of quality of life in cancer patients, in *Quality of Life in Cancer Patients: A Current Topic in Cancer Treatment and Care*, Takeda, F., Ed., Office of the Organizing Committee of the Workshop on Quality of Life in Cancer Patients, Saitama, Japan, 1984, 55.
4. **deHaes, J. C. J. M. and van Knippenberg, F. C. E.**, The quality of life of cancer patients: a review of the literature, *Soc. Sci. Med.*, 20, 809, 1985.
5. **Brinkley, D.**, Quality of life in cancer trials, *Br. Med. J.*, 291, 685, 1985.
6. **Yancik, R. and Yates, J. W.**, Quality of life assessment of cancer patients: conceptual and methodologic challenges and constraints, *Cancer Bull.*, 38, 217, 1986.
7. **deHaes, J. C. J. M. and van Knippenberg, F. C. E.**, Quality of life of cancer patients: a review of the literature, in *The Quality of Life of Cancer Patients*, Aaronson, N. K. and Beckman, J. H., Eds., Monogr. Ser. European Organization for Research and Treatment of Cancer, Raven Press, New York, 1987.
8. **de Haes, J. C. J. M.**, Quality of life: conceptual and theoretical considerations, in *Psychosocial Oncology*, Watson, M. and Greer, S., Eds., Pergamon Press, Oxford, 1985, 61.
9. **van Knippenberg, F. C. E. and deHaes, J. C. J. M.**, Measuring the quality of life of cancer patients: psychometric properties of instruments, *J. Clin. Epidemiol.*, 1043, 1988.
10. **Frank-Stromberg, M.**, Single instruments for measuring quality of life, in *Instruments for Clinical Nursing Research*, Frank-Stromberg, M., Ed., Appleton and Lange, Norwalk, CT, 1988, 79.
11. **Dean, H.**, Multiple instruments for measuring quality of life, in *Instruments for Clinical Nursing Research*, Frank-Stromberg, M., Ed., Appleton and Lange, Norwalk, CT, 1988, 97.
12. **Moinpour, C. M., Feigl, P., Metch, B., Hayden, K. A., Meyskens, F. L., Jr., and Crowley, J.**, Quality of life end points in cancer clinical trials: review and recommendations, *J. Natl. Cancer Inst.*, 81, 485, 1989.
13. **Skeel, R. T.**, Quality of life assessment in cancer clinical trials — it's time to catch up, *J. Natl. Cancer Inst.*, 81, 472, 1989.
14. **Donovan, K., Sanson-Fisher, R. W., and Redman, S.**, Measuring quality of life in cancer patients, *J. Clin. Oncol.*, 7, 959, 1989.
15. **Maguire, P. and Selby, P.**, Assessing quality of life in cancer patients, *Br. J. Cancer*, 60, 437, 1989.

16. **Barofsky, I. and Sugarbaker, P. N.**, Cancer, in *Quality of Life Assessments in Clinical Trials*, Spilker, B., Ed., Raven Press, New York, 1990, 419.
17. **Levine, M. N.**, Incorporation of quality of life assessment into clinical trials, in *Effect of Cancer on Quality of Life*, Osoba, D., Ed., CRC Press, Boca Raton, FL, 1991, chap. 8.
18. **Guyatt, G. H., Veldhuyzen Van Zanten, S. J. O., Feeney, D. H., and Patrick, D. H.**, Measuring quality of life in clinical trials: a taxonomy and review, *Can. Med. Assoc. J.*, 140, 1441, 1989.
18. **Helmstadter, G. C.**, *Principles of Psychological Measurement*, Appleton-Century-Crofts, New York, 1964.
20. **Orr, S. T. and Aisner, J.**, Performance status assessment among oncology patients: a review, *Cancer Treat. Rep.*, 70, 1423, 1986.
21. **Ruckdeschel, J. C. and Piantadosi, S.**, Assessment of quality of life (QL) by the Functional Living Index-Cancer (FLIC) is superior to performance status for prediction of survival in patients with lung cancer, *Proc. Am. Soc. Clin. Oncol.*, 8, 311, 1989 (abstr. 1209).
22. **von Neumann, J. and Morgenstern, O.**, *Theory of Games and Economic Behaviour*, 2nd ed., Princeton University Press, Princeton, NJ, 1947.
23. **Torrance, G. W.**, Utility approach to measuring health-related quality of life, *J. Chronic Dis.*, 40, 593, 1987.
24. **Feeney, D., Barr, R. D., Furlong, W., Torrance, G. W., and Weitzman, S.**, Quality of life of the treatment process in pediatric oncology: an approach to measurement, in *Effect of Cancer on Quality of Life*, Osoba, D., Ed., CRC Press, Boca Raton, FL, 1991, chap. 10.
25. **Goodwin, P. J.**, Economic evaluations of cancer care—incorporating quality of life issues, in *Effect of Cancer on Quality of Life*, Osoba, D., Ed., CRC Press, Boca Raton, FL, 1991, chap. 10.
26. **Till, J.**, Uses (and some possible abuses) of quality of life measures, in *Effect of Cancer on Quality of Life*, Osoba, D., Ed., CRC Press, Boca Raton, FL, 1991, chap. 11.
27. **Deyo, R. A. and Centor, R. M.**, Assessing the responsiveness of functional scales to clinical change: an analogy to diagnostic test performance, *J. Chronic Dis.*, 39, 897, 1986.
28. **Guyatt, G., Walter, S., and Norman, J.**, Measuring change over time: assessing the usefulness of evaluative instruments, *J. Chronic Dis.*, 40, 171, 1987.
29. **Norman, G. R.**, Issues in the use of change scores in randomized trials, *J. Clin. Epidemiol.*, 42, 1097, 1989.
30. **Jaeschke, R., Singer, J., and Guyatt, G. H.**, Measurement of health status. Ascertaining minimal clinically important difference, *Controlled Clin. Trials*, 10, 407, 1989.
31. **Sugarbaker, P. H., Barofsky, I., Rosenberg, S. A., and Gianola, F. J.**, Quality of life assessment of patients in extremity sarcoma trials, *Surgery*, 91, 17, 1982.
32. **Coates, A., Gebski, V., Bishop, J. F., Jeal, P. N., Woods, R. L., Snyder, R., Tattersall, M. H. N., Byrne, M., Harvey, V., Grantley, G., Simpson, J., Drummond, R., Browne, J., van Cooten, R., and Forbes, J. F.**, Improving the quality of life during chemotherapy for advanced breast cancer. A comparison of intermittent and continuous treatment strategies, *N. Engl. J. Med.*, 317, 1490, 1987.
33. **Wood-Dauphinee, S. and Williams, J. I.**, The Spitzer Quality of Life Index: its performance as a measure, in *Effect of Cancer on Quality of Life*, Osoba, D., Ed., CRC Press, Boca Raton, FL, 1991, chap. 13.
34. **Levine, M. N.**, Quality of life in breast cancer, in *Effect of Cancer on Quality of Life*, Osoba, D., Ed., CRC Press, Boca Raton, FL, 1991, chap. 8.
35. **Huisman, S. J., van Dam, F. S. A., Aaronson, N. K., and Hanewald, G. J. F. P.**, On measuring complaints of cancer patients: some remarks on the time span of the question, in *The Quality of Life of Cancer Patients*, Aaronson, N. K. and Beckman, J., Eds., Monogr. Ser. European Organization for Research and Treatment of Cancer, Raven Press, New York, 17, 101, 1987.
36. **Jaeschke, R., Singer, J., and Guyatt, G. H.**, A comparison of seven-point and visual analogue scales, *Controlled Clin. Trials*, 11, 43, 1990.
37. **Cronbach, L. J.**, Coefficient alpha and the internal structure of tests, *Psychometrika*, 16, 297, 1951.
38. **Priestman, T. S. and Baum, M.**, Evaluation of quality of life in patients receiving treatment for advanced breast cancer, *Lancet*, 1899, 1976.
39. **Baum, M., Priestman, T., West, R. R., and Jones, E. M.**, A comparison of subjective responses in a trial comparing endocrine with cytotoxic treatment in advanced carcinoma of the breast, in *Breast Cancer: Experimental and Clinical Aspects*, Mouridsen, H. T. and Palshof, T., Eds., Proc. 2nd EORTC Breast Cancer Working Conf., Pergamon Press, Oxford, 1980, 223.
40. **Padilla, G. V., Pesant, C., Grant, M. M., Metter, G., Lipsett, J., and Heide, F.**, Quality of life index for patients with cancer, *Res. Nurs. Health*, 6, 117, 1983.
41. **Schipper, H., Clinch, J., McMurray, A., and Levitt, M.**, Measuring the quality of life of cancer patients: The Functional Living Index-Cancer: development and validation, *J. Clin. Oncol.*, 2, 472, 1984.
42. **Selby, P. J., Chapman, J.-A.W., Etazadi-Amoli, J., Dalley, D., and Boyd, N. F.**, The development of a method for assessing the quality of life of cancer patients, *Br. J. Cancer*, 50, 13, 1984.
43. **Boyd, N. F., Selby, P. J., Sutherland, H. J., and Hogg, S.**, Measurement of the clinical status of patients with breast cancer: evidence for the validity of self assessment with linear analogue scales, *J. Clin. Epidemiol.*, 41, 243, 1988.

44. Aaronson, N. K., Bakker, W., Stewart, A. L., van Dam, F. S. A. M., van Zandwijk, N., Yarnold, J. R., and Kirkpatrick, A., Multidimensional approach to the measurement of quality of life in lung cancer clinical trials, in *The Quality of Life of Cancer Patients*, Aaronson, N. K. and Beckmann, J. H., Eds., Monogr. Ser. European Organization for Research and Treatment of Cancer, Raven Press, New York, 17, 63, 1987.

45. Aaronson, N. K., Bullinger, M., and Ahmedzai, S., A modular approach to quality of life assessment in cancer clinical trials, in *Cancer Clinical Trials: A Critical Appraisal*, Scheurlen, H., Kay, R., and Baum, M., Eds., *Rec. Res. Cancer Res.*, Springer-Verlag, Berlin, 111, 213, 1988.

46. Aaronson, N. K., Ahmedzai, S., Bullinger, M., Crabeels, D., Estape, J., Filiberti, A., Flechtner, H., Frick, U., Hurny, C., Kaasa, S., Klee, M., Mastilica, M., Osoba, D., Pfausler, B., Razavi, D., Rofe, P. B. C., Schraub, S., Sullivan, M., and Takeda, F., The EORTC quality of life questionnaire: interim results of an international study, in *Effect of Cancer on Quality of Life*, Osoba, D., Ed., CRC Press, Boca Raton, FL, 1991, chap. 14.

47. Karnofsky, D. A. and Burchenal, H. H., The clinical evaluation of chemotherapeutic agents in cancer, in *Evaluation of Chemotherapeutic Agents*, McLeod, C. M., Ed., Columbia University Press, New York, 1949, 191.

48. Zubrod, C. G., Schneiderman, M., Frei, E., et al., Appraisal of methods for the study of chemotherapy of cancer in man: comparative therapeutic trial of nitrogen mustard and triethylene thiophosphoramide, *J. Chronic Dis.*, 11, 7, 1960.

49. Spitzer, W. O., Dobson, A. J., Hall, J., Chesterman, E., Levi, J., Shepherd, R., Battista, R. N., and Catchlove, B. R., Measuring the quality of life of cancer patients. A concise QL-index for use by physicians, *J. Chronic Dis.*, 34, 585, 1981.

50. Levine, M. N., Guyatt, G., Gent, M., De Pauw, S., Goodyear, M. D., Hryniuk, W., Arnold, A., Findlay, B., Skillings, J. R., Bramwell, V. H., Levin, L., Bush, H., Abu-Zarra, H., and Kotalik, J., Quality of life in stage II breast cancer: an instrument for clinical trials, *J. Clin. Oncol.*, 6, 1798, 1988.

Chapter 8

INCORPORATION OF QUALITY-OF-LIFE ASSESSMENT INTO CLINICAL TRIALS

Mark N. Levine

TABLE OF CONTENTS

I. INTRODUCTION

Outcome measures in cancer clinical trials have traditionally been tumor response and survival. Recently, increasing attention has been given to the assessment of quality of life because many of our therapeutic modalities are associated with substantial morbidity with often minimal gains in response and survival.[1-4] The importance of this outcome measure is reflected by recent policy statements by both the Eastern Cooperative Oncology Group (ECOG) and the Southwest Oncology Group (SWOG) in support of quality of life as an outcome measure in their multicenter trials.[5-6]

Although the ultimate desire of a physician is to cure the patient of his/her cancer, more importantly, it is the physician's role to relieve discomfort and suffering from the disease. Historically, the measurement of quality of life has been in the domain of the psychologist, sociologist, and epidemiologist. However, if quality of life is to be relevant to patient care, quality-of-life assessment needs: (1) to be incorporated into clinical trials by those investigators who write protocols, (2) to be accepted enthusiastically by participating physicians who enroll study patients, and (3) to provide relevant information that can be used at the bedside by the patient and physician in clinical decision making. This chapter will focus on issues relevant to the incorporation of quality of life measurement into cancer clinical trials. It is not intended to be an in-depth methodologic review of this area, but to provide the clinician (physician or nurse) with a working knowledge of issues related to the use of quality of life in cancer clinical trials, so that ultimately the information so gained can be introduced into clinical practice.

II. DEFINITION OF QUALITY OF LIFE

The definition of quality of life has led to much debate over the years because it is an abstract concept[7,8] (see Chapter 3). However, for the interested clinician it is sufficient to recognize that quality of life encompasses aspects (jargon word that has been used is "domains") of physical, social and emotional health that are relevant and important to the patient.

The measurement of quality of life can be used for different purposes.[9] It can be used to (1) discriminate different health states between populations, (2) predict patient outcome, and (3) evaluate the effect of a therapeutic or diagnostic test on a patient over time. Although there are examples where an instrument can predict for outcome in the cancer patient, e.g., Karnofsky Performance Status, it is the third reason that is most relevant to the use of quality of life in cancer clinical trials.

In a trial when evaluating patients over time, quality-of-life assessment can be used to monitor the individual patient, thereby leading to a potential intervention to improve that patient's care and it can be used as an outcome measure for groups of patients to assess the overall effectiveness of an intervention.

III. WHEN TO USE QUALITY OF LIFE IN A CLINICAL TRIAL

The answer to this question is difficult. There are those who advocate the use of quality of life as an outcome measure in all clinical trials. However, it is important to recognize that the formal measurement of quality of life in a trial adds considerable complexity and expense to the study. If an intervention has a clearly established large clinical benefit with minimal morbidity, then most would agree that quality of life as an outcome measure would be unnecessary. However, we have reached the stage in cancer clinical research where most clinical trials, phase II and phase III, are being conducted to evaluate either new drugs, new combinations of established drugs, new fractionation schemes in radiation therapy, or new surgical or diagnostic techniques. Although such studies may lead to important advances in the understanding of the biology of cancer and management of the population of cancer patients, in many instances the benefits to the individual patient in terms of survival or palliation of symptoms may be small. Thus, in a clinical trial if either an intervention has a potential impact on the physical, emotional, or social function of the patient, or if the scientific question involves a substantial trade-off between quantity and quality of life, then common sense would dictate that quality of life could be used as an outcome measure.

IV. WHICH INSTRUMENT TO USE

The clinician who wishes to use quality of life as an outcome in a cancer clinical trial is faced with a wide array of instruments.[10,11] Some of these are generic, that is they have been designed to be applicable in a wide variety of populations because they cover the complete spectrum of function, disability and distress that is relevant to quality of life. Examples of this type might include the Sickness Impact Profile (SIP)[12] and the instrument developed by the Rand Corporation.[13] The SIP has been used in studies of cardiac rehabilitation, hip surgery, and treatment of back pain.[11] Generic instruments for the cancer population have been developed in order to be used in patients with different types of malignancies, e.g., Spitzer Quality of Life Index[14] and the Functional Living Index-Cancer (FLIC).[15]

Generic instruments save the investigator and patient time because they are designed for a wide variety of conditions and they may permit comparison across studies. However, they may not focus on the aspects of quality of life of particular interest for the question in the trial and thus could result in an instrument which might miss clinically important changes in quality of life.[16]

An alternate type of instrument is disease specific, that is, it has been developed to focus specifically on the condition or clinical question of interest.[11] The rationale for this approach lies in its potential to measure clinically important change in the patient.[16] The disadvantage is that such instruments may not be comprehensive and cannot be used for comparison between different conditions.

It is of interest that Aaronson et al., from the EORTC, have recently developed an instrument which combines the two approaches.[17] They employ a core generic instrument which can be used in different types of cancer, and specific modules which are added for specific conditions.

It is not our intention to debate which type of instrument, generic or specific, is better. Both can be appropriate, but it is important that the clinician recognize that the instrument be relevant to the question posed in the clinical trial and that it be able to measure whether a patient has changed, for better or worse, as a result of an intervention. For those not experienced in instrument development or use, a reasonable approach might be to seek the advice of a colleague who has experience in health status measurement, or failing this, contact the authors of one of the many published papers on quality of life in the cancer patient.[18,19]

V. PRINCIPLES OF INSTRUMENT-DEVELOPMENT

When selecting an instrument for use in a clinical trial, the clinician should check that the instrument satisfies a number of methodologic criteria (see Chapter 3):[8-11]

1. Physical, emotional, and social well-being. It is important to measure effects in all of these dimensions because therapy can have a profound impact on emotional and social function as well as physical function.
2. Importance to patients. Items must reflect areas of function that are important to cancer patients.

3. Quantifiable. The questionnaire must result in summary scores amenable to statistical analysis.
4. Validity. The questionnaire should truly be measuring the impact of an intervention on quality of life. The determination of validity can be problematic because there is no gold standard for quality of life. Convergent validity, i.e., the extent to which a questionnaire is consistent with other established instruments, is often used as supporting evidence for validity.
5. Reproducibility. Reassessment in stable patients should yield similar results.
6. Responsiveness. The questionnaire should be able to measure and detect clinically important change. The importance of this criterion for clinical trials has recently been recognized.[16,20,21]
7. Simplicity and convenience. Considerations of cost and respondent burden dictate that the questionnaire be relatively short.

VI. PRACTICAL ASPECTS

The use of questionnaires administered by personal interview, as compared with those that are self-administered, is controversial.[22-24] Interviewer-administered questionnaires are more expensive to use, and with such questionnaires it has been suggested that a patient may respond more favorably than truth in order to please the interviewer.[22-24] On the other hand, compliance may not be as good with a self-administered questionnaire and an interviewer (e.g., nurse) may occasionally identify particular treatment-related problems amenable to intervention, because of the personal interview. In a recently reported randomized trial in patients in a physiotherapy clinic, the mode of administration of a health status questionnaire did not influence its ability to measure change in a patient's health status.[23] Finally, if an interviewer is to administer a questionnaire, then a trained research assistant or nurse should perform this function. Physicians may not have the time to administer a questionnaire and patients may not respond in a "true" fashion to a physician-administered questionnaire because they want to please their physician.

Another area of controversy is whether the format of the questionnaire should be a visual analog scale (VAS) or a Likert scale (categorical) with multiple options.[22,24,25] Both approaches have their proponents, but there is no evidence to support one over the other. However, the patient may have difficulty abstracting with a VAS and the requirement to physically measure each response on the scale may complicate data management. Thus, a Likert scale is potentially the simplest format for large scale trials. Similarly, the optimal number of response options for a Likert scale is unclear, but seven response options seems reasonable.[25]

The optimum frequency of administration of a questionnaire in a clinical trial is unknown. The more often a questionnaire is completed, the more likely that a true picture of a patient's health status over a study period will be obtained. However, this must be balanced against the increased financial cost for the trial and potential inconvenience to the patient. Less frequent questionnaire administration is required for "stable" conditions; while if the patient's disease status is not stable, then more frequent questionnaire administration is optimal. No matter what the frequency of questionnaire administration is, the execution of the clinical trial should be conducted with rigorous quality control of the data to ensure maximum compliance.

Quality-of-life assessment is now being used in clinical trials of adjuvant therapy.[26] Questionnaires are often administered during the period of adjuvant chemotherapy or radiation, when the maximum impact of this treatment on quality of life is anticipated. In order for any quality of life instrument to be useful in clinical decision making in the evaluation of adjuvant therapy, assessments must be made not only during adjuvant therapy, but also later in the course of the disease, i.e., through disease recurrence if not to death.[27,28]

The timing of administration of a questionnaire in relation to an intervention may also be important. For example, it is possible that a patient would score a questionnaire differently if it were administered pre- or post-chemotherapy. Often, however, practical aspects such as space in a busy cancer clinic or time of day of chemotherapy treatment dictate when a questionnaire is administered. The time frame that a questionnaire refers to must be specified. The optimal period is unclear. If a questionnaire asks a patient to consider how they feel "at the present moment", then the adverse effect of an intervention 2 weeks previously will be missed. On the other hand, if the patient is asked to consider the previous 3 month period, then many changes in the patient's condition may have occurred and the patient may have difficulty responding. A time frame of 2 to 4 weeks seems to be a practical compromise.

If quality of life is to be used as a major outcome measure for a clinical trial, then it is imperative that there be strict compliance with completion of specified scheduled assessments. Failure to pay attention to this important issue, could potentially invalidate the study results. In a recently reported trial in which continuous chemotherapy was compared with intermittent chemotherapy in patients with Stage IV breast cancer, only 44% of the randomized patients completed quality-of-life assessments at both baseline and after three cycles of chemotherapy.[27] Similarly, Ganz et al. reported that only 58% of patients in a trial of chemotherapy for lung cancer were able to complete specified assessments.[29] Satisfactory compliance can only be ensured by the enthusiasm of trial investigators for quality of life measurement, by the strict adherence of study nurses and physicians to the protocol, and by thorough and complete data monitoring by the trial coordinators.

Another problem in using quality of life as an outcome in clinical trials is how to derive a simple summary score for an instrument which has many questions. Individual questions usually have response options on a numerical scale, for example, from 1 (no difficulty) to 7 (extreme difficulty). In some instruments the sum of the individual question responses is used as the summary score, while sometimes the mean of each of the question responses is used. Furthermore, it is unclear whether a simple mean of individual questions, or whether a weighted mean, based on the relative importance of each question to the patient, should be used. A potential drawback of employing a mean value as a summary score is that it may show very little change over time because individual question change scores (of opposite direction) may cancel each other out. For certain questions, however, there may be large change scores which would be missed if the mean change score is used. As more experience is gained with the use of quality-of-life questionnaires, more information should emerge on optimal methods of deriving aggregate scores.

A related issue is what change in score is meaningful and clinically important to patients. If a change of 1.0 units is observed, is this clinically significant? Guyatt and colleagues have recently described a method to determine the minimal clinically important difference for a quality-of-life questionnaire for patients with chronic lung disease and suggested that this value may be as low as 0.5 units on a seven-point Likert scale.[30] The minimal clinically important difference, as well as the between-subject variability in within person change in score may have important implications for sample size determination for clinical trials.[16] By using these parameters to calculate sample size, many fewer patients are required to detect differences in quality of life than for the more traditional cancer outcomes of response rate or survival.

Despite the best efforts of trial participants, there is always the problem of how to handle missing data in the analysis. It is possible, and even likely, that patients who are extremely ill will be unable to attend clinic for an assessment, and thus the quality of life information for that visit will be unavailable. This would tend to dampen the ability of any questionnaire to measure clinical change. Thus, the problem with ignoring missing data in the analysis is that the power to detect clinically important differences between treatments could be lessened. Sophisticated statistical modeling techniques have been suggested as potential ways of handling missing data in the analysis of quality of life outcomes for such trials.[30,31]

VII. QUALITY OF LIFE: THE FUTURE

Although quality of life questionnaires are now being widely used in cancer clinical trials, they continue to exist as research instruments. Little information is available, however, on how such quality of life information from clinical trials can be incorporated into routine patient and physician clinical decision making. There are examples in the cancer literature where quality-of-life assessments performed in a clinical trial have influenced clinical practice. Sugarbaker et al. measured quality of life in their patients with sarcoma who underwent limb-sparing surgery and these assessments led to refinements in the adjunctive radiation therapy administred to these patients.[33,34] Coates et al. demonstrated that by continuing maintenance chemotherapy in patients with metastatic breast cancer who have had an initial response to chemotherapy, quality of life is improved compared to a policy of stopping chemotherapy and only resuming it at disease progression.[27] The field of decision analysis in medicine has developed in order to help physicians develop conceptual frameworks for incorporating quality of life, as reflected by utilities into decision making.[35] Finally, the challenge in coming years involves developing methods for incorporating quality of life information from clinical trials into routine clinical practice.

REFERENCES

1. **Bernheinm, J. L.**, Measurement of quality of life: an imperative for experimental cancer medicine in *The Quality of Life of Cancer Patients*, Monogr. Ser. European Organization for Research and Treatment of Cancer, Aaronson, N. K. and Beckman, V., Eds., Raven Press, New York, 1987, 11.
2. **Van Dam, F. S. A. M., Linssen, C. A., and Couzijn, A. L.**, Evaluating quality of life in cancer clinical trials, in *Cancer Clinical Trials, Methods and Practice*, Buyse, M. E., Staquet, M. J., Sylvester, R. J., Eds., Oxford University Press, Oxford, 1984, 26.
3. **Schipper, H. and Levitt, M.**, Measuring quality of life: risks and benefits, *Cancer Treat. Rep.*, 69, 1115, 1985.
4. **Tannock, I. F.**, Treating the patient, not just the cancer, *N. Engl. J. Med.*, 317, 1534, 1987.
5. **Moinpour, C. M., Feigl, P., Metch, B., Hayden, A., Meyskens, F. L., and Crowley, J.**, Quality of life end points in cancer clinical trials: review and recommendations, *J. Natl. Cancer Inst.*, 81, 485, 1989.
6. **Skeel, R. T.**, Quality of life assessment in cancer clinical trials — it's time to catch up, *J. Natl. Cancer Inst.*, 81, 472, 1989.
7. **Calman, K. C.**, Definitions and dimensions of quality of life, in *The Quality of Life of Cancer Patients*, Monogr. Ser. European Organization for Research and Treatment of Cancer, Aaronson, N. K. and Beckman, J., Eds., Raven Press, New York, 1987, 1.
8. **Guyatt, G. H., Van Zanten, S., Feeney, D. H., and Patrick, D. L.**, Measuring quality of life in clinical trials: a taxonomy and review, *CMAJ*, 140, 1441, 1989.
9. **Kirshner, B. and Guyatt, G.**, A methodologic framework for assessing health indices, *J. Chronic Dis.*, 38, 27, 1985.
10. **Patrick, D. L. and Deyo, R. A.**, Generic and disease-specific measures in assessing health status and quality of life, *Med. Care*, 27 (Suppl.), 217, 1989.
11. **Guyatt, G. H., Bombardier, C., and Tugwell, P. X.**, Measuring disease-specific quality of life in clinical trials, *CMAJ*, 134, 889, 1986.
12. **Bergner, M., Bobbitt, R. A., Carter, W. B., et al.**, The sickness impact profile: development and final revision of a health status measure, *Med. Care*, 19, 787, 1981.
13. **Ware, J. E., Brook, R. H., and Davies-Avery, A.**, Conceptualization of measurement of health for adults in the health insurance study, in *Model of Health and Methodology*, Vol. 1, Rand Corporation, Santa Monica, CA, 1980.
14. **Spitzer, W. O., Dobson, A. J., Hall, et al.**, Measuring the quality of life of cancer patients, *J. Chronic Dis.*, 34, 585, 1981.
15. **Schipper, H., Clinch, J., McMurray, A., et al.**, Measuring the quality-of-life of cancer patients. The functional living index—cancer: development and validation, *J. Clin. Oncol.*, 2, 472, 1984.
16. **Guyatt, G., Walter, S., and Norman, G.**, Measuring change over time: assessing the usefulness of evalutive instruments, *J. Chronic Dis.*, 40, 171, 1987.

17. Aaronson, N. K., Bullinger, M., and Ahmedzai, S., A modular approach to quality of life assessment in cancer clinical trials, *Rec. Results Cancer Res.*, 111, 231, 1988.
18. Van Knippenberg, F. C. and DeHaes, J. C., Measuring the quality of life of cancer patients: psychometric properties of instruments, *J. Clin. Epidemiol.*, 41, 1043, 1988.
19. Donovan, K., Sanson-Fisher, R. W., and Redman, S., Measuring the quality of life in cancer patients, *J. Clin. Oncol.*, 7, 959, 1989.
20. Deyo, R. A. and Centor, R. M., Assessing the responsiveness of functional scales to clinical change: an analogy to diagnostic test performance, *J. Chronic Dis.*, 39, 879, 1986.
21. Norman, G. R., Issues in the use of change scores in randomized trials, *J. Clin. Epidemiol.*, 42, 1097, 1989.
22. Downie, W. W., Leatham, R. A., Rhind, V. M., et al., Studies with pain rating scales, *Ann. Rheum. Dis.*, 37, 378, 1978.
23. Chambers, L. W., Haight, M., Norman, G., et al., Sensitivity to change and the effect of mode of administration of health status measurement, *Med. Care*, 25, 470, 1987.
24. Deyo, R. A. and Patrick, D. L., Barriers to the use of health status measures in clinical investigation, patient care and policy research, *Med. Care*, 27 (Suppl.), 254, 1989.
25. Jaeschke, R., Singer, J., and Guyatt, G. H., A comparison of seven-point and visual analogue scales, *Controlled Clin. Trials*, 11, 43, 1990.
26. Levine, M. N., Guyatt, G. H., and Gent, M., Quality of life in stage II breast cancer: an instrument for clinical trials, *J. Clin. Oncol.*, 6, 1798, 1988.
27. Coates, A., Gebski, V., Stat, M., et al., Improving the quality of life during chemotherapy for advanced breast cancer. A comparison of intermittent and continuous treatment strategies, *N. Engl. J. Med.*, 317, 1490, 1987.
28. Gelber, R. D. and Goldhirsch, A., A new endpoint for the assessment of adjuvant therapy in postmenopausal women with operable breast cancer, *J. Clin. Oncol.*, 4, 1772, 1986.
29. Ganz, P. A., Haskell, C. M., Figlin, R. A., LaSoto, N., and Siau, J., Estimating the quality of life in a clinical trial of patients with metastatic lung cancer using the Karnofsky performance status and the functional living index-cancer, *Cancer*, 61, 849, 1988.
30. Jaeschke, R., Singer, J., and Guyatt, G. H., Measurement of health status. Ascertaining the minimal clinically important difference, *Controlled Clin. Trials*, 10, 407, 1989.
31. Potthoff, R. F. and Roy, S. B., A generalized multivariate analysis of variance model useful especially for growth curve problems, *Biometrika*, 51, 313, 1964.
32. Geisser, S., Growth curve analysis, in *Handbook of Statistics*, Vol. 1, Krishaiah, P. R., Ed., North-Holland, Amsterdam, 1980, 89.
33. Sugarbaker, P. H., Barofsky, I., Rosenberg, S. A., et al., Quality of life assessment of patients in extremity sarcoma clinical trials, *Surgery*, 91, 17, 1982.
34. Weddington, W. W., Segraves, K. B., and Simon, M. A., Psychological outcome of extremity sarcoma survivors undergoing amputation or limb salvage, *J. Clin. Oncol.*, 3, 1393, 1985.
35. Torrance, G. W., Measurement of health state utilities for economic appraisal, *J. Health Econ.*, 5, 1, 1986.

Chapter 9

STATISTICAL ANALYSIS OF TRIALS ASSESSING QUALITY OF LIFE

B. Zee and J. Pater

TABLE OF CONTENTS

I. INTRODUCTION

The importance of establishing the reliability, validity, and responsiveness to change of quality-of-life instruments before they are recommended for use in clinical trial protocols has regularly been emphasized. However, there has been little discussion in the clinical trials literature of the statistical methods to be used in the analysis of trials incorporating quality-of-life end-points.

Most commonly, these instruments are used to assess quality of life over time, i.e., in a longitudinal manner, which is the context we will discuss here. In general, there are two types of longitudinal studies. The first outcome of interest is the time until occurrence of an event. Such studies can be analyzed with the familiar lifetable methods. A prominent example in this context is the TWiST methodology of Gelber et al.,[1-3] where the length of a defined lifetime without symptoms of disease and toxicity of treatment is used as an outcome to describe patient's quality of life. The second type of longitudinal study employs the numerical results from quality-of-life questionnaires as outcome measures, which is more commonly used in other disciplines. The role of the analysis for this type of study is to summarize in some fashion the quality of life experience of groups of individuals over time. The following sections will discuss approaches to the analysis of these two types of studies. The discussions will emphasize on famigliarizing the reader with statistical techniques appropriate for the second type of longitudinal study, where results are obtained from quality-of-life questionnaires.

II. TIME TO EVENT END-POINTS

A. TIME WITHOUT SYMPTOMS AND TOXICITY (TWiST)

A quality-of-life end-point was developed by Gelber and Goldhirsch[1] in the assessment of adjuvant therapy in postmenopausal women with operable breast cancer. This end-point is defined as the time without symptom of disease and toxicity of treatment (TWiST), and was obtained by subtracting the amount of time of poor quality of life from each unit of time interval to adjust the measure of benefit. An example of how the time units were coded can be found in Gelber and Goldhirsch.[1] In a more recent paper, Goldhirsch et al.[2] extended their methodology to allow for the quality-weighted subtraction of time with symptoms or toxicity. Gelber et al.[3] have suggested using the Kaplan-Meier[4] method to estimate the survivor function of TWiST for the observed data.

It was pointed out by Gelber et al.[3] that the subtraction of the duration of toxicity from the time patients start receiving treatment to the time of first relapse induces a dependence between TWiST and the censoring mechanism. As a result, the Kaplan-Meier estimation is biased and overestimated the true TWiST. They also noted that the duration of TWiST should not be estimated unless all study patients have been followed past the time when subjective toxic effects might be observed.

TWiST appears to be useful for the comparison of survival with adjustment for patients' quality of life and has the advantage of using relatively familiar statistical methodology. However, it does not incorporate, except in an indirect way, the potentially important information obtainable by administering quality-of-life questionnaires to trial subjects. Furthermore, the application of Kaplan-Meier methods to data of this type does not appear to have been fully justified.

III. SUMMARIZATION OF DATA FROM QUALITY-OF-LIFE QUESTIONNAIRES

The usual approach to incorporating quality-of-life end-points into clinical trials is to administer quality-of-life questionnaires at multiple points in time before, during, and after the intervention being studied with the goal of portraying in a longitudinal fashion the patients' status over time. As has recently been pointed out by Matthews et al.,[5] the analysis of such serial data is often inadequate in that account is not taken of the fact that the multiple measurements at different time points are from the same patients. Successive observations on a given patient are likely to be correlated and separate significance tests at different time points cannot, thus, be interpreted as if they gave independent information. Further, if multiple tests are made, the problem of multiple comparisons must be accounted for.

A simple way to look at such serial data is by what Matthews et al.[5] called summary measures. The method considers individual patients as units and uses the responses for each individual to construct a single statistic which summarizes some aspect of that patient along time. One choice of response is the peaked response. For example, in a current melanoma trial where patients are randomized to receive either levamisole or interferon-gamma, a quality-of-life questionnaire will be administered every 16 weeks for the first year and every 32 weeks thereafter until the end of the third year. Following Matthews et al.,[5] a legitimate approach to the analysis would be to use the maximum change in overall quality-of-life scores as a summary response.

In most cases, however, the data will contain more information than could be summarized by one summary statistic. In such circumstances, a better approach is to employ a method of analysis which uses all observations on individual subjects in the comparison of the two groups, i.e., a repeated measures analysis. There are a number of ways to analyze data with repeated measurements. Our discussion will focus on three commonly used methods. The first of these is the univariate mixed model, which has been widely used and studied in psychologic and education research. The second is the multivariate analysis of variance method, where repeated measurements are being treated as a vector of responses. The relationship between the repeated measures within a patient can be described by the covariance matrix. This is considered to be the most direct approach to the repeated measures problem. The third approach is the polynomial growth curve method, which is an extension of the multivariate analysis of variance model. The parameters of a polynomial mean function are estimated instead of the actual mean values for each time point.

IV. METHODS OF ANALYSIS

A. UNIVARIATE ANALYSIS OF VARIANCE (ANOVA)

Univariate repeated measures analysis and the split-plot design[6] are very similar. The two have almost identical analysis of variance models. In a split-plot design, a factor A is randomly assigned to each subject (i.e., the whole plots), and these subjects are further divided into smaller portions (i.e., the subplots) where a factor B is randomly assigned to these sub-plots. In an univariate repeated measures model, treatments are randomly assigned to patients. Outcomes for each patient, e.g., quality of life, are then measured repeatedly over time. Therefore, time becomes the second factor analogous to factor B in the split-plot design. However, the two models differ in that the factor, time, cannot be randomized in a repeated measures design. If certain assumptions are fulfilled, the method of analysis for a split-plot design can be applied. Otherwise, a correction factor will have to be used to adjust for the degrees of freedom of the test statistic. The repeated measures analysis of variance model can be written in the following form:

$$y_{ijk} = u + a_i + b_{ij} + t_k + (at)_{ik} + \epsilon_{ijk}; \quad i = 1, \ldots, I$$

$$j = 1, \ldots, n_i$$

$$k = 1, \ldots, K$$

where a_i is the ith treatment effect; b_{ij} is the random effect of the jth patient in the ith treatment group; t_k is the effect of the kth time interval; and $(at)_{ik}$ is the ik^{th} interaction effect. The ϵ_{ijk} is the random error term assumed to be normally distributed with mean 0 and variance σ^2. The b_{ij} term is also assumed to be normally distributed with mean 0 and variance σ_b^2.

The sum of squares can be partitioned and their F-ratios can be determined as shown in the following ANOVA table:

Source	d.f.	Sum of squares	F
Treatment	$I - 1$	$Q_1 = K \sum_{i=1}^{I} n_i (\bar{y}_{i..} - \bar{y}...)^2$	F_1
Time	$K - 1$	$Q_2 = N \sum_{k=1}^{K} (\bar{y}_{..k} - \bar{y}...)^2$	F_2
Interaction	$(I - 1)(K - 1)$	$Q_3 = \sum_{i=1}^{I} \sum_{k=1}^{K} n_i (\bar{y}_{i.k} - \bar{y}_{i..} - \bar{y}_{..k} + \bar{y}...)^2$	F_3
Error (patient)	$(N - I)$	$Q_4 = K \sum_{i=1}^{I} \sum_{j=1}^{n_i} (\bar{y}_{ij.} - \bar{y}_{i..})^2$	
Error (time)	$(N - I)(K - 1)$	$Q_5 = \sum_{i=1}^{I} \sum_{j=1}^{n_i} \sum_{k=1}^{K} (\bar{y}_{ijk} - \bar{y}_{ij.} - \bar{y}_{i.k} - \bar{y}_{i..})^2$	
Total	$NK - 1$	$Q_6 = \sum_{i=1}^{I} \sum_{j=1}^{n_i} \sum_{k=1}^{K} (\bar{y}_{ijk} - \bar{y}...)^2$	

The average over the population from which the subjects are drawn may be denoted by $E(y_{ijk}) = u + a_i + t_k + (at)_{ik}$. The variance-covariance matrices associated with each level of treatment i, Σ_i are assumed to be common to all I population denoted by Σ. Huynh and Feldt[7] found a general condition under which the mean square ratios in repeated measurement design have an exact F-distribution, that is, the elements of the covariance matrix can be expressed in the form of

$$\sigma_{ij} = \gamma_i + \gamma_j + \lambda\delta_{ij}; \quad \text{where } \delta_{ij} = \begin{cases} 1 & \text{if } i = j \\ 1 & \text{if } i \neq j \end{cases}$$

In a typical two-arm study $I = 2$, and $N = n_1 + n_2$. Compound symmetry, as described by Geisser[8] is a special case of the above Huynh-Feldt condition when the covariance matrix Σ can be expressed as follows:

$$\Sigma = \sigma^2 \begin{pmatrix} 1 & \rho & \cdots & \rho \\ \rho & 1 & \cdots & \rho \\ \vdots & \vdots & \ddots & \vdots \\ \rho & \rho & \cdots & 1 \end{pmatrix}$$

where ρ is the correlation between two time intervals. The compound symmetry condition implies that the random variables are equally correlated and have equal variance. The F-tests following a usual split-plot analysis of variance is valid in this situation. However, the condition of compound symmetry may not be satisfied in real study. Box[9] derived a correction factor e for adjusting the numbers of degrees of freedom for the mean square ratios. When the data do not satisfy the compound symmetry assumption, the mean square ratios for time effect becomes $F[(K - 1)e, (N - I)(K - 1)e]$, and Geisser and Greenhouse[10] had shown that the mean square ratios for the treatment by time interaction effect is $F[(I - 1)(K - 1)e, (N - I)(K - 1)e]$. It can be seen that when e approaches unity, the F-ratios approach that of the split-plot design.

$$e = \frac{K^2(\bar{\sigma}_{ii} - \bar{\sigma}..)^2}{(K - 1)(\sum\limits_{i=1}^{K} \sum\limits_{j=1}^{K} \sigma_{ij}^2 - 2K \sum\limits_{i=1}^{K} \bar{\sigma}_i^2. + K^2\bar{\sigma}^2..)}$$

Geisser and Greenhouse[10] also showed that the lower bound for the correction factor e is $1/(K-1)$. The most conservative adjustment in the degrees of freedom of the mean square ratios is by substituting the lower bound to the corresponding F-distribution. The F-distribution using the conservative adjustment for time effect and treatment by time interaction effect becomes $F[1, I(J-1)]$ and $F[(I-1), I(J-1)]$, respectively.

Investigators who wish to keep the analysis as simple as possible may not be willing to apply a data-dependent correction factor. In this case, the conservative correction may be used without estimate e. For those who are willing to apply this correction factor, Greenhouse and Geisser[11] suggested a three-step procedure:

1. The mean square ratio of interest is first tested with the conventional degree of freedom. If the F ratio is not significant, the analysis stops for the null hypothesis would not be rejected by reducing the degrees of freedom.
2. If the F ratio is significant, the conservative test is performed with the degrees of freedom reduced by the value of the lower limit of e. If the F ratio is larger than this conservative critical value, it may be declared significant.
3. If the conservative test is not significant, then the correction factor e will be estimated from the sample covariance matrix and the F ratio be tested with degree of freedom reduced by the estimate.

Collier et al.[12] examined the effect of using the e correction factor estimated from the data. They found that the e-adjustment provides a test with a type I error close to that of the nominal level. The size of the conservative test, on the other hand, was shown to be low in comparison with the nominal level.

The statistical analysis of the univariate analysis of variance can be performed by using SAS[13] procedure GLM. SAS calculates all test statistics with respect to the residual mean square. For a proper assessment of the time and treatment by time interaction effects, we must also calculate the variance component of the patient effect. This can be done by specifying the RANDOM statement in the SAS GLM procedure.

B. MULTIVARIATE ANALYSIS OF VARIANCE (MANOVA)

Continuous quality-of-life outcomes measured repeatedly over time can be analyzed using the univariate analysis of variance approach with compound symmetry assymption for the covariance structure. However, observations on successive measurements from the same patient are often highly correlated. The assumption that the covariance matrix is in the form of compound symmetry may not be valid in practice. On the other hand, repeated measures from the same patient can be arranged in the form of a vector of responses, where each element in the response vector is correlated to the other elements. The analysis of this kind of multiresponse data is termed multivariate analysis. Cole and Grizzle[14] suggested that multivariate analysis of variance is more suitable when a univariate method is inappropriate. Both univariate and multivariate approaches rest on the assumption that the population random error components follow a normal distribution. Unlike the univariate analysis of variance model which stipulates a particular form of the population covariance matrix, the multivariate method makes no assumption to the form of the covariance matrix. A discussion of multivariate analysis can be found in classical texts such as Timm,[15] Morrison,[16] and Anderson.[17] Discussion of the within subjects hypotheses relevant in repeated measures data can be found in Timm,[18] Rogan et al.,[19] and Fleiss.[20] We will introduce several hypotheses that are of interest and show how they can be formulated in the multivariate analysis of variance model.

H_{01}: Are there differences in the quality of life outcomes between treatment groups?
H_{02}: Are there any differences in quality of life outcomes over time?
H_{03}: Are differences in quality of life outcomes between the two treatments consistent at every time interval?

The quality of life outcomes can be arranged in the form of a matrix. Let y_{ijk} be the quality of life outcome for the jth patient in the ith treatment group measured at the kth time point, where y_{ij} is a K-dimension vector of quality of life outcomes for each patient. Suppose $y_{i1}, y_{i2}, ..., y_{in}$ are independently and identically distributed as a normal distribution $N(\mu,\Sigma)$. A general multivariate linear model, for the case of a two arm study, can be written in the following form:

$$y_{ijk} = \mu_{ik} + \epsilon_{ijk} \quad i = 1, 2.$$

$$j = 1, 2, ..., n_i.$$

$$k = 1, 2, ..., K.$$

This model can be written in matrix notation for convenience, i.e.,

$$E(Y) = XB$$

where Y is an N by K matrix ($N = n_1 + n_2$) of quality-of-life outcomes, each row of Y has a multivariate normal distribution with mean vector μ and covariance matrix Σ; X is an N by 2 matrix of indicator variables representing the treatment groups; B is a 2 by K matrix of unknown parameters of population means.

$$Y = \begin{pmatrix} y_{111} & y_{112} & \cdots & y_{11K} \\ \vdots & \vdots & \cdots & \vdots \\ y_{1n_11} & y_{1n_12} & \cdots & y_{1n_1K} \\ y_{211} & y_{212} & \cdots & y_{21K} \\ \vdots & \vdots & \cdots & \vdots \\ y_{2n_21} & y_{2n_22} & \cdots & y_{2n_2K} \end{pmatrix}$$

$$X = \begin{pmatrix} 1 & 0 \\ \vdots & \vdots \\ 1 & 0 \\ 0 & 1 \\ \vdots & \vdots \\ 0 & 1 \end{pmatrix} \qquad B = \begin{pmatrix} \mu_{11} & \mu_{12} & \cdots & \mu_{1K} \\ \mu_{21} & \mu_{22} & \cdots & \mu_{2K} \end{pmatrix}$$

The hypothesis H_{01} to H_{03} among the cell means may be written in a general form:

$$H_0: LBM = 0$$

Hypothesis H_{01} to H_{03} can be tested by modifying the matrix L and M in H_0. The test statistics for the above hypotheses are functions of the characteristic roots of $S_H S_E^{-1}$ where

$$S_H = M'B'L'[L(X'X)^{-1}L']^{-1} LBM$$

$$S_E = M'Y'[I - X(X'X)^{-1}] YM$$

Discussion of the test statistics in this type of analysis can be found in most multivariate analysis texts.[15-17]

The following example will be used to illustrate this method. If continuous quality-of-life scores were measured every month for 4 months, the difference between the two treatment groups can be tested by using:

$$L = (1 \quad - \quad 1) \qquad M = \begin{pmatrix} 1/4 \\ 1/4 \\ 1/4 \\ 1/4 \end{pmatrix}$$

i.e.,

$$H_{01}: (\mu_{11} + \mu_{12} + \mu_{13} + \mu_{14})/4 = (\mu_{21} + \mu_{22} + \mu_{23} + \mu_{24})/4$$

The difference over time can be tested by averaging the effect of treatment and testing an orthogonal contrast of time points. This can be done by changing the L and M matrices into the following form:

$$L = \begin{pmatrix} 1 & 1 \\ 2 & 2 \end{pmatrix} \qquad M = \begin{pmatrix} 1 & 1 & 1 \\ -1 & 0 & 0 \\ 0 & -1 & 0 \\ 0 & 0 & -1 \end{pmatrix}$$

i.e.,

$$H_{02}: (\mu_{11} + \mu_{21})/2 = (\mu_{12} + \mu_{22})/2,$$

$$(\mu_{11} + \mu_{21})/2 = (\mu_{13} + \mu_{23})/2,$$

$$(\mu_{11} + \mu_{21})/2 = (\mu_{14} + \mu_{24})/2.$$

The hypothesis that the differences between two treatments are consistent at every time point is equivalent to testing the interaction effect by specifying the L and M matrices in the following form:

$$L = (1 \quad - \quad 1) \qquad M = \begin{pmatrix} 1 & 1 & 1 \\ -1 & 0 & 0 \\ 0 & -1 & 0 \\ 0 & 0 & -1 \end{pmatrix}$$

i.e.,

$$H_{03}: \mu_{11} + \mu_{21} = \mu_{12} + \mu_{22};$$

$$\mu_{11} + \mu_{21} = \mu_{13} + \mu_{23},$$

$$\mu_{11} + \mu_{21} = \mu_{14} + \mu_{24}.$$

If there is no interaction effect, hypothesis H_{01} is a legitimate question to ask. However, if there is a significant interaction, the differences between the two treatment groups will not be consistent. In this situation, it may be of interest to identify the time intervals where departures between treatments occur. For example, we may want to test whether the difference between treatments at the third time interval is the same as the differences between treatments in the first and second time intervals. This can be done with the following L and M matrices:

$$L = (1 \quad -1) \qquad M = \begin{pmatrix} 1/2 \\ 1/2 \\ -1 \\ 0 \end{pmatrix}$$

i.e.,

$$H_0: ((\mu_{11} + \mu_{12}) - (\mu_{21} + \mu_{22}))/2 = \mu_{13} - \mu_{23}$$

If quality-of-life outcomes over time is significant, it may be of interest to determine whether they follow a linear trend, a quadratic trend, or a cubic trend by modifying the L and M matrices.

$$L = \begin{pmatrix} \frac{1}{2} & \frac{1}{2} \end{pmatrix} \qquad M = \begin{pmatrix} -3 \\ -1 \\ 1 \\ 3 \end{pmatrix} \qquad M = \begin{pmatrix} 1 \\ -1 \\ -1 \\ 1 \end{pmatrix} \qquad M = \begin{pmatrix} -1 \\ 3 \\ -3 \\ 1 \end{pmatrix}$$

$$\text{linear} \qquad \text{quadratic} \qquad \text{cubic}$$

A choice between the multivariate test and the univariate test depends upon whether the assumption of compound symmetry is valid. Davidson[21] had shown that the univariate test is more powerful when the covariance is in the form of compound symmetry. When this assumption is violated, the e-adjusted and conservative univariate approaches or the multivariate analysis of variance approach can be used. The statistical analysis of the multivariate analysis of variance can be performed by using SAS procedure GLM. A MANOVA statement or REPEATED statement can be used to test the hypotheses of interest.

C. GROWTH CURVE MODEL

A growth curve model is usually applied to the situation in which we have a moderate number of serial measurements on each patient, where interest in the study is to investigate changes of quality-of-life scores over time. This method allows us to fit an overall polynomial curve for patients being allocated to the same treatment. In practice, first or second degree polynomial function usually fits the data fairly well. A second degree polynomial function for a growth curve model will require us to estimate only three parameters for the mean polynomial functions in each treatment group. This formulation of repeated measures may reduce the number of estimated parameters. For example, we will obtain a total of eight quality-of-life outcomes of each patient in the melanoma study. Using the multivariate analysis of variance method, we will have to estimate eight parameters for each treatment mean vector. However, if the quality of life along time in both treatment groups is either flat in shape or increasing in a linear fashion, a linear polynomial function with two parameters in the growth curve model is sufficient to summarize the mean vector. Comparison between treatments can be made by testing the parameters of the growth curves.

There is an extensive body of literature available on this subject. We will focus on the approach along the lines of the development by Potthoff and Roy.[22] The growth curve model developed by Potthoff and Roy[22] is a generalization of the multivariate analysis of variance model. It can be written in the following form:

$$E(Y) = XBP$$

where Y is an N by K matrix of quality of life outcomes, X is an N by 2 matrix of indicator variables representing treatment groups; B is a 2 by q matrix of unknown parameters representing a $(q-1)$ degree of polynomial function; and P is a q by K matrix of known constants of time intervals where the quality-of-life questionnaires were administered.

$$Y = \begin{pmatrix} y_{111} & y_{112} & \cdots & y_{11K} \\ \vdots & \vdots & \cdots & \vdots \\ y_{1n_11} & y_{1n_12} & \cdots & y_{1n_1K} \\ y_{211} & y_{212} & \cdots & y_{21K} \\ \vdots & \vdots & \cdots & \vdots \\ y_{2n_21} & y_{2n_22} & \cdots & y_{2n_2K} \end{pmatrix}$$

$$X = \begin{pmatrix} 1 & 0 \\ \vdots & \vdots \\ 1 & 0 \\ 0 & 1 \\ \vdots & \vdots \\ 0 & 1 \end{pmatrix} \qquad B = \begin{pmatrix} \mu_{11} & \cdots & \mu_{1q} \\ \mu_{21} & \cdots & \mu_{2q} \end{pmatrix}$$

$$P = \begin{pmatrix} 1 & \cdots & 1 \\ t_1 & \cdots & t_K \\ & \cdots & \\ t_1^{q-1} & & t_K^{q-1} \end{pmatrix}$$

It is obvious that the degree in the polynomial function cannot exceed the number of repeated measures, i.e., $q < K$, otherwise the parameters are not estimable. In order to obtain an unbiased estimate of B and to test the hypothesis that $LBM = 0$ as in the multivariate analysis of variance, Potthoff and Roy[22] recommended a transformation of the response matrix Y using:

$$Z = Y\,G^{-1}P'(PG^{-1}P')^{-1}$$

where G is any K by K symmetric positive definite matrix such that $PG^{-1}P'$ exists. After transformation, the model becomes:

$$E(Z) = (XB)$$

Hence, the hypothesis may be tested using the previous multivariate analysis of variance test criteria after determining the characteristic roots of $S_H S_E^{-1}$ where:

$$S_H = M'BL'[L(X'X)^{-1}L']^{-1}\,LBM$$

$$S_E = M'Z'(I - X(X'X)^{-1}X')\,ZM$$

and B can be estimated by:

$$B = (X'X)^{-1}X'YG^{-1}P(PG^{-1}P')^{-1}$$

Potthoff and Roy[22] argued that the choice of G is arbitrary and a simple way of choosing G is to set G to be the identity matrix, $G = I$. He also showed that the estimate B is always unbiased. However, Rao[23] gave an alternative reduction of the model leading to a conditional model which gives the same estimate for B. He showed that the best linear unbiased estimator of B is obtained only when G is equal to the population covariance matrix Σ. He further suggested that instead of using an arbitrary G matrix, an estimate S of the population covariance matrix calculated from the data should be used.

$$S = Y'[I - X(X'X)^{-1}X'] \, Y$$

Khatri[24] also obtained a maximum likelihood estimate of B which is identical in form to that of Rao[23] and Potthoff and Roy.[22]

$$B = (X'X)^{-1}X'YS^{-1}P(PS^{-1}P')^{-1}$$

The statistical analysis of growth curve modelling can be performed using BMDP 5V.[25] Other statistical packages designed to do matrix operations can also be used to do the transformation (e.g., SAS/IML).

D. MISSING OBSERVATIONS

The problem of missing data is likely to arise in practice for a clinical trial which requires long-term follow-up on patients.

In the univariate analysis, the mixed analysis of variance model discussed in the previous section involves the variances of the random error σ^2 as well as the variance of the random patient effect σ_b^2. With missing observations in the data, these variances will affect the estimated of the fixed effects in the model. The estimation problem for the variance component terms itself is not trivial. One may use the maximum likelihood method as described in Harville[26] or the restricted maximum likelihood method in Patterson and Thompson[27] to tackle this problem. However, both these methods require interative computation and can be treated as special cases of the multivariate approach.

The missing data problem in growth curve model can be approached by using the approach of Kleinbaum.[28] He partitioned the data into a number of disjoint subsets where each set of patients has observations at exactly the same set of time points. He then transforms the multivariate data to a univariate form and estimates the parameters by univariate linear models theory. The drawback to this approach is that when the missing data occur at different time points, the number of subsets may be large, and some subsets may have small numbers of patients. Also, the behavior of the test statistics in moderate size samples is not known. Another approach to missing data in both multivariate analysis of variance and the growth curve model is by using the EM (Expectation-Maximization) algorithm to obtain maximum likelihood estimates. The E step consists of calculating the means and covariance including missing observations by estimated values from the observed data. The parameters of interest will then be estimated. Assuming the new parameters are correct, we re-estimate the missing values to generate another set of parameters. This iterative process will continue until convergence. In-depth discussion of the theory of the EM Algorithm and its applications can be found in Dempster et al.,[29] Beale and Little,[30] and Orchard and Woodbury.[31] Jennrich and Schluchter[32] described methods of analysis for both structured and unstructured covariance Σ in multivariate analysis of variance and growth curve model. If a structured covariance, such as intraclass correlation or autoregressive correlation between measures, is acceptable, explicit likelihood functions can be written for the growth curve model and the parameters can be solved by Newton-Raphson algorithm as described in Seth and Mazumdar.[33]

V. DISCUSSION

As we hope is evident from the preceding sections, the approach to the analysis of studies incorporating quality-of-life end-points needs to be given almost as careful consideration as the development and testing of the instruments used. While methods other than those we have discussed can clearly be used, we agree with Matthews et al.[5] that approaches which do not take into account the special characteristics of serial data should be avoided, as they may lead to erroneous conclusions. We have emphasized repeated measures methods because they are appropriate to the circumstances and seem to have been somewhat neglected by investigators in this area. We hope our presentation will stimulate attempts to apply these techniques to quality-of-life studies.

REFERENCES

1. **Gelber, R. and Goldhirsh, A.,** A new endpoint for the assessment of adjuvant therapy in postmenopausal women with operable breast cancer, *J. Clin. Oncol.*, 4, 1772, 1986.
2. **Goldhirsh, A., Gelber, R., Simes, R., Glasziou, P., and Coates, A.,** Costs and benefits of adjuvant therapy in breast cancer: a quality-adjusted survival analysis, *J. Clin. Oncol.*, 7, 36, 1989.
3. **Gelber, R., Gelman, R., and Goldhirsh, A.,** A quality-of-life oriented endpoint for comparing therapies, *Biometrics*, 45, 781, 1989.
4. **Kaplan, E. L. and Meier, P.,** Nonparametric estimation from incomplete observations, *J. Am. Stat. Assoc.*, 53, 457, 1958.
5. **Matthews, J. N. S., Altman, D., Campbell, M. J., and Royston, P.,** Analysis of serial measurements in medical research, *Br. Med. J.*, 300, 230, 1990.
6. **Cochran, W. G. and Cox, G. M.,** *Experimental Designs*, 2nd ed., John Wiley & Sons, New York, 1957.
7. **Huynh, H. and Feldt, L. S.,** Conditions under which mean square ratios in repeated measurements designs have exact F-distributions, *J. Am. Stat. Assoc.*, 65, 1582, 1970.
8. **Geisser, S.,** Multivariate analysis of variance for a special covariance case, *J. Am. Stat. Assoc.*, 58, 660, 1963.
9. **Box, G. E. P.,** Some theorems on quadratic forms applied in the study of analysis of variance problems. I. Effects of inequality of variance and correlation between errors in the two-way classification, *Ann. Math. Stat.*, 25, 484, 1954.
10. **Geisser, S. and Greenhouse, S.,** An extension of Box's results on the use of F distribution in multivariate analysis, *Ann. Math. Stat.*, 29, 855, 1958.
11. **Greenhouse, S. and Geisser, S.,** On methods in the analysis of profile data, *Psychometrika*, 24, 95, 1959.
12. **Collier, R. O., Jr., Baker, F. B., Mandeville, G. K., and Hayes, T. F.,** Estimates of test size for several test procedures based on conventional variance ratios in the repeated-measurements experiments, *Biometrics*, 16, 547, 1967.
13. Statistical Application Software, SAS Institute Inc., Cary, NC, 1985.
14. **Cole, J. W. L. and Grizzle, J. E.,** Applications of multivariate analysis of variance to repeated measurements experiments, *Biometrics*, 22, 810, 1966.
15. **Timm, N. H.,** *Multivariate Analysis with Applications in Education and Psychology*, Brooks/Cole, Monterey, CA, 1975.
16. **Morrison, D. F.,** *Multivariate Statistical Methods*, McGraw-Hill, New York, 1967.
17. **Anderson, T. W.,** *An Introduction to Multivariate Statistical Analysis*, 2nd ed., John Wiley & Sons, New York, 1984.
18. **Timm, N. H.,** Multivariate analysis of variance of repeated measurements, in *Handbook of Statistics*, Vol. 1, Krishnaiah, P. R., Ed., North-Holland, New York, 1980, 41.
19. **Rogan, J. C., Keselman, H. L., and Mendoza, J. L.,** Analysis of repeated measurements, *Br. J. Math. Stat. Psychol.*, 32, 269, 1979.
20. **Fleiss, J.,** Repeated measurements studies, in *The Design and Analysis of Clinical Experiments*, John Wiley & Sons, New York, 1986, chap. 8.
21. **Davidson, M. L.,** Univariate versus multivariate tests in repeated-measures experiments, *Psychol. Bull.*, 77, 446, 1972.
22. **Potthoff, R. F. and Roy, S. N.,** A generalized multivariate analysis of variance model useful especially for growth curve problems, *Biometrika*, 51, 313, 1964.

23. **Rao, C. R.,** The theory of least square when the parameters are stochastic and its application to the analysis of growth curves, *Biometrika*, 52, 447, 1965.

24. **Khatri, C. G.,** A note on a MANOVA model applied to problems in growth curve, *Ann. Inst. Stat. Math.*, 18, 75, 1966.

25. BMDP Statistical Software, Berkeley, CA, 1988.

26. **Harville, D. A.,** Maximum likelihood approaches to variance component estimation and to related problems, *J. Am. Stat. Assoc.*, 72, 320, 1977.

27. **Patterson, H. D. and Thompson, R.,** Recovery of interblock information when block sizes are unequal, *Biometrika*, 58, 545, 1971.

28. **Kleinbaum, D.,** A generalization of the growth curve model which allows missing data, *J. Multivar. Anal.*, 3, 117, 1973.

29. **Dempster, A. P., Laird, N. M., and Rubin, D. B.,** Maximum likelihood from incomplete data via the EM algorithm (with Discussion), *J. R. Stat. Soc.*, B39, 1, 1972.

30. **Beale, E. M. L. and Little, R. J. A.,** Missing values in multivariate analysis, *J. R. Stat. Soc.*, B37, 129, 1975.

31. **Orchard, T. and Woodbury, M. A.,** A missing information principle: theory and applications, in *Proc. 6th Berkeley Symposium Math. Stat. Probability*, Vol. I, 1972, 697.

32. **Jennrich, R. and Schluchter, M.,** Unbalanced repeated-measures models with structured covariance matrices, *Biometrics*, 42, 805, 1986.

33. **Seth, A. K. and Mazumdar, S.,** Estimation of parameters of a polynomial model under intraclass correlation structure for incomplete longitudinal data, *Commun. Stat. — Theory Meth.*, 15(5), 1549, 1986.

Chapter 10

ECONOMIC EVALUATIONS OF CANCER CARE — INCORPORATING QUALITY-OF-LIFE ISSUES

Pamela J. Goodwin*

TABLE OF CONTENTS

* Dr. Goodwin is a Career Scientist of the Ontario Ministry of Health.

I. INTRODUCTION

Cancer is a major cause of morbidity and mortality in Western society. In recent decades, the number of new cases of cancer has increased dramatically, largely due to the aging of the population and the rapid increase in tobacco-related cancers.[1] During the same time, the costs of caring for these patients have increased, due in part to the absolute increase in the number of new cases and also to the fact that treatments have become more complex (and expensive). To assist policy makers allocate health care resources optimally, economic evaluations can be conducted to relate the costs of treatments to their beneficial effects. Assessments of the effects of treatment on quality-of-life (QOL) can be incorporated into these evaluations, a process that is discussed in considerable detail in this chapter. It must be emphasized that the information obtained from economic evaluations is intended for use in policy making and not for use in making decisions regarding individual patients. This information should be considered in conjunction with other relevant data when decisions are made regarding resource allocation.

This chapter will describe the types of economic evaluation that exist, review their potential role in the care of cancer patients and discuss the important methodologic issues and unresolved problems relating to the incorporation of QOL measurements into these evaluations. Sufficient information regarding the methodology used in economic evaluations will be presented to allow readers to understand the factors involved in incorporation of QOL into these evaluations but specific techniques will not be discussed in detail. Readers are referred to standard texts if additional information is desired.[2,3]

II. WHAT ARE ECONOMIC EVALUATIONS?

Considerable confusion exists in the literature regarding the terminology used to describe economic evaluations. Many authors use the terms "cost-benefit" and "cost-effectiveness" interchangeably when, in fact, they refer to techniques that are quite different. The differences between the techniques will be described in detail in Section II.B and will be considered only briefly here. The major difference relates to the way health outcomes are valued. In cost benefit analysis (CBA) health outcomes are valued in monetary units, such as dollars, while in cost-effectiveness analysis (CEA) they are valued in natural units, such as years of life gained. Use of the former technique often involves putting a dollar value on a year of life whereas the latter does not. Drummond et al., in their book on methods of economic evaluation,[2] have provided an excellent description of the appropriate use of these terms and have presented a readily understandable classification of the different types of health care evaluations that appear in the medical literature.

A. RELATIONSHIP TO OTHER HEALTH CARE EVALUATIONS

All health care evaluations have the potential to include two major components. The *first* is an evaluation of the outcomes or consequences of the health care program(s). These consequences are variable and they may include, for example, the effect of the program on survival, quality adjusted survival or tumor response to treatment. The choice depends on the purpose of the evaluation, the specific program(s) being studied and the type of evaluation being conducted. The *second* major component is the cost of the program(s) being studied. The specific items to be included in this costing depend on the viewpoint or perspective of the evaluation (see Section III.A), the purpose of the study, as well as the period of time being costed. The latter is called the horizon of the study and it may vary considerably from study to study. For example, when an evaluation is conducted from the viewpoint of the treating hospital only costs of a given treatment from the time of admission to the time of discharge will be included. When a more comprehensive societal viewpoint is taken, all costs incurred from the time of diagnosis to the time of death should be included. Independent of the horizon of the study, the specific costs included may consist of direct costs (such as operating costs within the health care sector or out of pocket expenses to patients), indirect

TABLE 1
Classification of Health Care Evaluations

No. of programs evaluated	Components Examined in the Evaluation		
	Consequences only	Costs only	Both costs and consequences
One	Outcome description	Cost description[a]	Cost-outcome description[a]
More than one	Efficacy of effectiveness evaluation	Cost analysis[a]	Cost-minimization analysis, cost-effectiveness analysis, cost-benefit analysis, cost-utility analysis[b]

[a] Partial economic evaluation.
[b] Complete economic evaluation.

Adapted from Drummond, M. F., Stoddart, G. L., and Torrance, G. W., *Methods for the Economic Evaluation of Health Care Programmes,* Oxford Medical Publications, Oxford, 1987. With permission.

costs (such as time lost from work) or intangible (psychic) costs. Further information on costing is contained in Drummond et al.[2] In addition to these two major components all health care evaluations may compare two or more programs or treatments or simply describe a single program.

These factors can be incorporated into the classification of health care evaluations shown in Table 1. Although there may be a role for partial economic evaluations in certain circumstances, complete economic evaluations provide the most comprehensive information and are usually the preferred type of evaluation. Because of this, the remainder of this chapter will deal with complete economic evaluations only.

B. CLASSIFICATION OF COMPLETE ECONOMIC EVALUATIONS

Complete economic evaluations identify and compare both the costs and consequences of two or more programs and their results are usually expressed as a cost per unit of consequence for one program in relation to the other. Four major types of complete economic evaluations are described below. The approach to costing is similar in all of these techniques. They differ in major ways with respect to the measurement of consequences.

Cost-minimization analysis (CMA) is the simplest type of complete economic evaluation. In CMAs the health care programs being evaluated have outcomes that have been demonstrated to be identical in all relevant aspects. A classical example of this is the comparison of the same surgical procedure performed on an in-patient vs. out-patient basis. Because outcomes are identical, this type of evaluation simply compares the costs of the programs being evaluated. It is considered complete because the equivalence of outcomes of the programs being evaluated has been clearly demonstrated. A recent example of a CMA found that surgical treatment of esophageal cancer resulted in an additional cost of $10,105 (Australian) per patient when compared to the use of radical radiation treatment.[4]

CEA identifies the outcome of the programs being evaluated in natural units such as years of life gained or tumor response to treatment. To compare two programs, their outcomes must have the same units. The costs of each program are identified and the incremental (or additional) cost of one program relative to the other is compared to the incremental change in outcome for that program relative to the other and the results expressed as a ratio. For example, a recently published CEA found that screening mammography performed every 2 years in asymptomatic women over 50 years of age cost $4850 (American) per year of life gained when compared to a policy of routine care.[5] When a program is both more effective and less costly (or vice versa), the choice of one program over the other is clear. When the difference in benefits and costs are in the same direction, for example, if one program is both more effective and more costly, the choice is less obvious and it may depend on the magnitude of the incremental cost in relation to the incremental benefit or on one of the other factors described in Section III.C.

CBA values the consequences of programs in monetary units such as dollars and then subtracts the incremental costs (in dollars) from the incremental benefits (also in dollars) to arrive at a net cost for one program over another. Although this approach is theoretically attractive it requires that health outcomes, such as years of life gained, be valued in dollars. This process is not straightforward and may not be acceptable to many health care professionals. One recent CBA valued life according to the present value of future earnings and found that the use of cisplatin-based combination chemotherapy in patients with advanced testicular cancer resulted in a net saving of $150,000,000 per year in the US.[6] Because testicular cancer is a disease that occurs predominantly in working men this approach to the valuation of the benefits of treatment was feasible (although not without problems). Difficulties arise when this approach is attempted in the unemployed, homemakers, or the elderly and when comparisons are made between diseases that occur with different frequencies in high and low income earners. In these situations, some lives are valued more highly than others and low income earners may be discriminated against. Of greater importance in these evaluations is the fact that the impact of the disease and its treatment on quality of life is ignored. Because of these limitations, CBAs of health care programs are not commonly performed.

The final type of complete economic evaluation, cost-utility analysis (CUA), also places a value on the program outcomes. The valuation procedure used incorporates QOL into the outcomes but it does not place a dollar value on them. In CUAs the outcomes must be expressed in units of time, for example life years, and this time must be adjusted for value, or quality, using utility techniques (described in Section IV). CUAs provide an estimate of the cost of one program relative to another per healthy day or quality-adjusted life year (QALY) gained. An example of this type of evaluation recently published by our group demonstrated that the use of one form of chemotherapy compared to another in patients with extensive small cell lung cancer resulted in both improved survival and improved quality adjusted survival at a cost of $4495 (Canadian) per QALY gained.[7] CUA is the only type of economic evaluation that incorporates the effect of health care programs on QOL.

In all types of complete economic evaluations, data regarding program effectiveness and patterns of resource utilization are most reliable when obtained prospectively in the context of a randomized clinical trial. This approach may also facilitate collection of data regarding QOL and should be used whenever possible.

III. THE ROLE OF ECONOMIC EVALUATIONS IN HEALTH CARE

A. THE NEED FOR ECONOMIC EVALUATIONS

Economic evaluations are performed when demands for the use of health care resources exceed the available supply and decisions must be made regarding resource allocation. If these decisions are not made explicitly, allocation will occur on an *ad hoc* basis and inefficiency may result. In some health care systems these *ad hoc* decisions may result in the provision of care to those most able to pay while in others, resources may be allocated on a first come, first served basis. With either approach, some resources will likely be allocated to services that are either of marginal benefit or extremely costly rather than to more effective and less costly services.

Economic evaluations provide information that assists policy makers allocate resources in the most efficient manner possible.[2] They identify relevant alternative programs that are competing for the same health care resources. When identifying alternatives it is important to remember that, although a "no treatment" option may exist, it cannot be assumed that a policy of "no treatment" will not be associated with significant resource utilization. Individuals who are ill (particularly those who have malignant disease) consume resources even if they do not receive active treatment, and the costs of these resources may exceed those of active treatment. This was recently demonstrated in an economic evaluation of the use of chemotherapy in patients with unresectable non-small cell lung cancer by our group in which the use of cyclophosphamide, adriamycin, and cisplatin chemotherapy resulted in increased survival and cost $949 (Canadian) less per patient compared to a policy of best supportive care.[8]

These evaluations also provide a framework for the identification of costs from different viewpoints, that is, from the perspective of different groups or individuals who are responsible for payment of these costs. These viewpoints can include, among others, the treating institution, the patient and/or his family, government, third party health insurance programs and society. When a societal viewpoint is taken all relevant costs and consequences are considered. This is the most comprehensive viewpoint and many feel it should be taken whenever possible. When the viewpoint is more restrictive care must be taken that a new program does not appear to make more efficient use of resources simply because costs are shifted from one source to another with no overall saving. For example, a policy decision by a tertiary care cancer center not to offer treatment to patients with metastatic lung cancer might shift the burden of care (and the associated costs) to primary care community hospitals with no overall saving to the health care system.

Finally, economic evaluations provide an estimate of the magnitude of the costs associated with the adoption of a new program. The magnitude of these costs may not have been intuitively obvious as is clear from the economic evaluation of the approach to the management of patients with carcinoma of unknown primary reported by Levine et al.[9] When they compared an aggressive approach to the management of patients with carcinoma of unknown primary to a less aggressive approach they found this cost $1,570,000 (Canadian) per additional patient alive at one year, an amount that was considerably higher than most oncologists would have anticipated.

B. INFORMATION OBTAINED FROM ECONOMIC EVALUATIONS

Complete evaluations provide estimates of the relative costs and consequences of one health care program in comparison to another. As noted above, when the consequences of a program are expressed in units of time they can be adjusted for QOL using the techniques outlined in Section IV. The resulting CUA can then provide an estimate of costs in relation to effects on both quality and quantity of life.

C. OTHER FACTORS TO BE CONSIDERED WHEN MAKING POLICY DECISIONS

Economic factors should never be considered in isolation when policy decisions are made regarding specific treatments, even when these economic factors include the effects of the treatments being evaluated on the QOL of those who receive them. Treatment efficacy must continue to be a major factor when decisions are made regarding new treatments. This is particularly true in oncology where diseases are often fatal and even small increments in survival can be important. Other considerations include patient, physician, and societal preferences regarding alternative treatments, as well as the availability and acceptability of treatments. The effect of the treatment on QOL may be overshadowed by one of these other factors when policy decisions are made.

IV. INCORPORATION OF QUALITY OF LIFE INTO ECONOMIC EVALUATIONS

The approaches taken to measurement of QOL in CUAs may differ from those in the clinical setting. These differences occur because QOL information is used for different purposes in the two situations. As discussed in other chapters,[10,11] QOL measures can be used to evaluate change in QOL over time, to predict outcome or prognosis or to discriminate between individuals with respect to QOL. It is primarily the latter application that is relevant in economic evaluations.

In clinical settings QOL measurements are often conducted to determine specific aspects of QOL (for example, effect of pain, nausea, or shortness of breath on QOL) and measurements obtained in individual patients are of primary importance. When QOL measures are used in CUAs the effects of treatment on individuals are of less importance than effects on groups and only effects on overall QOL are considered. This is because the results of CUAs are not applied to individual patients and they are not intended to address the impact of treatment on specific symptoms. Instead, they provide information on the overall impact and costs of different treatments in groups of patients.

In CUAs QOL is measured using the utility approach. Much of the developmental work regarding the use of utilities in CUAs has been done at McMaster University by a group headed by George Torrance;[2] the work of this group will be referred to extensively. In addition, a recent series of articles provides an excellent review of utilities.[12-15] Some of these concepts are also discussed by Till in Chapter 11.[10]

A. THEORETICAL BASIS FOR THE USE OF UTILITIES

The term *utility* refers to the preference that subjects exhibit for a given health state. It does not refer to the usefulness of the health state. The absolute value of a utility is a measure of the strength of the preference for the health state and it is usually expressed on a scale of 0 to 1 where 0 represents death and 1 represents perfect health. The use of utilities to measure QOL is based on the work of von Neumann and Morgenstern[16] who developed modern utility theory. This theory is based on a set of five axioms that govern the behavior of individuals presented with a series of lotteries and it describes a method of decision making under uncertainty. According to this theory, when individuals are faced with a series of gambles they will act in such a manner that they maximize the expected utility of the outcomes. The axioms upon which the theory is based have considerable face validity and they provide a strong theoretical basis for the use of utilities in this situation. For a detailed discussion of utility theory readers are referred to Schoemaker et al.[17] or Hershey et al.[18] Utilities have been used to obtain information regarding QOL in individual patients to assist in making treatment decisions as well as in groups of subjects to assist in the making of policy decisions. The discussion that follows relates primarily to the latter use of utilities and it is not intended to be a comprehensive review of the use of utilities to measure QOL in all situations.

Utilities have several important characteristics that make them useful in economic evaluations. First, they measure QOL on a scale that is anchored by death and perfect health. The values obtained are therefore generalizable across different health states and different evaluations. Second, utilities can provide comprehensive information on all aspects of QOL including physical, emotional, sensory, cognitive, and self-care function. Inclusion of social functioning in the determination of utilities in economic evaluations is controversial and some authors believe that only health-related factors should be included when these evaluations are conducted in the health care sector.[19]

Third, the number of health states that can be assessed using utilities is often greater than can be assessed using other methods.[19] This is because it is theoretically not necessary for subjects to experience a health state in order to provide a utility value. The health state may simply be described to them in a standard scenario that includes information on all important health attributes. It should be noted that prognosis is not considered part of a health state and should not be included in the health state description — the time spent in a health state and the risk of death are defined during the measurement procedure. Thus, it is possible to measure utilities for health states that are uncommon or in which disability is so profound it is otherwise difficult to apply the measures. Fourth, utilities can be determined using different subjects having different viewpoints. For example, it may be considered appropriate to measure the utility of living in a given health state in members of the general population if the viewpoint of the CUA is a societal one and society is required to pay for the health care intervention being evaluated. In other situations other subjects may be more appropriate. There are some concerns about the measurement of utilities in subjects who have not experienced a given health state that will be discussed below in Section IV.E.

A final characteristic of utilities that is essential for their use in CUA is that, because they are measured on a 0 to 1 scale anchored by death and perfect health, they can be used to incorporate the effects of treatment on both morbidity and mortality into a single weighted outcome measure, QALYs. The manner in which this is done will be described in Section IV.D.

B. MEASUREMENT TECHNIQUES

Utilities can be measured using one of several techniques or they can simply be assigned using judgment.[20,21] The latter approach involves the estimation of a utility or range of plausible values of a utility for a given health state without a formal measurement process. This approach provides only a rough estimate of the utility value and the potential effects of uncertainty in these estimates on the results of the CUA should be assessed. This approach has been used by Weinstein et al.[22] in the assessment of postmenopausal estrogen replacement and other commonly used therapies in nonmalignant disease. Because of the nonrigorous nature of this approach it will not be discussed further.

The classic method for measuring utilities is the standard gamble (SG).[21] This technique is derived directly from the axioms underlying the von Neumann-Morgenstern model and as such it is felt by some[21,23] but not all[17,25] investigators to have criterion validity. The method is widely used and it has often served as a reference for other techniques. The technique involves the presentation of a series of paired gambles to a subject. For a permanent health state, the subject is asked to choose between the certainty of living in a given health state for the remainder of his natural life vs. a gamble with a given probability (X) of living for the same period of time in perfect health vs. a given risk of immediate death (1-X). When the probability of living with perfect health approaches 1, most subjects will choose the gamble for most health states. When it approaches 0 the certainty of living in the health state under consideration will be preferred for most health states. As X is varied, a point is reached where the individual is indifferent to the choice being presented. The value of X at that point represents the utility of the health state being measured. Slight modifications of this technique are used to measure temporary health states and health states worse than death.[20]

Because many individuals have difficulty dealing with numerical probabilities visual props can be used to provide a graphic representation of probabilities. Additional problems may be encountered in risk averse individuals who avoid options involving a gamble simply because they involve risk. Use of the SG is time consuming and it probably requires a certain minimal level of intelligence for its successful completion.[24]

A second technique for the measurement of utilities is the time trade-off (TTO). This technique was developed by Torrance et al.[26] specifically for use in health care settings. When this technique is used subjects are presented with a choice. They may choose to live for a given life expectancy (T) in a specified chronic health state and then die or to live in a healthy state for time X (<T) and then die. The time X is varied and when the subject is indifferent to the choice, the utility of the health state is obtained as X/T. Health states worse than death and temporary health states can also be measured using modifications of this technique. The use of the TTO is time consuming but it is simpler to use than the SG.[19] The technique can be made more understandable when visual props are used.

A third technique, the category rating scale (CRS), is extremely simple to use and measures utilities directly. The scale consists of a straight line, usually anchored by death at one end and by perfect health at the other. Subjects are asked to place a mark on this line in a position that represents their preference for the health state being evaluated relative to these anchors. When more than one health state is measured simultaneously subjects are asked to ensure that the marks for each health state are in order of preference and that the distances between marks represent differences in preference for the health states. Both permanent and temporary health states can be assessed using this technique, although they should be measured separately. Visual aids can be used to simplify the method even further. Modifications of this technique require subjects to group health states into a series of discrete, equally spaced categories anchored by death and perfect health as before rather than to indicate their preferences on a continuous scale.

Four additional techniques have been described to measure preferences for health states. These include an equivalence technique,[27,28] ratio scaling,[29] magnitude estimation,[30] and willingness to pay.[31] The latter values preferences in dollar amounts or as a proportion of annual income and may prove to have some applicability to economic evaluations. These have not been commonly used in economic evaluations and will not be discussed in detail here.

An alternate approach to the measurement of utilities uses any of the three major methods described above to determine utilities for individual attributes of QOL (for example, physical, emotional, sensory, and cognitive function) and then aggregates these values to obtain utilities that reflect overall QOL.[12,32] The utilities obtained using this approach can then be combined in different ways to obtain overall utility values for a large number of health states. The techniques used to measure individual utilities are similar to those described above but formulae must be developed to combine the utilities in an appropriate way. The use of this technique is most appropriate when the utilities of a large number of health states must be determined and it is not feasible to measure each individually. When smaller numbers of health states are involved, it is probably more appropriate to measure their utilities individually. Although this multiattribute approach has not been used extensively in economic evaluations in the past, its use in the measurement of health preferences has been favored over the holistic approach outlined above in a recent review.[12]

C. VALIDATION OF MEASUREMENT TECHNIQUES

The reproducibility of utility measurements obtained using the three major techniques described above has been examined; findings that are most relevant to their use in economic evaluations are described below.

Torrance et al.[24] studied the intra-test reliability of the SG and TTO techniques as well as the test-retest reliability of all three techniques. They found the intra-test reliability coefficient (r) to be 0.77 for both SG and TTO, and acknowledged that these results might underestimate the reliability of the techniques because of problems with the replication procedure during their testing. Other work by this group has identified higher reliability coefficients — 0.77 to 0.92 for the SG, 0.77 to 0.88 for TTO, and 0.86 to 0.94 for the CRS.[24,32] These values suggest that the intra-test reliability of all three techniques is acceptable. Test-retest reliability has been reported to be somewhat lower (r = 0.53, 0.62, 0.49 for SG, TTO, CRS, respectively, for measurements taken 1 year apart).[24] Slightly better agreement for TTO (r = 0.63 to 0.80) was reported by Churchill et al.[33] when tests were conducted 6 weeks apart and for all three techniques (r = 0.77 to 0.87) when tests were conducted 1 week apart.[34] At least part of the difference in repeated measurements may have been due to changes in preference over time and not to measurement error.[24] It should be noted that these coefficients all refer to the reliability of individual measurements and not to group means which may be more stable. The latter are used in economic evaluations and it is possible their reliability is better.

Because the SG is derived directly from the fundamental axioms of decision theory it is felt by some to have criterion validity and has been used as a reference for the assessment of the convergent validity of the other techniques.[21,24] There is some evidence that the underlying axioms of decision theory are violated when SG is used to measure health preferences,[17,25] therefore other approaches to validation have also been used.

When utility values obtained using the TTO technique were compared to those obtained using the SG, Torrance et al.[24] found good agreement of individual measurements (coefficients of validity 0.65 and 0.84 before and after correction for internal unreliability). When population means were compared, the results obtained using TTO were found to be equivalent to those obtained using SG (r = 0.98). Similar results were obtained by Detsky et al.[35]

In contrast, utility values obtained using the CRS correlated poorly with those obtained using SG. When individual values are used, the coefficient of validity was only 0.36 in one study by Torrance et al.[24] Similar results were obtained when population means were compared. Utility values obtained using CRS were systematically lower than when SG was used in four studies.[36-39] Torrance et al.[24] examined these differences further and found that the population means obtained using CR could be related to those obtained using TTO by means of a power function. When this transformation was performed, r increased to 0.82, a more acceptable level.

Additional support for the validity of measurements obtained using these three techniques comes from observations that values are similar when measurements are made on both patients and physicians (see below) and from the observation that utility values differ in predictable ways for different health states.[33,40,41]

Thus, it appears that all three methods provide satisfactory estimates of mean utility values in populations, although the results obtained using the CRS may require transformation. The use of group means also improves precision, particularly when sample sizes are large.

D. INCORPORATION OF UTILITIES INTO ECONOMIC EVALUATIONS

As outlined in Section II.B, the incorporation of QOL into CUAs allows the effects of treatment programs on both morbidity and mortality to be combined into a single outcome measure, QALYs. This outcome measure is obtained by multiplying the time spent in a given health state by the utility of that health state measured on a scale of 0 to 1.[2] Thus, 2 years spent in a health state that has a utility of 0.5, are equivalent to one QALY. It then follows that living 2 years in a health state with a utility of 0.5 is equivalent to living 4 years in a health state with a utility of 0.25, both being equal to one QALY. If more than one health state exists in a treatment program, the time spent in each health state is multiplied by the utility of that health state and the resulting quality-adjusted life years are added together to obtain a total number of QALYs for that treatment program.

This approach assumes that time spent in a health state is valued linearly, an assumption that may not be true.[26,42,43] It also assumes that individuals are truly prepared to "trade-off" more time in a less than perfect health state for less time in a state of perfect health. While this may be correct in some situations, in others increased duration of survival may be preferred to increased quality of survival. It is possible that utility values obtained using TTO will be the most appropriate for this application, however, this has not been conclusively demonstrated. This approach to combining quality and quantity of life also involves ethical dilemmas that have been discussed by Till in Chapter 11.[10]

E. LIMITATIONS AND PROBLEMS

It has been shown in the preceding sections that it is possible to measure utilities using one of three commonly used measurement techniques and that the values obtained in these measurements are reasonably reliable and valid. It has also been shown that it is possible to use these utility values to obtain a measure of quality adjusted survival that can be used in economic evaluations. In spite of the demonstrated feasibility of this approach, there are many issues regarding the measurement of utilities and their incorporation into economic evaluations that are yet to be resolved.

Several of these issues relate to the selection of subjects for the measurement of utilities and others relate to the procedures used to measure or aggregate them. In regard to the selection of subjects, factors that need to be clarified include whose utilities should be measured and at what time these measurements should be performed. The former uncertainty arises because utilities can be measured in individuals who have never experienced the health state being evaluated. Potential subjects include the general public, health care professionals and patients. Some investigators have found little difference in the values obtained when different groups are assessed[7,33,39,42,44] but others have obtained different results.[42,45] Overall, it appears two characteristics of the subjects (age and experience of the health state) exert effects on health preferences as measured using utilities.[14] Although the most appropriate choice of subjects may be dictated by the viewpoint of the study, research is needed to understand the differences that may exist in utility values among groups and to identify the impact of these differences on the results of the CUA. If large differences exist among groups of subjects, particularly between those who have and have not experienced a given health state, ethical issues regarding the use of surrogates to obtain utility values will have to be addressed. Some of these issues are addressed in Chapter 11.[10]

An additional problem relates to the timing of utility measurements. Womens' preferences for anesthesia during labor have been shown to be dramatically different before, during, and after labor[46] by one group of investigators, although others[47] have found preferences to be stable before and after treatment. These observations raise the issue of when utilities should be measured and whether the effects of changing utilities should be examined in CUAs. It also raises the issue of whether utilities for a given health state may change as adaptation to the health state occurs and whether this factor should be considered in economic evaluations.

Utility values may also be dependent on certain features of the measurement procedure. Independent of the technique used, the amount of detail provided in the health state description or the situation of the patient to whom the description applies has had a significant effect on the utility value obtained in some reports[36,49] as has the order of the methods used to measure them.[36] Similarly, the manner in which health state descriptions are framed and the anchors used appear to influence results.[14,49,50] Controversy also exists regarding the most appropriate method for aggregating utility values for use in CUAs.[12,20] Currently, mean values are most commonly used. This may be appropriate in some economic evaluations, although differential weighting of individual preferences may also be appropriate at times. Finally, the assumption that quantity of survival can be adjusted for quality using a simple mathematical procedure and that patients are truly willing to trade off time in a less desirable health state remains unproven. These assumptions are fundamental to the methods described in this chapter and they require urgent investigation.

Clearly, additional research is needed to determine the importance of each of these issues in CUA and to investigate the validity of the assumptions that are made when survival is adjusted for quality as discussed in Section IV.D. Prior to the resolution of these issues it would be prudent to measure utilities in a variety of groups using a variety of techniques and to examine the effect of uncertainty in these measurements on the results of the economic evaluation to ensure that they do not change significantly.

V. CONCLUDING REMARKS

It cannot be denied that economic factors are becoming increasingly important in the assessment of programs for the care of cancer patients and a considerable literature is developing in this area. The techniques described in this chapter have been developed to allow a determination of program costs and to allow the effects of programs on both quality and quantity of life to be incorporated into a single outcome variable, quality adjusted survival, which is then related to program costs. Unfortunately, many unresolved issues exist regarding the use of these techniques.

The work that has been performed thus far has occurred in response to a need to combine quality and quantity of survival into a single variable in a consistent and meaningful way. Such a variable would have potential use in clinical settings as well as in the development of health policy. With respect to the latter, the ability to relate the costs of health care programs to their effect on quality adjusted survival would facilitate decisions regarding the equitable distribution of available health care resources. Although the QALY may ultimately prove to be an appropriate approach the unresolved issues relating to the assumptions underlying QALYs and the methodology used to measure utilities must be addressed. In the meantime, investigators who incorporate QOL into economic evaluations should examine the effects of these unresolved methodologic issues on their results and readers of these evaluations should be aware of the limitations of the technique.

ACKNOWLEDGMENTS

The author gratefully acknowledges the helpful comments and criticisms provided by Dr. P. Warde during the preparation of this manuscript.

REFERENCES

1. Bailar, J. C. and Smith, E. M., Progress against cancer?, N. Engl. J. Med., 314, 1226, 1986.
2. Drummond, M. F., Stoddart, G. L., and Torrance, G. W., Methods for the Economic Evaluation of Health Care Programmes, Oxford Medical Publications, Oxford, 1987.
3. Warner, K. E. and Luce, B. R., Cost-Benefit and Cost-Effectiveness in Health Care: Principles, Practice, and Potential, Health Administration Press, Ann Arbor, MI, 1982.
4. Walker, Q. J., Salkeld, G., Hall, J., O'Rourke, I., Bull, C. A., Tiver, K. W., and Langlands, A. O., The management of oesophageal carcinoma: radiotherapy or surgery? Cost considerations, Eur. J. Cancer Clin. Oncol., 25, 1657, 1989.
5. Van der Maas, P. J., de Koning, H. J., van Ineveld, B. M., van Oortmarssen, G. J., Habbema, J. D. F., Lubbe, K. T. N., Geerts, A. T., Collette, H. J. A., Verbeek, A. L. M., Hendriks, J. H. C. L., and Rombach, J. J., The cost-effectiveness of breast cancer screening, Int. J. Cancer, 43, 1055, 1989.
6. Shibley, L., Brown, M., Schuttinga, J., Rothenberg, M., and Whalen, J., Cisplatin-based combination chemotherapy in the treatment of advanced-stage testicular cancer: cost-benefit analysis, J. Natl. Cancer Inst., 82, 186, 1990.
7. Goodwin, P. J., Feld, R., Evans, W. K., and Pater, J., Cost-effectiveness of cancer chemotherapy: an economic evaluation of a randomized trial in small-cell lung cancer, J. Clin. Oncol., 6, 1537, 1988.
8. Jaakkimainen, L., Goodwin, P. J., Pater, J., Warde, P., and Rapp, E., Counting the costs of chemotherapy in a National Cancer Institute of Canada randomized trial in non-small cell lung cancer (NSCLC), J. Clin. Oncol., 8, 1301, 1990.
9. Levine, M. N., Drummond, M. F., and Labelle, R. J., Cost-effectiveness in the diagnosis and treatment of carcinoma of unknown primary origin, Can. Med. Assoc. J., 133, 977, 1985.
10. Till, J. E., Uses (and some possible abuses) of quality of life measures, in Effect of Cancer on Quality of Life, Osoba, D., Ed., CRC Press, Boca Raton, FL, 1991, chap. 11.
11. Osoba, D., Aaronson, N., and Till, J. E., A practical guide to selecting quality of life measures in clinical trials and practice, in Effect of Cancer on Quality of Life, Osoba, D., Ed., CRC Press, Boca Raton, FL, 1991, chap. 7.
12. Froberg, D. G. and Kane, R. L., Methodology for measuring health state preferences. I. Measurement strategies, J. Clin. Epidemiol., 42, 345, 1989.
13. Froberg, D. G. and Kane, R. L., Methodology for measuring health-state preferences. II. Scaling methods, J. Clin. Epidemiol., 42, 459, 1989.
14. Froberg, D. G. and Kane, R. L., Methodology for measuring health-state preferences. III. Population and context effects, J. Clin. Epidemiol., 42, 585, 1989.
15. Froberg, D. G. and Kane, R. L., Methodology for measuring health-state preferences. IV. Progress and a research agenda, J. Clin. Epidemiol., 42, 675, 1989.
16. von Neumann, J. and Morgenstern, O., Theory of Games and Economic Behaviour, 3rd ed., John Wiley & Sons, New York, 1953.
17. Schoemaker, P. J., The expected utility model: its variants, purposes, evidence and limitations, J. Econ. Lit., 20, 529, 1982.
18. Hershey, J. C., Kunreuther, H. C., and Schoemaker, P. J. H., Sources of bias in assessment procedures for utility functions, Manage. Sci., 28, 936, 1982.
19. Torrance, G. W., Utility approach to measuring health related quality of life, J. Chronic. Dis., 6, 593, 1987.
20. Torrance, G. W., Measurement of health state utilities for economic appraisal, J. Health Econ., 5, 1, 1986.
21. Weinstein, M. C. and Fineberg, H. V., Clinical Decision Analysis, W. B. Saunders, Philadelphia, 1980.
22. Weinstein, M. C., Economic assessments of medical practices and technologies, Med. Decision Making, 1, 309, 1981.

23. Holloway, C. A., *Decision Making Under Uncertainty: Models and Choices*, Prentice-Hall, Englewood Cliffs, NJ, 1979.

24. Torrance, G. W., Social preferences for health states: an empirical evaluation of three measurement techniques, *Socioecon. Planning Sci.*, 10, 129, 1979.

25. Llewellyn-Thomas, H., Sutherland, H. J., Tibshirani, R., Ciampi, A., Till, J. E., and Boyd, N. F., The measurement of patients' values in medicine, *Med. Decision Making*, 2, 449, 1982.

26. Torrance, G. W., Thomas, W. H., and Sackett, D. L., A utility maximization model for evaluation of health care programs, *Health Serv. Res.*, 7, 118, 1972.

27. Berg, R. L., Establishing the values of various conditions of life for a health status index, in *Health Status Indices*, Berg, R. L., Ed., Hospital Research and Education Trust, Chicago, 1973, 120.

28. Bush, J. W., Chen, M. M., and Patrick, D. L., Health status index in cost-effectiveness: analysis of PKU program, in *Health Status Indices*, Berg, R. L., Ed., Hospital Research and Education Trust, Chicago, 1980, 172.

29. Rosser, R. M. and Kind, P., A scale of valuations of states of illness: Is there a social consensus?, *Int. J. Epidemiol.*, 7, 347, 1978.

30. Stevens, S. S., Issues in psychosocial measurement, *Psychol. Rev.*, 78, 426, 1971.

31. Thompson, M. S., Willingness to pay and accept risks to cure chronic disease, *Am. J. Public Health*, 76, 392, 1986.

32. Torrance, G. W., Boyle, M. H., and Horwood, S. P., Application of multiattribute utility theory to measure social preferences for health states, *Oper. Res.*, 30, 1043, 1982.

33. Churchill, D. N., Morgan, J., and Torrance, G. W., Quality of life in end-stage renal disease, *Peritoneal Dialysis Bull.*, 4, 20, 1984.

34. O'Connor, A. M., Boyd, N. F., and Till, J. E., Influence of elicitation techniques, position order and test-retest error on preferences for alternative cancer drug therapy, *Proc. 10th Natl. Nursing Res. Conf.*, Toronto, 1985.

35. Detsky, A., McLaughlin, J. R., Abrams, B., L'Abbe, A., Whitwell, J., Bombardier, C., and Jeejeebhoy, K. N., Quality of life of patients on long-term total parenteral nutrition at home, *J. Gen. Intern. Med.*, 1, 26, 1986.

36. Llewellyn-Thomas, H., Sutherland, H. J., Tibshirani, R., Ciampi, A., Till, J. E., and Boyd, N. F., Describing health states. Methodologic issues in obtaining values for health states, *Med. Care*, 22, 543, 1984.

37. Read, J. L., Quinn, R. J., Berwick, D. m., Fineberg, H. V., and Weinstein, M. C., Preferences for health outcomes: comparison of assessment methods, *Med. Decision Making*, 4, 315, 1984.

38. O'Connor, A. M., Boyd, N. F., Warde, P., Stolbach, L., and Till, J. E., Eliciting preferences for alternative drug therapies in oncology: influence of treatment outcome description, elicitation technique and treatment experience on preferences, *J. Chron. Dis.*, 40, 811, 1987.

39. Wolfson, A. D., Sinclair, A. J., Bombardier, C., and McGeer, A., Preference measurements for functional status in stroke patients: interrater and intertechnique comparisons, in *Values and Long Term Care*, Kane, R. L. and Kane R. A., Lexington Books, Lexington, MA, 1982.

40. Kind, P., Rosser, R., and Williams, A., Valuation of quality of life: some psychometric evidence, in *The Value of Life and Safety*, Jones-Lee, M. W., North-Holland, Amsterdam, 1982, 159.

41. Thompson, M. S., Read, J. L., and Liang, M., Feasibilty of willingness-to-pay measurement in chronic arthritis, *Med. Decision Making*, 4, 195, 1984.

42. Sackett, D. L. and Torrance, G. W., The utility of different health states as perceived by the general population, *J. Chron. Dis.*, 31, 697, 1978.

43. Sutherland, H. J., Llewellyn-Thomas, H., Boyd, N. F., and Till, J. E., Attitudes toward quality of survival. The concept of maximal endurable time, *Med. Decision Making*, 2, 299, 1982.

44. Kaplan, R. M. and Bush, J. W., Health related quality of life measurement for evaluation research and policy analysis, *Health Psychol.*, 1, 61, 1982.

45. Boyd, N. F., Sutherland, H., Heasman, K. Z., Tritchler, D. L., and Cummings, B., Whose utilities for decision analysis?, *Med. Decision Making*, 10, 58, 1990.

46. Christensen-Szalansi, J. J. J., Discount functions and the measurement of patients' values. Women's decisions during childbirth, *Med. Decision Making*, 4, 47, 1984.

47. Llewellyn-Thomas, H. A., Sutherland, H. J., Ciampi, A., Etezadi-Amoli, J., Boyd, N. F., and Till, J. E., The assessment of values in laryngeal cancer: reliability of measurement methods, *J. Chron. Dis.*, 37, 283, 1984.

48. Ciampi, A., Silberfeld, M., and Till, J. E., Measurement of individual preferences: the importance of "situation-specific" variables, *Med. Decision Making*, 2, 483, 1982.

49. Sutherland, H. J., Dunn, V., and Boyd, N. F., Measurement of values for states of health with linear analog scales, *Med. Decision Making*, 3, 477, 1983.

50. Kahneman, D. and Tversky, A., The psychology of preferences, *Sci. Am.*, 1960, 1982.

Chapter 11

USES (AND SOME POSSIBLE ABUSES) OF QUALITY-OF-LIFE MEASURES

James E. Till

TABLE OF CONTENTS

I. INTRODUCTION

In clinical oncology, the end-points physicians use to judge the results of treatment are sometimes ill defined, but the primary aim is usually to try to maximize the duration of disease-free or recurrence-free survival.[1] However, there is also an appreciation that there is more to life than not dying. Because cancer and its treatment can have major impacts on quality of life (QOL), clinical oncologists are fully aware of the potential usefulness of meaningful quantitative measures of QOL.[1] This interest in measurement of QOL of cancer patients is not confined to recent years. For example, in 1934, Roberts[2] presented a hypothetical plot of "general health" vs. time of a kind remarkably analogous to those shown below (see Figure 1).

What has, at least until recently, limited the practical usefulness of QOL measurement has been a paucity of well-characterized measures that are rooted in sound philosophical concepts, have been subjected to rigorous scientific evaluation, and have stood the test of time in a variety of situations that are both of practical importance, and of continuing interest to oncologists.

A. DEFINITION OF QOL

A central issue in all considerations of QOL is the definition being used. As indicated elsewhere in this volume, there is wide acceptance of the highly subjective nature of the concept. Here, the concept of QOL as a subjective expression or evaluation of an individual's physical, mental, and social situation will be emphasized (cf. the definitions of QOL provided by Jonsen et al.[3]).

B. ETHICAL CONSIDERATIONS

There are a number of ethical issues and problems that are raised by the use of QOL assessments. The potential for discrimination is one of them, as discussed in Section IV. No extensive consideration of the ethical issues involved in evaluating QOL will be attempted here. It should be noted, however, that ethical considerations are vital even at the outset of any protocol for assessing QOL.[4] The choice of measures or end-points involves value assumptions, and therefore involves subtle, yet not insignificant, ethical choices. Bioethics can provide insight into the uses of QOL data. It also has important contributions to make to research ethics, in relation to the design, review, conduct, interpretation, and reporting of research protocols for assessing QOL, whether or not these contributions are explicitly recognized.

C. USES OF QOL ASSESSMENTS

Research on quantitative assessments of QOL has received an impetus over the past decade from a desire to assess the QOL of patients entered into randomized prospective clinical trials. The intent is usually to obtain data on QOL either during the treatment process[5] or subsequently as end-points. In addition, the usual assessments of response to therapy and duration of survival are carried out.

There are other uses of QOL assessments in addition to their use as process or outcome measures in clinical trials. Three uses will be considered below, and some of their possible ramifications and pitfalls will be reviewed and discussed. A few examples will be cited to illustrate particular points, but a comprehensive review of all the reported examples of uses of QOL measures in oncology is beyond the scope of this chapter.

Three major uses of QOL assessments are (cf. Guyatt et al.[6]):

1.   To evaluate the extent of change in the QOL of an individual or group, across time. This is the main focus for those interested in the measurement of QOL in clinical trials.

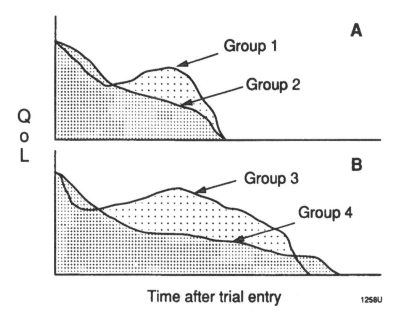

FIGURE 1.   Each profile represents a quantitative assessment of a defined aspect of quality of life, plotted across time, for a hypothetical "typical" patient enrolled in a clinical trial. A: Quality-vs.-quality comparison. B: Quality-vs.-quantity comparison (cf. Bush,[1] Roberts[2]).

2. To predict outcome or prognosis. An example is the use of QOL information as a stratifying variable for patients entering clinical trials.
3. To discriminate between individuals differing significantly in one or more measures of QOL. Such information could be used in clinical decision making, for example in relation to withholding or withdrawing treatment.

The third use of QOL data, in relation to discrimination between individuals, can pose some difficult ethical problems. It is generally assumed that the availability of QOL measures is a "good thing", in that attention to the quality as well as the quantity of survival would be expected to lead to improved patient care. However, it is now well recognized that the application of research results can sometimes pose unexpected problems. The application of the results of research on QOL measures is no exception.[7] It will be argued in Section IV that, when QOL measures are used as a basis for "labeling" individual patients, rather than for assessing interventions, ethical difficulties may then arise.

The major emphasis in this chapter will be on possible impacts of the application of QOL assessments to situations of practical interest for oncologists. However, it will be apparent that the concepts and methods currently being used in the development of innovative approaches to the quantitative measurement of QOL are still quite unfamiliar to many oncologists, as are some of the underlying ethical issues. It will be predicted, in some concluding comments, that an increasing familiarity with these approaches will provoke shifts in attitudes, and that such attitudinal shifts are likely to have more impact on the care of cancer patients than will the QOL assessments themselves.

II. ASSESSMENTS TO EVALUATE EXTENT OF CHANGE IN QOL

Evaluations of QOL across time are useful in clinical trials, or in studies of the natural history of disease.[6] The former use (in clinical trials) is of particular interest in oncology.

The latter use (in studies of the natural history of disease) is important, for example, for chronic illnesses that do not require a preoccupation with death or survival.[8] Quality-of-life issues (and cost issues) are likely to play a major role in the long-term management of most chronic diseases, irrespective of the preferred approach to management, be it "watchful waiting", lifestyle changes, or pharmacological interventions.[8,9]

Yates[10] has suggested some situations where QOL studies are indicated, including high risk treatments with a low probability of cure, intensive screening procedures for moderate-risk individuals, and prophylaxis in asymptomatic individuals.

A. AN EXAMPLE OF QOL ASSESSMENTS IN CLINICAL TRIALS

Studies of limb-sparing therapy in patients with extremity soft-tissue sarcomas provide an illustration of some issues that may arise when QOL assessments are included in clinical trials.

Current management achieves local control of disease in a high proportion of patients.[11] Local methods to conserve limb function have largely replaced traditional approaches of ablative surgery.[11,12] Frequently, these methods employ conservative surgery with pre- or postoperative radiotherapy.[11,13]

In 1982, Sugarbaker et al.[14] reported on a study designed to test the hypothesis that limb-sparing surgery plus radiation would provide improved QOL when compared with amputation, for 26 patients with soft-tissue sarcoma. The members of the research team reported that, at the beginning of the study, they had a definite bias; they were convinced that sparing a limb as opposed to amputating it offered a QOL advantage (that is, less extensive loss of function). The results of the QOL assessment did not support the hypothesis. Indeed, some evidence was obtained that there may actually have been a deterioration in QOL, as assessed by an apparent increase in sexual dysfunction for patients who received limb-sparing treatment (surgery, radiation therapy, and chemotherapy), when compared with amputees who received surgery and radiotherapy.

It should be noted, however, that two different methods of eliciting data about sexual function yielded different results. When patients were interviewed, subtest analysis (that is, an analysis of results for the individual components of a multifaceted QOL assessment) suggested that there was statistically significant sexual dysfunction for patients who received the limb-sparing treatment regimen, compared with the amputees. However, self-reports of sexual dysfunction did not reveal a statistically significant difference between groups. A similar degree of sexual dysfunction was reported in both types of assessments, for patients who received limb-sparing treatment. In contrast, less sexual dysfunction was reported for some of the amputees in interviews than in self-report assessments, especially for one male and one female amputee. The unexpected results reported by Sugarbaker et al.[14] on sexual dysfunction need to be interpreted cautiously. The number of patients studied was not large, and subtest analysis was required for statistically significant differences to emerge.

It should also be noted that limb salvage is a more complex surgical procedure than amputation, and that salvaged limbs vary as to their degree of function; there is often limitation of motion, instability, and discomfort.[15]

It was postulated that any sexual dysfunction detected after limb-sparing treatment may have been a result of the combined effects of the radiation therapy and chemotherapy on testicular or ovarian dysfunction. Alternatively, decreased limb function associated with radiation fibrosis may have interfered with normal sexual activity.

In 1985, Weddington et al.[15] evaluated the impact of limb-sparing surgery vs. amputation on psychological outcomes. They compared 14 amputees and 9 patients with salvaged limbs, using a battery of assessment instruments. They failed to demonstrate a significant difference between these two treatments. Most patients revealed only minor psychological symptoms, and 55% demonstrated good to excellent adjustment to their surgery and disease. The

TABLE 1
Changes in QOL, for Patients with Extremity Sarcomas, at 12 Months Compared with Pretreatment Evaluations

Parameter	Number of patients				p
	Same	Increased	Decreased	Total	
Joint motion assessment[a]	19	8	21	48	<0.05
Performance of daily activities[a]	28	8	8	44	>0.25
Employment status[b]	36	2	17	55	<0.01
Frequency of intercourse[b]	18	6	23	47	<0.01
Pain (McGill Questionnaire)[b]	17	23	14	54	<0.25
Global QOL (FLIC)[b]	10	25	9	44	<0.01

[a] Results for 56/88 patients with any functional information recorded at 12 months, who had pretreatment data for the parameter of interest.

[b] Results for 57/88 patients with any psychosocial information recorded, pretreatment and at 12 months.

From Chang, A. E., et al., *J. Clin. Oncol.*, 7, 1217, 1989. With permission.

authors[15] concluded that a psychological outcome advantage of limb-salvage surgery compared to amputations has yet to be demonstrated.

It was not clear whether the unexpected results from the studies of Sugarbaker et al.[14] and Weddington et al.[15] reflected difficulties in measuring QOL (including difficulties in relation to the statistical power of the analyses of the data), or the effective rehabilitation of the amputees, or difficulties in the rehabilitation of patients who had multimodal limb-sparing treatment.[16]

Recently, Chang et al.[16] have prospectively evaluated changes in QOL that occurred across time in patients with extremity sarcomas who underwent limb-sparing therapy. Their study provides a good example of the state of the art in the use of QOL assessments.

Among the 88 patients studied by Chang et al.,[16] 60 had high grade sarcomas, with 33 randomized to receive radiation therapy in addition to postoperative chemotherapy. Of the 88 patients, 28 who had low grade or desmoid tumors did not receive chemotherapy; 15 of the 28 were randomized to receive radiotherapy after limb-sparing surgery.

These patients were evaluated over a 3.5 year period. Data from preoperative baseline assessments and the 6- and 12-month periods postoperatively were the most complete. Selected QOL data obtained at 12 months are shown in Table 1. Several aspects of the study deserve mention:

1. *Incompleteness of the data:* At 12 months, only 57 (65%) and 56 (64%) of the 88 patients had provided both pre- and post-treatment data for at least one item of the psychosocial and functional evaluations, respectively.

    As pointed out below (Table 2, item 4), special procedures are needed to minimize missing data. To date, in oncology, gaps in the information are a constant source of concern in the use of QOL assessments; they could introduce bias into the results. It seems unlikely that missing responses would be randomly distributed across the distribution of QOL scores.

2. *Limb function:* A variety of parameters were used to assess limb function. One of these, joint motion assessment, is included in Table 1. A significant proportion of patients showed a decline in joint motion at 12 months. Nonetheless, the performance of daily activities was not impaired in a significant number of patients at 12 months (Table 1). It was not possible to demonstrate from all the data that radiation therapy was the sole factor contributing to changes in limb function. Perhaps the technique of radiation therapy that was used in this study did not contribute to changes in limb

function more than did surgery alone. Alternatively, perhaps the smaller number of patients in each subgroup reduced the power of subgroup comparisons. This study illustrates how the results of subgroup analysis need to be interpreted with caution.

3. *Psychosocial parameters:* Declines were observed in employment status and sexual function. However, the overall QOL, as measured by the Functional Living Index-Cancer (FLIC) of Schipper et al.,[17] was found to be increased (Table 1). It appears that, despite declines in limb function, employment status, and sexual function, patients reported an improved overall QOL. This may be a reflection of an improved outlook on life arising from expectations of cure from disease, not detected by the other measures. However, most measures of overall QOL, such as the FLIC, are designed to describe physical and psychosocial functioning, but do not necessarily provide much information about the underlying reasons for any changes in functioning.

These results illustrate that QOL cannot be defined by a single test. On the one hand, the measures need to be customized to the patients being studied and the research questions being asked. On the other hand, there is likely to be a set of "core" questions about general health status that should normally be considered, if only to screen for unexpected impacts on general health, and especially physical and psychosocial functioning (see below, Table 3, item 6). In addition, it is useful to have one global scale for an overall assessment of QOL. Such global "uniscales"[18-21] are less able to discriminate between groups and are less sensitive to change than are composite measures,[22] but they are simple to use, and may incorporate aspects of a patient's experience not assessed by more specific measures.

B. USES OF QOL DATA OBTAINED FROM CLINICAL TRIALS

When the results of QOL assessments have been obtained within clinical trials, how is that information likely to be used? The long-term goal of QOL assessments should always be to find ways to improve the care of patients. This goal is in accord with the ethical principle of beneficence, that is, the obligation to improve the patient's welfare and well-being.[23] However, another ethical principle also should be taken into account. The ethical principle of respect for the autonomy of the patient requires that the patient's preferences be given a high priority in decision making.[23] Efforts to improve the care of patients should include, to some extent, the involvement of the patients themselves, particularly if QOL assessments are at least partially influenced by patients' perspectives and values about QOL (see also Section II.D).

The results of studies of limb-sparing surgery vs. amputation for patients with soft-tissue sarcoma summarized above illustrate why comparative studies are among those with the greatest potential for QOL assessments (cf. Section II.C). QOL information may be particularly useful in the medical decision-making process when two different treatment modalities can be compared in phase III trials, as is the case for limb-sparing approaches for sarcoma,[16] and also for radical surgery vs. more conservative operations for breast cancer.[24,25] In such situations, where questions about possible differences in QOL are a central feature of the study, the same measures can be used in the same ways to evaluate the QOL of similar groups of patients randomized to one treatment modality or the other.

Taken together, the results illustrate how QOL assessments may be used in attempts to optimize therapies for the treatment of various malignancies. However, comparisons of treatment modalities which merely describe their outcomes, and do not pay specific attention to possible improvements in these modalities in order to minimize any negative impacts on QOL, represent a passive acceptance of such impacts.

A more active stance involves the use of QOL assessments as aids in the development of interventions designed to ameliorate the impacts that cancer (or cancer treatments) may have on quality of life.[25-27] In the case of limb-sparing approaches for sarcoma, as in conservative operations for breast cancer (or, indeed, any other approach to the management

TABLE 2
Strategies for the Incorporation of QOL Assessments into Clinical Trials[a]

1. Select protocols with the greatest potential for the inclusion of QOL assessments.
2. Choose measures with appropriate characteristics (see Table 3).
3. Pay careful attention to the timing of the administration of QOL instruments,[28,75,76] based on features of the protocol design, such as the time of occurrence of treatment toxicity. The frequency of measurement should not be too high, e.g., once every 4 or 5 weeks.[76] It is critical that, regardless of the times chosen for QOL assessments, all patients in the study be assessed at the same times.[28]
4. Use special procedures to minimize missing data, and to maximize quality control and feasibility.[10,28,76-80] Major deterrents include patient burden and staff burden[80] (see also Table 3). For example, a key person, someone who is specially trained and enthusiastic, should be responsible for the collection of QOL data.[76,77] It is particularly noteworthy that patients are often very pleased that someone has finally paid attention to their circumstances and emotions, and discussions may ensue that raise the question of referral to a social worker, psychologist, or psychiatrist.[76] Such discussions, though almost always beneficial, may markedly increase the time required for data collection. They also may occasionally pose unexpected challenges to the professional skills and responsibilities of the data collectors, e.g., by occasionally revealing sensitive issues about quality of patient care and the confidentiality of QOL data collected for research purposes.

[a] Based on the SWOG guidelines.[28] See also Aaronson and Beckman.[81]

of cancer), this involves a continuing effort to find ways to improve QOL, while still trying to maximize the duration of disease- or recurrence-free survival. Of course, oncologists have always had these objectives; QOL assessments simply attempt to provide a more quantitative approach.

C. STRATEGIES FOR QOL ASSESSMENTS IN CLINICAL TRIALS

In this section, some strategies relevant to the incorporation of QOL assessments in clinical trials research will be reviewed briefly. They are summarized in Table 2. Particular emphasis will be placed on the policy recommendations developed recently by the Southwestern Oncology Group (SWOG) to guide the inclusion of quality-of-life end-points in large-scale multi-institutional trials carried out by cancer clinical trials groups.[28]

The primary strategy is only to select protocols with the greatest potential for QOL assessments, because resources are unlikely to permit the inclusion of QOL assessments in every clinical trial. Two practical considerations can serve as useful guides:[28]

- First, is the disease one for which impacts on QOL are widely recognized?
- Second, is there substantial interest in including QOL end-points into the trial?

It should be noted that the SWOG guidelines include a recommendation that only certain classes of phase III studies have the greatest potential for meaningful QOL assessments.[28] High priority studies would include the following:

1. Those studies involving adjuvant therapy for patients at risk of recurrence. QOL assessments are needed to ascertain the extent to which any delays in recurrence which may be achieved by the use of adjuvant therapy may be offset by deterioration in one or more aspects of QOL.
2. Those involving disease sites with an extremely poor prognosis. If there is little realistic prospect of any improvements in duration of survival, then QOL, during the treatment process or subsequently, may be of primary interest.
3. Those comparing different treatment modalities. Comparisons of the risks and benefits of the differing treatment modalities could be misleading, unless the same set of measures is used to evaluate the impact on QOL of the differing treatments, during the treatment process or subsequently.

4. Those involving treatments of different intensities and/or durations. Again, any improvements in conventional outcome measures which may be gained by the use of more intensive therapy may be offset by deterioration in one or more aspects of QOL, during the treatment process or subsequently.

5. Those in which survival is expected to be equivalent, but QOL is expected to show treatment differences. In such studies, QOL during the treatment process or subsequently, is clearly of primary interest.

The priorities listed above are all in relation to phase III trials. The SWOG recommendation that QOL assessments be centered on phase III studies is based on the view that phase II studies are not considered appropriate for assessment of QOL, because they are not comparative. Their purpose is to assess the biological effectiveness of a particular intervention. In comparative studies, the extent of any differences in QOL is compared across groups, and across time. Although the interpretation of apparent differences in the QOL for different groups may pose difficulties (see Section II.D), these difficulties may be less severe than those that may arise when attempts are made to interpret the QOL profile for a single group, in the absence of any control.

However, it could be argued that QOL assessments also should be included in some phase II studies, either in those situations where an impact on quality of life is expected, or when it is anticipated that the main benefit of the intervention will be to quality of life.[29] Indeed, at present, phase II studies of interventions that have some potential to improve QOL may receive a low priority simply because no survival benefit is anticipated. Even in the absence of any comparison, the assessment of QOL in these situations would not only provide systematically collected quantitative data about QOL, but would also have educational value in giving more prominence to QOL issues in the thinking of investigators. It would also provide them with an opportunity to become more familiar with QOL measures, and thus would prepare them to undertake comparative QOL studies in phase III trials.[29]

The SWOG guidelines recommend that QOL measurement instruments for use in clinical trials have several properties. The characteristics of desirable measures are summarized in Table 3. A similar, but more extensive, table of properties has been described by Donovan et al.[26] Neither these characteristics, nor other strategies for the incorporation of QOL assessments into clinical trials (Table 2), will be considered further here, because they are dealt with in detail in other chapters.

D. QUALITY-QUALITY COMPARISONS

QOL data may be used for two main kinds of comparisons. The first is for "quality vs. quality" comparisons; the second for "quality vs. quantity" (quality of survival vs. duration of survival) comparisons. In the first case, survival times are assumed to be equivalent. The "area under the curve" for some measure of QOL, plotted as a function of time, is compared for the groups (Figure 1A). These comparisons depend on the assumptions that the appropriate components of QOL are being compared, and that the groups perceive these components in similar ways. It is also assumed that the QOL measures used yield reliable and valid data and are sensitive enough to reveal clinically interesting differences. In particular, it is assumed that any aggregation of the data done to facilitate plotting of the results has neither obscured relevant differences, nor weighted the various dimensions of QOL in inappropriate ways.[30]

The assumption that the members of the groups being compared perceive the components of QOL in similar ways is unlikely to be a strong one. The relative values placed upon different aspects of QOL may depend on a number of factors,[31] possibly including the experience of the groups during and after treatment. For example, perhaps patients who have experienced more severe treatment toxicity might alter their perception of the severity of any subsequent toxicity, relative to patients who have not previously experienced such toxicity (see, for example, Reference 32).

TABLE 3
Characteristics of Appropriate QOL Measures[a]

1. Assessments should be provided by the patients themselves.
2. Brief questionnaires should be used, e.g., ones that take no longer than 15 to 20 min to complete, and are easy to check for omitted questions, mistakes, etc. immediately after completion.[76]
3. Assessment instruments should have well-established measurement properties, especially in relation to evidence of sensitivity to change (responsiveness).
4. The time frame to be imposed on each item in the questionnaire should be clearly defined, e.g., experience over the past day, past week, or longer? The longer the time frame, the more likely that enduring responses rather than transient variations will be detected, but problems about recall will become more acute as the time frame widens.
5. Use of a categorial response format minimizes the labor involved in processing questionnaires.
6. Measures of physical functioning, emotional functioning, and general symptoms should always be included, along with a global measure of QOL.
7. Additional protocol-specific measures may be required, e.g., tests for social, sexual, or cognitive functioning, although sensitive issues such as prognosis or sexuality should be avoided unless they are specifically required by the protocol.

[a] Based on the SWOG guidelines.[28] See Also Aaronson and Beckmann.[81]

For comparisons of differences in QOL, it would be convenient if a single meaningful holistic score for QOL could be obtained. "Utility-based" QOL assessments have been used in this way for studies in areas other than oncology, such as a trial of an oral gold compound for arthritis.[33] Utility-based approaches have their origins in a theory of decision making under uncertainty described by von Neumann and Morgenstern.[34] The aggregation of scores among persons depends on assumptions about interpersonal comparisons of utilities,[33] which pose difficulties;[35] however, some form of consistency of preferences underlies any valid measure of QOL.[33] The measurement techniques involved in utility-based approaches have been explored in an oncology context,[36,37] but these techniques have not yet been widely used in clinical trials in oncology (see, for example, Reference 38).

Utility-based assessments are particularly useful when attempts are made to combine duration of survival and QOL into a single variable, such as "quality-adjusted life years" (QALYs, see Section IV.B).

Another attractive feature of utility-based QOL assessments is that they provide a systematic, axiomatically based approach to the elicitation of a patient's preferences. They also facilitate patient involvement in clinical decision making.[39] How best to incorporate individual preferences into decision making raises a variety of challenging ethical and methodological issues. Although they will not be considered in any detail here, they form an active area of current research.[39-42]

"Preference utilitarianism", where what is ethically acceptable is determined by the extent to which one's preferences are satisfied, is an underlying ethical issue.[4] Preference utilitarianism has been suggested as a logical next step, supplanting classical "act" and "rule" utilitarianism.[42]

E. QUALITY-QUANTITY COMPARISONS

A second use of QOL data from clinical trials is for "quantity vs. quality" comparisons (Figure 1B). In this case, survival times are *not* assumed to be equivalent. The "area under the curve" for a selected measure of QOL (such as a "utility-based" holistic score, see Section II.D), plotted across time, is combined in some way with survival data. The two sets of combined data are then compared for the groups.

An issue arises when trade-offs between quantity and quality must be made. Such comparisons require the important assumption that it is appropriate to trade-off some specified decrease in quality of life in order to seek some specified increase in duration of life, or vice versa. There is evidence in the literature (see, for example, References 32 and 43) that volunteers, who are not personally involved in such trade-offs, consider them acceptable. There is very little evidence that patients, faced with such trade-offs in considering real-life decisions, would accept such trade-offs to the same extent.

Recent work illustrates the need to examine this issue further.[44] Cancer patients (56 patients with breast, lung, gastrointestinal, or other types of cancer) who had recently agreed to undergo chemotherapy were interviewed prior to their first treatment. They were interviewed again 6 weeks following the initiation of treatment, when they had personally experienced some of the side effects of chemotherapy. The purpose of the study was to test whether or not personal experience with the effects of chemotherapy would influence attitudes toward trade-offs between QOL and duration of survival. The results were unexpected; these particular patients indicated a reluctance to trade off more than a very minor decrease in duration of survival in order to achieve an improved QOL. They showed a similar reluctance whether or not they had experienced the side effects of chemotherapy. Their extreme reluctance to make trade-offs, in comparison with volunteers who participated in other studies,[32,43] raises questions about the extent to which patients close to the time of decision making are willing to trade off survival rate for better quality of life.

Ideally, in this study,[44] the first assessment of these patients' willingness to accept trade-offs should have been done prior to the decision to undergo chemotherapy. It is possible that the patients who participated in this study simply expressed preferences that were consonant with a treatment decision that had already been made, and remained consonant with this decision even after experiencing treatment toxicity. However, the important question of the extent to which willingness to accept QOL-vs.-duration of survival trade-offs is situation dependent still needs to be raised. Suppose that, in general, patients are extremely reluctant to trade-off survival for QOL at the time of decision making, but indicate a willingness to do so if interviewed at other times. If the patient's preferences are to be given a high priority in decision making (see Section II.B), how should this objective best be met? In this example, which preference should predominate? The one expressed at the time of decision making, which would favor aggressive treatments in which prolongation of survival is sought even at the cost of markedly reduced quality of life? Or, the one expressed at other times, which would indicate a less aggressive treatment that would place less emphasis on survival and more on QOL? For clinical decision making, truly relevant preferences, from that patient (or, if necessary, an appropriate surrogate), and expressed close to the time of the actual decision, are likely to predominate.

III. USE OF QOL ASSESSMENTS TO PREDICT OUTCOME OR PROGNOSIS

To illustrate a predictive use of QOL measures, one example will be mentioned briefly. It shows the potential of QOL information for use as stratifying variables for patients entering clinical trials. The example is provided by the results of a quality of life study initiated by the Lung Cancer Study Group (LCSG) in 1985.[45] The purpose of the study was to test and refine the measurement of QOL in lung cancer patients, and to study the relationship of QOL measurement to other clinical parameters, especially recurrence and survival. The QOL instrument used was the Functional Living Index-Cancer (FLIC).[17] The Karnofsky Performance Status[46] was also assessed.

Only preliminary results have been published, but these indicate that the baseline QOL score was a strong and statistically significant prognostic indicator for survival, comparable in predictive power to the extent of disease. In contrast, the Karnofsky Performance Status demonstrated only a marginally significant effect. Similarly, the baseline QOL score was highly prognostic for recurrence, even when the results were adjusted for the influence of other prognostic factors using a multivariate statistical model. These results provide preliminary evidence that QOL scores may be (at least in clinical trials for patients with lung cancer) an important prognostic variable, more suitable for use as a stratifying variable than the Karnofsky Performance Status. It remains to be determined whether or not a baseline QOL score will be useful as a stratifying variable for other disease sites, including those for which the prognosis is not extremely poor.

IV. USE OF QOL MEASURES TO DISCRIMINATE BETWEEN INDIVIDUALS

A major potential use of QOL assessments is within the context of clinical decision making in relation to individual patients. It seems likely that, as the results of QOL measures become more acceptable to practicing clinicians, these measures will increasingly be used in making clinical decisions about withholding or withdrawing treatment. For example, QOL data could provide strong support for the view that a particular patient has a very poor prognosis. If, for medical reasons, or for reasons based on a scarcity of resources, consideration is already being given to limitations on care, then quantitative QOL data are likely to tip the balance.

At the present stage in the development of QOL measures, this type of use is likely to be premature. There are technical reasons for this, in that the sensitivity and specificity of present measures are usually such that they are useful only when results are averaged over the members of a group. They are likely to be misleading if applied to individuals. Unless the sensitivity and specificity of the measures are high, too many false conclusions may be drawn.[47]

A. AN ETHICAL ISSUE

There are other considerations in addition to technical ones that enter into the use of QOL data in clinical decision making. The use of QOL data to discriminate among individuals also has the potential to raise ethical problems. This potential can be illustrated by results obtained from a study designed to measure the extent to which individual differences and situations influence preferences about a medical treatment.[7,48] In this study, 226 women in two Ontario cities were asked for their views about a hypothetical medical decision. In the study design, the disease, a form of malignant lymphoma, did not vary, nor did the proposed choice between a conservative and a radical treatment. What did vary was the description of the hypothetical patient's situation before the onset of disease. The participants in the study each received different situational descriptions, selected randomly from a set of eight; the descriptions ranged from quite favorable to quite unfavorable situations. It was expected that the perceived desirability of the radical treatment relative to the conservative one would be influenced by the situation of the hypothetical patient prior to treatment. A method of utility assessment, based on the "standard gamble",[33,34,36,49] was used to obtain a quantitative assessment of the perceived desirability of the radical treatment, and to express it in terms of a mean desirability score. The "standard gamble" is a utility-based approach[34] (see Section II.D) in which, in essence, the utility of the outcome of a particular option is assessed in terms of the risk of harm one is willing to accept in order to try to obtain (or, alternatively, to avoid) that particular outcome. The desirability scores were averaged across all the participants who received a particular one of the eight situational descriptions.

The results agreed with expectation, in that the respondents showed a statistically significant tendency to be influenced by the characteristics that distinguished one patient from another. The results also indicated that the respondents, on the average, were more likely to advocate gambling on the risky radical treatment in unfavorable situations, and especially when the fictitious patient was physically handicapped, socially isolated, and lacking in the

TABLE 4
Synopsis of One of Eight Descriptions of the Distinguishing Characteristics of Fictitious Patients, Used to Assess Effects of Such Characteristics on Preferences in a Hypothetical Medical Decision[7,48]

Patient A is a 35-year-old unmarried woman who lives in a nursing home for handicapped adults .... She suffered from polio as a child and is crippled for life .... Her adoptive parents are dead and she has become suspicious of people .... She has lost motivation and spends most of her time watching television.

motivation to improve their situation. Some respondents suggested that such patients had "nothing to lose" (see Table 4 for a synopsis of the description of this fictitious patient[48]).

There are several possible interpretations of the results.[7,48] The one that is disturbing from an ethical point of view is that, when the results for the participants were averaged, there emerged a consensus that patients who are physically handicapped, socially isolated, and lacking in motivation to improve their situation, should be advised to accept the greater risk of radical treatment. This apparent consensus brings to mind the ways in which vulnerable groups have been exploited for risky experimental purposes in the past.[50-52] The results of this study illustrate the way that the results of quantitative techniques of QOL assessment could be used to justify, at one extreme, the selection of vulnerable individuals to receive risky radical treatments. At the other extreme, particularly when resources are constrained, QOL assessments could also be used as a justification for withholding treatment from some vulnerable groups, while making the same treatment available to others whose situation or prognosis is assessed to be more favorable. The ethical issue is one of "justice".[23]

The ethical principle of justice also raises fundamental questions about access to health care. There may be vulnerable patients who need treatment but do not receive it. There may also be a risk that all patients will lose some of their dignity and worth through other related applications of QOL to decision making. An example is the incorporation of QOL assessments into decisions about the desirability of different health care programs. This example is considered further in the next section. This is a version of the principle of justice, referred to as "fairness". It refers not only to micro-allocation decisions (involving direct patient care), but also meso- (institutional) and macro- (governmental) decisions about resource allocation. In short, if misused, QOL measures could discriminate not only against individuals, but also against classes of individuals and, potentially, the larger community.[4]

From an optimistic point of view, QOL assessments provide a means to foster improvements in physical and psychosocial health, by recognizing ill-defined problems and focusing attention on them. In doing so, they may contribute to efforts to provide more humane health care. From a pessimistic point of view, however, they do have the potential to contribute to the development of a new social ethic, one which could be used to justify discrimination against those deemed to be "unfit", that is, below some predetermined quality threshold.[7] This warning should be borne in mind whenever the use of QOL measures to "label" individuals is being considered. Decisions to limit care are happening now. There are clear dangers inherent in anyone except the patient making decisions related to his or her personal quality of life.[59]

B. QUALITY-ADJUSTED LIFE YEARS

Measures of duration of life which fail to take into account quality of life are widely assumed to be inadequate as a basis for decisions about the desirability of different health care programs. It is also widely accepted, at least by health economists, that 1 year spent in a particular health state may be preferred to 1 year spent in another state. The concept of quality-adjusted life years (QALYs) has been developed as a means to combine duration of survival and quality of survival into a single variable. The basic idea is that, for any individual, the prospect of living Y years in less than full health may be considered equivalent to the prospect of living X years in perfect health, when $X < Y$.[53-56] When different health care programs are expected to yield different combinations of duration and quality of survival, QALYs provide a simple way to compare them.

As previously discussed (Section II.E), the assumption that people are willing to consider trade-offs between quality and duration of survival is supported by empirical data derived from presumably healthy volunteers.[32,43] Corresponding data about the willingness of patients to consider such trade-offs is lacking.[44] However, it has been argued (e.g., Reference 57) that, for planning decisions about alternative uses of resources, it is the views of the larger population who must pay for the programs, rather than those of the smaller population who will benefit from them, that should be given the greatest weight. Also, initiating a program now, such as a program for cancer prevention, may affect the QOL of anonymous future beneficiaries, for whom "general public" QOL evaluations may be reasonable ones to use. Only for clinical decision-making purposes would it be the patients' views that are clearly the most important.[57,58]

Any separation of "planning decisions" from "clinical decision making" raises concerns about its possible consequences. "Distancing" from the ill may make the planner's job less difficult, but might it impair just and compassionate decision making?[59]

It is beyond the scope of this chapter to discuss the QALY concept in any detail. It will be noted only that there have been objections to the concept on ethical grounds. For example, it has been argued[60,61] that QALYs (1) fallaciously value time lived instead of individual lives; (2) take an excessively narrow view of what quality of life might be; and (3) are unjust. A contrary view[62] is that (1) health care priorities should be influenced by our capacity both to increase life expectation and to improve people's quality of life; (2) a particular improvement in health should be regarded as of equal value, no matter who gets it, and should be provided unless it prevents a greater improvement from being offered to someone else; (3) it is the responsibility of everyone to discriminate (between people) whenever necessary to ensure that our limited resources go where they will do the most good. However, as pointed out earlier (Section IV.A), discrimination between people on the basis of QOL measurements can be a major source of ethical problems. These problems may become even more acute for physicians if the domain of medicine is not limited to the biomedical aspects of the disease (see Section V).

These two positions differ sharply in relation to the importance assigned to keeping people alive, irrespective of how poor their prognosis is, and no matter what sacrifices others have to bear as a consequence. They also differ in the importance assigned to not discriminating between people, not even according to their differential capacity to benefit from treatment.[62] The clash between these two positions is likely to assume much more prominence as concerns about cost containment intensify.

The QALY concept is considered here only because it is being used increasingly as a tool for economic evaluations of different therapeutic options. If this concept is to be used extensively, its apparent simplicity should not be allowed to obscure the methodological and philosophical difficulties it entails.

Some methodological issues involved in the use of QALYs in health care decision making have been reviewed by Loomes and McKenzie,[55] Gafni,[63] and Mehrez and Gafni[64] in articles written for readers familiar with the methodologies used for measuring health state preferences (for reviews of these methodologies, see References 65 to 68). Some of the philosophical difficulties have been mentioned above.

It should be stressed that the purpose of QALYs is to provide an index for combining duration and quality of life, and that the aggregation of scores for different individuals is done on the basis of some explicit algorithm ("social welfare function") which provides weights for each individual. It is not essential to adopt a particular algorithm in which a year of healthy life is weighed equally regardless of who consumes it. For reasons of ethics or policy, or for some other reason, a different algorithm may be preferred, such as one that gives heavier weight to the elderly, or the young, or sufferers from a particular disease. From the viewpoint of the analyst, the choice of algorithm is essentially arbitrary. One needs only to be aware of the implications of the algorithm that has been selected.[69]

Clearly, some rational and justifiable way of incorporating QOL information into policy decisions about health care programs is badly needed, in an era of increasing concern about cost containment. For the purposes of this chapter, all that is required is a warning: the kinds of analyses, such as "cost-utility analysis",[57,58] for which the QALY concept was designed, are not self-contained mathematical analyses that can deliver an objective answer to questions about the cost or worth of programs for health care. These methods of analysis are based on assumptions, and on sets of values, that may not be readily apparent to anyone other than experts in the field. These methods could be manipulated or applied in an inappropriate manner.[70]

V. CONCLUDING COMMENTS

The growing interest in quantitative approaches to QOL assessment in oncology could be regarded as one example of a more general trend of considerable significance. In developed countries, the aging of the population, the increased importance of long-term illnesses, and changes in the economics and organization of health care delivery are posing vexing problems.[71,72] Research focused solely on the biomedical aspects of disease has, by itself, been insufficient to deal with all of these problems. Attention is increasingly being paid to the "clinical basic sciences" (e.g., References 47, 71, and 73), defined here as the "basic" (conceptual or analytic) contributions made by epidemiology, biostatistics, clinical decision making, bioethics, health economics, health psychology, and other aspects of the behavioral and social sciences concerned with the health-related behavior of individuals and groups. These sciences provide an approach to the economic, behavioral and social issues that are relevant to human health.

It has been argued[74] that the domain of medicine should be limited to the biomedical aspects of disease. Nonphysiological factors, such as personal or social factors related to etiology or management, should be left to others. The contrary view is that, if nonphysiological factors are excluded from consideration, important aspects of cancer control may be neglected.[80] A long-standing exposure to the impacts of cancer and its treatment on the quality as well as the duration of survival means that oncologists are likely to be aware of limitations of an exclusive focus on physiological factors, and willing to pay attention to nonphysiological aspects of patient care and cancer control.

It has been pointed out that, if medicine is defined narrowly, others will take up the challenge to wrestle with the broader issues whose resolution is crucial to meeting the whole range of health needs of the general population.[71] Those who accept such a challenge are much more likely to be allocated the resources than those who reject it!

QOL assessment can be regarded as one important step in the direction of a less-narrowly defined research model, e.g., in relation to controlled clinical trials. Some exposure to the "clinical basic sciences" is essential if well-designed QOL assessments are to be carried out. The range of variables to be examined should take into account psychosocial factors as well as physical factors and symptoms. Analysis of the results of QOL studies requires some sophistication in biostatistical methods. Uses of the data involve considerations about clinical decision making and bioethics; examples of these latter considerations have been outlined above.

It may be concluded that the development and use of QOL measures provides a vital link between the traditional emphasis in clinical investigation on the application of biomedical concepts and techniques, and the emerging need for a familiarity with the content and applications of the more broadly based "clinical basic sciences". In the longer term, this linkage, and the shifts in attitudes that it provokes, may prove to have more impact on health care than will the QOL assessments themselves.

ACKNOWLEDGMENTS

The author thanks N. F. Boyd, D. R. Carlow, D. H. Feeney, R. Feld, P. J. Goodwin, E. M. Meslin, D. Osoba, K. I. Pritchard, J. S. Senn, H. J. Sutherland, and D. Warr for their helpful comments and criticisms. The usual disclaimer about responsibility of anyone but the author for errors or faulty interpretations applies. Career support through the Ontario Cancer Treatment and Research Foundation, and grant support from the National Cancer Institute of Canada and the Medical Research Council of Canada, are gratefully acknowledged.

REFERENCES

1. Bush, R. S., *Malignancies of the Ovary, Uterus and Cervix*, Edward Arnold, London, 1979, sect. I.
2. Roberts, F., The radiation treatment of neoplasms. VI, *Br. J. Radiol.*, 7, 151, 1934.
3. Jonsen, A. R., Siegler, M., and Winslade, W. J., *Clinical Ethics: A Practical Approach to Ethical Decisions in Clinical Medicine*, 2nd ed., MacMillan, New York, 1986, chap. 3.
4. Meslin, E. M., personal communication.
5. Feeny, D. H., et al., chapter 6, this volume.
6. Guyatt, G. H., Van Zanten, S. J. O. V., Feeny, D. H., and Patrick, D. L., Measuring quality of life in clinical trials: a taxonomy and review, *Can. Med. Assoc. J.*, 140, 1441, 1989.
7. Till, J. E., Quality-of-life assessment: beware the tyranny of the majority, *Humane Med.*, 2, 100, 1986.
8. Taylor, T. R., Commentary, *J. Fam. Practice*, 28, 407, 1989.
9. DeBoer, G., Bean, H., Brazier, T., Elhakim, T., Elliott, J., Howatson, A., McCartney, M., and Till, J., Evaluation of cancer treatment: use of a medical info system to compare costs of alternative modes of treatment for advanced indolent malignant lymphoma, in *MEDINFO-83*, North-Holland, Amsterdam, 1983, 233.
10. Yates, J. W., Quality of life assessment and health policy decisions, in *Assessment of Quality of Life and Cancer Treatment*, Ventrafridda, V., van Dam, F. S. A. M., Yancik, R., and Tamburini, M., Eds., Excerpta Medica, Amsterdam, 1986, 211.
11. O'Sullivan, B., Limb-sparing measurement in extremity soft-tissue sarcomas in the adult, *Can. J. Surg.*, 31, 397, 1988.
12. Shibata, H. R., Definitive surgical management for soft-tissue sarcomas, *Can. J. Surg.*, 31, 407, 1988.

13. Temple, W. J., Bramwell, V., Eisenhauer, E., Jenkin, R. D. T., Langer, F., and Worth, A. J., Guidelines for the surgical management of soft-tissue sarcoma, Report of the Canadian Sarcoma Group, *Can. J. Surg.*, 31, 410, 1988.

14. Sugarbaker, P. H., Barofsky, I., Rosenberg, S. A., and Gianola, F. J., Quality of life assessment of patients in extremity sarcoma trials, *Surgery*, 91, 17, 1982.

15. Weddington, W. W., Jr., Segraves, K. B., and Simon, M. A., Psychological outcome of extremity sarcoma survivors undergoing amputation or limb salvage, *J. Clin. Oncol.*, 3, 1393, 1985.

16. Chang, A. E., Steinberg, S. M., Culnane, M., Lampert, M. H., Reggia, A. J., Simpson, C. G., Hicks, J. E., White, D. E., Yang, J. J., Glatstein, E., and Rosenberg, S. A., Functional and psychosocial effects of multimodality limb-sparing therapy in patients with soft tissue sarcomas, *J. Clin. Oncol.*, 7, 1217, 1989.

17. Schipper, H., Clinch, J., McMurray, A., and Levitt, M., Measuring the quality of life of cancer patients: the Functional Living Index-Cancer: development and validation, *J. Clin. Oncol.*, 2, 472, 1984.

18. Spitzer, W. O., Dobson, A. J., Hall, J., Chesterman, E., Levi, J., Shepherd, R., Battista, R. N., and Catchlove, B. R., Measuring quality of life of cancer patients: a concise QL-Index for use by physicians, *J. Chronic Dis.*, 34, 585, 1981.

19. Selby, P. J., Chapman, J.-A. W., Etazadi-Amoli, J., Dalley, D., and Boyd, N. F., The development of a method for assessing the quality of life of cancer patients, *Br. J. Cancer*, 50, 13, 1984.

20. Gough, I. R., Furnival, C. M., Schilder, L., and Grove, W., Assessment of the quality of life of patients with advanced cancer, *Eur. J. Cancer Clin. Oncol.*, 19, 1161, 1983.

21. Coates, A., Dillenbeck, C. F., McNeil, D. R., Kaye, S. B., Sims, K., Fox, R. M., Woods, R. L., Milton, G. W., Solomon, J., and Tattersall, M. H. N., On the receiving end. II. Linear analogue self-assessment (LASA) in evaluation of aspects of the quality of life of cancer patients receiving therapy, *Eur. J. Cancer Clin. Oncol.*, 19, 1633, 1983.

22. Ciampi, A., Lockwood, G., Sutherland, H. J., Llewellyn-Thomas, H. A., and Till, J. E., Assessment of health-related quality of life: factor scales for patients with breast cancer, *J. Psychosoc. Oncol.*, 6, 1, 1988.

23. Beauchamp, T. L. and Childress, J. F., *Principles of Biomedical Ethics*, 3rd ed., Oxford University Press, New York, 1989.

24. Lasry, J.-C. M., Margolese, R. G., Poisson, R., Shibata, H., Fleischer, D., Lafleur, D., Legault, S., and Taillefer, S., Depression and body image following mastectomy and lumpectomy, *J. Chronic Dis.*, 40, 529, 1987.

25. Maguire, P., Using measures of psychological impact of disease to inform clinical practice, in *Assessment of Quality of Life and Cancer Treatment*, Ventrafridda, V., van Dam, F. S. A. M., Yancik, R., and Tamburini, M., Eds., Excerpta Medica, Amsterdam, 1986, 119.

26. Donovan, K., Sanson-Fisher, R. W., and Redman, S., Measuring quality of life in cancer patients, *J. Clin. Oncol.*, 7, 959, 1989.

27. Till, J. E., Quality of survival, in *Medical Radiology: Innovations in Radiation Oncology*, Withers, H. R. and Peters, L. J., Eds., Springer-Verlag, Berlin, 1988, 25.

28. Moinpour, C. M., Feigl, P., Metch, B., Hayden, K. A., Meyskens, F. L., Jr., and Crowley, J., Quality of life end points in cancer clinical trials: review and recommendations, *J. Natl. Cancer Inst.*, 81, 485, 1989.

29. Osoba, D., personal communication.

30. Till, J. E., McNeil, B. J., and Bush, R. S., Measurement of multiple components of quality of life, *Cancer Treat. Symp.*, 1, 177, 1984.

31. Culyer, A. J., *Measuring Health: Lessons for Ontario*, Ontario Economic Council, Toronto, 1978.

32. Sackett, D. L. and Torrance, G. W., The utility of different health states as perceived by the general public, *J. Chronic Dis.*, 31, 697, 1978.

33. Feeny, D. H. and Torrance, G. W., Incorporating utility-based quality-of-life assessment measures in clinical trials, *Med. Care*, 27, S190, 1989.

34. von Neumann, J. and Morgenstern, O., *Theory of Games and Economic Behavior*, 2nd ed., Princeton University Press, Princeton, NJ, 1947.

35. Arrow, K. J., *Social Choice and Individual Values*, 2nd ed., Yale University Press, New Haven, CT, 1963.

36. Llewellyn-Thomas, H., Sutherland, H. J., Tibshirani, R., Ciampi, A., Till, J. E., and Boyd, N. F., The measurement of patients' values in medicine, *Med. Decision Making*, 2, 449, 1982.

37. Llewellyn-Thomas, H., Sutherland, H. J., Tibshirani, R., Ciampi, A., Till, J. E., and Boyd, N. F., Describing health states: methodological issues in obtaining values for health states, *Med. Care*, 22, 543, 1984.

38. Dones, L., Wiltshaw, E., Birkhead, B. G., and Jackson, R. R. P., Towards an assessment of toxicity in the treatment of ovarian cancer, *Cancer Chemother. Pharmacol.*, 20, 213, 1987.

39. Schwartz, S. and Griffin, T., *Medical Thinking: The Psychology of Medical Judgment and Decision Making*, Springer-Verlag, New York, 1986, 227.

40. Sutherland, H. J., Llewellyn-Thomas, H. A., Lockwood, G. A., Tritchler, D. L., and Till, J. E., Cancer patients: their desire for information and participation in treatment decisions, *J. R. Soc. Med.*, 82, 260, 1989.

41. O'Connor, A. M. C., Boyd, N. F., Tritchler, D. L., Kriukov, Y., Sutherland, H. J., and Till, J. E., Eliciting preferences for alternative cancer drug treatments: the influence of framing, medium, and rater variables, *Med. Decision Making*, 5, 453, 1985.

42. Beauchamp, T. L., Ethical theory and bioethics, in *Contemporary Issues in Bioethics*, 3rd ed., Beauchamp, T. L. and Walters, L., Eds., Wadsworth, Belmont, CA, 1989.

43. Sutherland, H. J., Llewellyn-Thomas, H., Boyd, N. F., and Till, J. E., Attitudes toward quality of survival: the concept of "maximal endurable time", *Med. Decision Making*, 2, 299, 1982.

44. O'Connor, A. M. C., Boyd, N. F., Warde, P., Stolbach, L., and Till, J. E., Eliciting preferences for alternative drug therapies in oncology: influence of treatment outcome description, elicitation technique and treatment experience on preferences, *J. Chronic Dis.*, 40, 811, 1987.

45. Ruckdeschel, J. C. and Piantadosi, S., for the Lung Cancer Study Group, Assessment of quality of life (QL) by the Functional Living Index-Cancer (FLIC) is superior to performance status for prediction of survival in patients with lung cancer, *Proc. ASCO*, 8, 311, 1989.

46. Karnofsky, D. A. and Burchenal, J. H., The clinical evaluation of chemotherapeutic agents in cancer, in *Evaluation of Chemotherapeutic Agents*, Macleod, C. M., Ed., Columbia University Press, New York, 1949, 191.

47. Sackett, D. L., Haynes, R. B., and Tugwell, P., *Clinical Epidemiology*, Little, Brown, Boston, 1985.

48. Ciampi, A., Silberfeld, M., and Till, J. E., Measurement of individual preferences: the importance of "situation-specific" variables, *Med. Decision Making*, 2, 483, 1982.

49. Torrance, G. W., Social preferences for health states: an empirical evaluation of three measurement techniques, *Socioecon. Plann. Sci.*, 10, 129, 1976.

50. Beecher, H. K., *Research and the Individual: Human Studies*, Little, Brown, Boston, 1970.

51. Levine, R. J., *Ethics and Regulation of Clinical Research*, 2nd ed., Urban and Schwarzenberg, Baltimore, 1986, chap. 4.

52. Faden, R. R. and Beauchamp, T. L., *A History and Theory of Informed Consent*, Oxford University Press, New York, 1986, chap. 5.

53. Weinstein, M. C. and Stason, W. B., Foundations of cost-effectiveness analysis for health and medical practices, *N. Engl. J. Med.*, 296, 716, 1977.

54. Williams, A., The value of QALYs, *Health Soc. Serv. J.*, July, 1985, 5.

55. Loomes, G. and McKenzie, L., The use of QALYs in health care decision making, *Soc. Sci. Med.*, 28, 299, 1989.

56. Carr-Hill, R. A., Assumptions of the QALY procedure, *Soc. Sci. Med.*, 29, 469, 1989.

57. Drummond, M. F., Stoddard, G. L., and Torrance, G. W., *Methods for the Economic Evaluation of Health Care Programmes*, Oxford University Press, Oxford, 1987, 112.

58. Torrance, G. W., Measurement of health state utilities for economic appraisal, *J. Health Econ.*, 5, 1, 1986.

59. Senn, J. S., Advocate for all patients: the physician in health-policy formulation, *Humane Med.*, 4, 24, 1988.

60. Harris, J., Life: quality, value and justice, *Health Policy*, 10, 259, 1988.

61. Harris, J., QALYfying the value of life, *J. Med. Ethics*, 13, 117, 1987.

62. Williams, A., Response: QALYfying the value of life, *J. Med. Ethics*, 13, 123, 1987.

63. Gafni, A., The quality of QALYs (quality-adjusted-life-years): do QALYs measure what they at least intend to measure?, *Health Policy*, 13, 81, 1989.

64. Mehrez, A. and Gafni, A., Quality-adjusted life years, utility theory, and healthy-years equivalents, *Med. Decision Making*, 9, 142, 1989.

65. Froberg, D. G. and Kane, R. L., Methodology for measuring health-state preferences. I. Measurement strategies, *J. Clin. Epidemiol.*, 42, 345, 1989.

66. Froberg, D. G. and Kane, R. L., Methodology for measuring health-state preferences. II. Scaling methods, *J. Clin. Epidemiol.*, 42, 459, 1989.

67. Froberg, D. G. and Kane, R. L., Methodology for measuring health-state preferences. III. Population and context effects, *J. Clin. Epidemiol.*, 42, 585, 1989.

68. Froberg, D. G. and Kane, R. L., Methodology for measuring health-state preferences. IV. Progress and a research agenda, *J. Clin. Epidemiol.*, 42, 675, 1989.

69. Feeney, D. H., personal communication.

70. Emery, D. D. and Schneiderman, L. J., Cost-effectiveness analysis in health care, *Hastings Center Report*, 8, July/August 1989.

71. **Schroeder, S. A., Zones, J. S., and Showstack, J. A.,** Academic medicine as a public trust, *JAMA,* 262, 803, 1989.
72. **Mustard, J. F.,** in *Proceedings of the Conference on Health in the '80s and '90s and its Impact on Health Sciences Education, Council of Ontario Universities,* 1983, 3.
73. **Feinstein, A. R.,** Models, methods and goals, *J. Clin. Epidemiol.,* 42, 301, 1989.
74. **Seldin, D. W.,** The boundaries of medicine, *Trans. Assoc. Am. Physicians,* 94, lxxv, 1981.
75. **Fayers, P. M. and Jones, D. R.,** Measuring and analysing the quality of life in cancer clinical trials: a review, *Stat. Med.,* 2, 429, 1983.
76. **van Dam, F. S. A. M., Linssen, C. A. G., and Couzijn, A. L.,** Evaluating 'quality of life' in cancer clinical trials, in *Cancer Clinical Trials: Methods and Practice,* Buyse, M. E., Staquet, M. J., and Sylvester, R. J., Eds., Oxford University Press, Oxford, 1984, 26.
77. **Aaronson, N. K.,** Methodological issues in psychosocial oncology with special reference to clinical trials, in *Assessment of Quality of Life and Cancer Treatment,* Ventrafridda, V., van Dam, F. S. A. M., Yancik, R., and Tamburini, M., Eds., Excerpta Medica, Amsterdam, 1986, 29.
78. **Aaronson, N. K., Bullinger, M., and Ahmedzai, S.,** A modular approach to quality-of-life assessment in clinical trials, *Rec. Results Cancer Res.,* 111, 231, 1988.
79. **Aaronson, N. K., van Dam, F. S. A. M., Polak, C. E., and Zittoun, R.,** Prospects and problems in European psychosocial oncology: a survey of the EROTC Study Group on Quality of Life, *J. Psychosoc. Oncol.,* 4(4), 43, 1986.
80. **Yancik, R. and Yates, J. W.,** Quality-of-life assessment of cancer patients: conceptual and methodological challenges and constraints, *Cancer Bull.,* 38, 217, 1986.
81. **Aaronson, N. K. and Beckmann, J. H.,** Eds., *Quality of Life of Cancer Patients,* Raven Press, New York, 1987.

Chapter 12

CANCER PATIENTS' UNMET SUPPORT NEEDS AS A QUALITY-OF-LIFE INDICATOR

Vincent Mor, Edward Guadagnoli, and Rebecca B. Rosenstein

TABLE OF CONTENTS

I. INTRODUCTION

In recent years, consideration of individuals' quality of life as a dominant factor in case-specific treatment and health financing decisions has rapidly moved from the domain of health service researchers to the applied world of public policy makers and the popular press. Increasingly, advocates for new technologies and proponents of rationing life prolonging techniques rationalize their positions on the basis of estimated quality adjusted years of survival. The widespread adoption of this concept of quality of life for public policy development makes it incumbent upon researchers to both understand and report which aspect of quality of life they are studying. A number of general quality-of-life indices have been reported and repeatedly tested in the literature.[1-3] Disease-specific measures have also been developed and widely reported, particularly for oncology and advanced cardiac patient populations since the consequences of treatment choices for many of these patients are best assessed in terms of quality of life rather than survival.[4-8]

Although most can be summarized into a single aggregate score, quality-of-life indices have generally been constructed to be multidimensional. Analyses of the interrelationship among the separate dimensions has frequently found them to be strongly correlated.[6,9,10] The common underlying dimension of such scales is the patient's health status. Accordingly, quality-of-life measures are frequently characterized as capturing health-related quality of life.[11] The empirical basis for the dominant role of health status is demonstrated by the fact that the physical health items in scales such as the Spitzer Quality of Life Index[4] as well as Symptom Impact Profile[1] and the Quality of Well Being Scale[2] are strongly correlated with the other items which do not ostensibly measure health status. Even in the Functional Living Index-Cancer, which developed a factor based on differentiation between physical, emotional, and social subscales, these parameters are correlated.[6] The pre-eminence of health in such scales appears to be consistent with personal and public valuation of positive health states.

In spite of the importance of health, other aspects of life are surely relevant to the patient. In the cancer arena, Heinrich and colleagues have focused on the multiplicity of problems patients encounter that are attributable to the disease and its treatment.[12] The relevance of this approach as a measure of quality of life is that the more disease and treatment problems patients have, the less likely that they will be able to enjoy their lives. Such a measure has some advantages over standardized scales since patient's responses are also very useful for care planning. However, the definition of such problems is highly subjective. Analyses of the resulting Cancer Inventory of Problem Situations (CIPS) scale reveal that it is highly correlated with the Karnofsky Performance Status index and other physical measures among cancer patients undergoing treatment.

Another approach, derived from the gerontological literature, is to assess patients' need for services as well as whether those needs are being met.[13-15] This approach is relevant to care planning as is the CIPS, but it explicitly defines patients' needs on the basis of health-related functional deficits, making it less relativistic than the CIPS. Unmet need is present only if the patient cannot perform, or has difficulty performing, needed tasks independently *and* if the individuals' existing family network and/or formal services are insufficient to meet the patients' need. Considering the degree of *unmet* need as a measure of quality of life among cancer patients addresses the clinical utility aspects of quality-of-life measures originally suggested by Spitzer.[16] Unmet need for assistance with daily living could also be used as an outcome measure to assess the effect two different treatments have on patients' and families' ability to undertake everyday tasks of living that are complicated by disease advance, treatment toxicity, and associated demands such as special meals, homes, symptom management, etc.[17]

The purpose of this chapter is to introduce and operationalize the measurement of patients' unmet need for community support services as an indicator of patients' quality of life. Unmet need is conceptualized as a function of both the physiological effects of disease and treatment and the associated support pressures. We present data on the prevalence of cancer patients' need and unmet need for support services, the correlates of need and unmet need and the incidence of changes over a 6-month period among patients with advanced cancer.

II. METHODS

Data for the current study were derived from a large scale survey of medical oncology patients undergoing chemotherapy in Rhode Island. Data were obtained by telephone interview by trained interviewers with over 2 years experience interviewing cancer patients regarding their treatments and reactions. In order to increase our understanding of the natural history of needs among cancer outpatients, we interviewed a subsample of patients 6 to 9 months after their initial interview. We selected only patients with metastatic disease to observe a maximal amount of change in the level of reported need and unmet need. Given the progressive nature of the disease, we expected metastatic patients to be more likely to report a change in need status over time. The follow-up and baseline interviews were identical.

A. SAMPLE

Two of Rhode Island's five hospital-based oncology clinics and eight of the State's 19 private oncology practices provided names of patients undergoing active chemotherapy to study personnel. Study-eligible patients had to have been treated within 1 month of interview and were 21 years of age or older. There were no eligibility restrictions governing the type of chemotherapy received, nor the type of cancer.

Following patient identification, and with physician permission, patients were sent a letter describing the study which requested their participation and informed them that they would be telephoned soon to arrange a time for the proposed study interview. Provisions for a proxy respondent (in all cases a family member) were made in cases where the patient was either physically, cognitively, or emotionally unable to complete an interview.

B. INTERVIEW CONTENT

The 45- to 55-min telephone interview was designed to assess patients' daily living needs, symptom experience, and functional status as well as demographic characteristics and features of the social support available to them. The domains of specific interest for analyses reported here include patient need and unmet need, physical functioning, symptom, and social support. The measurement framework for each of these is described below.

C. FUNCTION BASED NEED DETERMINATION

We grouped patients' reports under three life-functioning domains (personal, intrumental, and administrative) that have been commonly reported in the gerontological literature.[13,14] We have found this approach useful in characterizing needs of cancer patients as well.[15,17] Bathing and mobility were the activities that comprised the personal care domain. Only these personal activities of daily living were selected because as out-patients we did not expect many in the sample to report need for assistance with activities that are lower on the activities of daily living hierarchy.[18,19] The instrumental domain included meal preparation, light housework, heavy housework, shopping, transportation to physician, and transportation for other purposes. Home health care, home chemotherapy, and child care were also independently assessed during the interview with virtually no patients reported to require assistance in any of these areas. Activities within the administrative domain included completing forms and paperwork such as insurance claims and applications for government assistance, financial counseling, legal counseling, and obtaining information about cancer treatment.

For each activity, we determined the patients' needs status in terms of whether they were able to independently perform all aspects of the specific activity. Independent performance of the activity, per se, meant that the individual had no need for assistance. Met need existed if an individual was unable to perform the activity independently and they received assistance for that activity and reported that no additional assistance was required. If the patient required assistance with the task and none was provided or if additional assistance was required, unmet need existed. We created separate dependent variables for each of these domains reflecting the number of areas of need or unmet needs present. Additionally, an overall summary indicator of needs and unmet needs across all domains was constructed.

D. MEASURES OF PHYSICAL HEALTH

Health status measures included in the interview were self-reported symptoms, recent hospitalizations, restricted activity days, bed days, and the Spitzer Quality of Life Index.[16] Patients reported whether they experienced any of 17 pre-defined symptoms (e.g., pain, nausea and vomiting, dry mouth, etc.) in the 2 weeks prior to the interview. We also asked patients whether they had been hospitalized in the month prior to the interview. Two other health status measures were obtained — number of days spent in bed and number of days patients cut down on activity normally performed due to illness or injury. Both of these questions were taken from standardized health interview survey items and reflect patients' reported status 2 weeks prior to the interview.

We also used the Spitzer Quality of Life Index in the self-report mode over the telephone. Previous research with this and similar samples of cancer patients suggest comparable levels of reliability and validity in using the telephone vs. in person interview format.[9] The QLI is a five-item instrument specifically designed to measure the health-related quality of life of patients receiving medical care and captures five domains of functioning (activity, physical health, emotional health, social interaction, and overall health). High scores indicate higher quality of life. Earlier research on this measure reveals that it is primarily associated with physical functioning.[9,20]

E. SOCIAL SUPPORT MEASURES

We included several measures of social support, specifically the size of the helping network and its perceived resiliency. Patients reported the number of people they felt were available to provide help to them, or the number that they could most rely on if they were to need help. The resiliency of the helping network was measured by patients' reported level of confidence (five levels: very confident to not at all confident) that others were available to provide, or to continue to provide, assistance with daily living needs.

F. ANALYTIC APPROACH

Our analyses were conducted in three stages. First, descriptive and correlational analyses of the need and unmet need variables within and across domains in relation to the social support characteristics of patients. Next, we related both need variables to survival among the metastatic patients selected for reinterview. Finally, we used the follow-up sample to assess the stability of need and unmet need over time in the population of surviving metastatic disease patients.

All bivariate relationships are assessed in terms of the Pearson chi-square statistic. In the case of ordinal measures, Kendalls tau and Spearman's rho are used as measures of association. In assessing the stability of reported need and unmet need, status over time, Cohen's kappa was calculated as a measure of stability for each individual activity area.

III. RESULTS

A. SAMPLE DESCRIPTION

A total of 597 patients were identified over a 6-month period beginning in April, 1986. Treating physicians denied permission to contact only 11 (1.8%) eligible patients in all participating practices. Prior to interview, 24 (4%) patients died, and we were unable to locate an additional 32 (5.4%) patients. Additionally, 119 (19.3%) patients refused to be interviewed either directly, or a family member refused. A total of 413 patients were interviewed. Those patients who refused to be interviewed did not differ from respondents with respect to gender and treatment location (hospital based clinic vs. private oncology office), however, refusers were older. Proxies responded more frequently for males (16%) than for females (4%; $p < 0.001$).

Table 1 presents the descriptive characteristics of the baseline sample of study subjects. Nearly half (47%) had a diagnosis of breast cancer which is consistent with the high proportion of females (71%) in the sample. The average patient age in this predominantly white sample was 60.3 years and ranged 21 to 91 years. Over half (63%) were married and 80% lived with at least one other person. A third of the patients were employed at the time of interview and most (54%) had been diagnosed for at least 1 year prior to the interview. Fifty-eight percent of the patients had metastatic disease based on medical record data and 63% were receiving a palliative regimen of chemotherapy at the time of identification for the study (treatment for symptom relief) while one quarter were receiving adjuvant treatment, with the remaining patients receiving treatment that had a curative intent. Proxy patients accounted for only 31 interviews.

Of the 220 metastatic patients initially interviewed, 71 or (32.3%) died before the second interview could be conducted, 25 (11.4%) refused to be reinterviewed or were lost to follow-up. The remaining 124 patients completed the second interview 6 to 8 months after the first.

Overall, only 14.3% of the patients needed assistance performing personal activities. In the instrumental domain 32% had a need of assistance in two or fewer areas, 42% needed assistance in three to five activities, and 26% needed help in six or more activities. The majority (57%) needed no assistance in administrative activities while 31% reported needing help in one activity and 12% reported needing help in two or more activities. Patients with need for assistance in personal and administrative activities were highly likely to have instrumental needs as well; 100% of patients with personal needs and 94% of those with administrative needs had at least one instrumental need. Although most patients with personal needs had administrative needs as well (70%), fewer than half (46%) of patients with instrumental needs had need for assistance with administrative activities.

Almost half of the sample reported they had five or fewer individuals available to help with their daily living (only 3% said no one was available) while one third reported having six to ten persons available and the remainder reported having more than ten helpers. With respect to perceived resiliency, 57% of the patients reporting maintained that they were extremely confident that their family and friends could help, or continue to help them. Only 22% of the sample maintained that they were only somewhat, or not at all, confident that they could continue to receive the assistance they needed. The amount of confidence patients expressed in the continued ability of their family and friends to assist them increased as the number of family members and friends available increased.

B. CORRELATES OF NEED

Table 2 presents the relationship between need for assistance and various measures of physical status. The total number of instrumental needs is highly correlated with the number of symptoms patients reported (Spearmans rho $= .49$ $p < 0.001$), the Spitzer QLI (Spearmans rho $= -.59$ $p < 0.001$), the number of days spent in bed and the number of days of

TABLE 1
Demographic Characteristics of
Sample

Variable	N	%
Age		
21—44	56	17.0
45—54	69	16.7
55—64	110	26.6
65—74	120	29.1
75—91	58	14.0
Sex		
Male	174	30.6
Female	291	71.3
Race		
White	401	97.6
Non-white	10	2.4
Marital status		
Married	257	62.2
Widowed	88	21.3
Divorced/separated	37	9.0
Never married	31	7.5
Education		
<High school	112	27.4
High school	144	35.2
Some college	64	15.6
College graduate	36	8.8
Postgraduate	53	13.0
Religion		
Protestant	119	30.2
Catholic	235	59.6
Jewish	18	4.6
Other/none	22	5.6
Employment status		
Not employed	278	67.3
Employed	135	32.7
Income		
$0 to $15,000	116	40.7
$15,000 to $30,000	84	29.5
$30,000 to $45,000	36	12.6
$45,001 +	49	17.2
Household composition		
Lives alone	83	20.2
Lives with one	171	41.6
Lives with two or more	157	28.2
Cancer type		
Breast	193	47.2
Lung	27	6.6
Colorectal	32	7.8
Gyn	20	4.9
Other	137	33.5
Intent of treatment		
Curative	49	12.1
Adjuvant	103	25.4
Palliative	254	62.6
Number of symptoms		
0—3	160	38.7
4—6	126	30.5
7—9	93	22.5
10+	26	6.3

TABLE 2
Physical Status and Needs

Measure of physical status	Percent with any personal need	Percent with 0—2, 3—5, 6—8 instrumental needs			Percent with 0, 1, 2+ administrative needs		
Number of Symptoms							
0—3	3.2	52.3	39.9	7.8	69.7	23.9	6.5
4—8	17.3	22.0	45.2	32.2	52.5	35.0	12.6
9—14	31.6	8.9	37.5	53.6	36.4	41.8	21.8
Days in Bed in Past 2 Weeks							
0	8.9	37.7	44.6	17.7	61.0	31.0	8.0
1—7	16.4	14.8	37.0	48.1	56.4	23.6	20.0
8—14	58.3	8.6	25.7	65.7	21.2	48.5	30.3
Hospitalization Past Month							
No	12.1	36.2	41.1	22.7	57.9	30.4	11.7
Yes	25.0	13.3	46.7	40.0	49.2	38.1	12.7
Activity Decrease Past Month							
No	12.7	44.7	37.7	17.7	61.9	27.5	10.6
Yes	15.7	16.9	46.6	36.5	50.8	36.5	12.7
Spitzer Quality of Life Index							
10	0.0	61.8	36.3	2.0	69.2	24.3	6.5
7—9	7.7	29.0	50.8	20.2	61.1	30.1	8.8
0—6	41.7	7.1	29.6	63.3	35.4	42.4	22.2

decreased activity in the preceding 2 weeks (Spearmans rho= .36 and .29, respectively, <0.001). Need was also related to disease characteristics. Breast cancer patients, those with metastatic disease and those receiving palliative treatment, were more likely to have instrumental needs than were those with other types of cancer (all p's <0.01).

Our examination of the relationship between social support measures and patients' level of reported need revealed that the number of helpers was not significantly correlated with the number of instrumental or administrative needs, but that the presence of personal needs appeared to be related to the number of helpers available (Kendalls tau = $-41.2\,p$ <0.002). On the other hand, patients' perceived resiliency of their helping network decreased as a function of the number of personal, instrumental, and administrative needs. For example, 60% of the patients with no personal needs were extremely confident of the continued ability of their family and friends to provide needed assistance, but only 37% of those with at least one personal need were extremely confident ($p = 0.001$). Similarly, the higher the number of instrumental needs, the less likely that patients reported that they were extremely confident of continued support; 62% of those with two instrumental needs vs. 44% of those with six to eight instrumental needs; ($p = 0.003$).

C. PREVALENCE AND CORRELATES OF UNMET NEED

Four and one half percent of study patients reported having had an unmet need for personal activities, 18.5% with instrumental activities, and 11.4% with administrative activities. Overall, 28.8% study patients reported having unmet needs in at least one area; 21% had unmet need in only one area, 6.5% in two, and 1.3% in all three domains.

TABLE 3
Proportion of Patients with Unmet Need by Social Support (Resiliency) and Number of Needs in Each Domain

Domain of need	Number of needs	N	Perceived resiliency of social support	
			Low	High
Personal	1	23	50.0	9.1
	2	15	58.3	66.7
Instrumental	1—2	79	22.2	0.0
	3—5	151	48.3	11.0
	6—8	73	39.0	3.1
Administrative	1	105	27.7	12.1
	2+	32	52.9	53.3
All types	1—3	107	28.6	9.7
	4—6	141	50.9	14.3
	7—8	42	55.6	13.3
	9+	19	72.7	50.0

Unmet need was partially related to patients' physical status. In general, the more needs a patient reported in a given area, the more likely at least one of those would be unmet. For example, 17% of patients with one, 49% of patients with two, and 60% of patients with three needs in the administrative domain reported an unmet need for at least one administrative activity. Similarly, among patients reporting only one or two needs in the instrumental domain, 7.5% reported an unmet need while of those reporting six or more areas of need activities in the instrumental domain, 26% had an unmet need.

Unmet need was particularly related to social support. Table 3 presents unmet need in relation to both the number of activities in which patients' needed assistance and social support as measured by patients' perceived resiliency of their helping network. For the most part, patients with higher perceived resiliency were less likely to have an unmet need at any given level of need for assistance in any need domain than were individuals without resilient systems. Major exceptions to this generalization are in the area of personal and administrative domains of individuals with two or more needs. In this small number of cases, the beneficial effects of a highly resilient support network seem to be overwhelmed by multiple needs. Within the instrumental activity areas, the proportion of people with highly resilient support networks having any unmet needs is substantially lower than is the case for persons without resilient networks. Across all areas, in general, those patients with resilient support networks are only one third as likely to have unmet needs as are those without resilient support networks, regardless of the level of need patients have.

We conducted loglinear analyses on the data presented in Table 3 to separately test the effect of the resiliency by needs interaction in predicting the level of unmet needs within each domain as well as for the summary measures of unmet need. For all four equations (personal, instrumental, administrative, and the summary) the level of need patients reported was a highly significant determinant of unmet. For the instrumental needs and the overall needs models the resiliency of the support network was also highly significant. In no case did we observe a significant interaction between resiliency and need level, suggesting that resiliency did not appear to arise as a function of the presence of patient need.

A similar pattern to that displayed in Table 3 was observed when the strength of the social support network was measured by the number of individuals available to help. For example, among patients with four to six needs overall, 42% of those with one to three helpers as opposed to 23% of those with seven to ten helpers had an unmet need. The

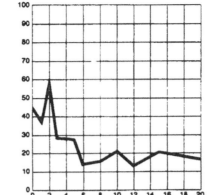

PERCENT WITH
UNMET NEEDS

NUMBER OF HELPERS

FIGURE 1.   Percentage of unmet patient needs in relation to number of helpers
(see text).

importance of helpers in mediating the effect of physical needs and deterioration on the likelihood of having unmet needs is exemplified in Figure 1 which relates the number of helpers to the percent of patients having at least one unmet need. Those with less than two helpers are substantially more likely to have at least one unmet need than were those with four, five, or six helpers.

D. CHANGES IN UNMET NEED

Of the 220 metastatic patients interviewed at baseline, 71 died before a second interview could be conducted, 25 refused to be reinterviewed or were lost to follow-up (in most cases, too sick or hospitalized) leaving 124 patients who were interviewed 6 to 9 months after the initial interview.

Table 4 compares the baseline physical and need characteristics of the metastatic patients with respect to their status at follow-up. Patients with low QLI, and high numbers of symptoms and need for assistance were also more likely to die before the follow-up interview ($p < 0.001$, $p < 0.001$, $p < 0.01$, respectively). While not as strongly related to mortality, patients with unmet need were more likely to die than to be reinterviewed (44 vs. 28%, $p < 0.04$). Clearly, those who died before the follow-up interview clearly represented the sickest and neediest subgroup of metastatic patients.

The presence of unmet need at the time of the baseline interview was a strong predictor of the presence of unmet need at follow-up. Nearly 60% of those with unmet need at the initial interview had an unmet need at follow-up, while 87% of those with no unmet need at baseline retained this favorable status 6 to 9 months later. In the areas of personal instrumental activities, 56.5% of those with at least one unmet need at baseline still had a least one unmet need at follow-up, whereas only 7.4% of those with no unmet personal or instrumental need at baseline had one later. This relationship was less pronounced for administrative needs. Indeed, only 33% of those with an unmet administrative need at baseline had an unmet need at follow-up. Only 6.1% of those with no unmet administrative needs at baseline had one at follow-up.

The incidence of new unmet needs in each need domain was fairly small (between 6 and 13%). However, over 1/3 of those with an unmet need in each area had resolved their unmet need 6 to 9 months later. Since the incidence rate is calculated based on the relatively large number of patients who did not have an unmet need at Time 1 whereas the "resolution"

TABLE 4

Relationship Between Follow-Up Outcome and Patient Condition at Baseline (Metastatic Patients Only)

	Reinterviewed	Died	Refused or lost
QLI			
10	66.7	25.6	7.7
7—9	65.4	22.4	12.1
0—6	37.0	50.7	12.3
Number of symptoms			
0—3	70.8	16.9	12.3
4—8	54.0	34.5	11.5
9—14	37.8	51.4	10.8
Total number of needs			
0—3	60.3	23.3	16.4
4—6	63.0	28.4	8.6
7—8	48.8	36.6	14.6
9+	36.0	64.0	0.0
Number of categories of unmet need			
None	60.4	28.1	11.5
One or more	51.1	40.4	8.5
2+	31.6	52.6	15.8

rate is calculated on the small number of cases that had an unmet need at Time 1, the proportion of surviving patients with unmet need at Time 2 is similar to that observed at Time 1. The percentage of patients with unmet personal needs at Time 2 is 2%, for instrumental needs it is 15%, and for administrative needs it is 8%.

Social support at baseline appeared to be related to unmet need in personal and instrumental activities at follow-up. Only 7% of patients who felt extremely confident that their family could continue to provide assistance had unmet personal or instrumental needs at follow-up, whereas 30.6% of those who felt less certain of support at baseline had an unmet need at follow-up ($p < 0.004$). The total number of personal and instrumental needs as well as social support resiliency were important determinants of the development of *new* unmet personal or instrumental needs. Among patients with three or fewer personal or instrumental needs at baseline, 6.3% of those who were extremely confident vs. 18.8% of those who were less confident had developed unmet personal or instrumental needs by follow-up; among those with more than seven personal or instrumental needs at baseline, the corresponding values were 14.3 and 33.3%, respectively.

IV. DISCUSSION

Our study of a large sample of active treatment chemotherapy patients found high levels of need, particularly in the instrumental activities arena. We observed substantially lower levels of unmet need, but still fairly prevalent overall (28%). We found that need was strongly related to traditional correlates of health-related quality of life such as the number of symptoms and the Quality of Life Index. The probability of having an unmet need increased as a function of the total need burden patients experienced, but was substantially modified as a function of the level of social support, measured either in terms of the number of helpers or the perceived resiliency of the helping network. Indeed, loglinear analyses revealed that positive social support was predictive of unmet needs largely independent of patients' functional level. As expected, total needs at baseline were strongly related to survival as was the case for the Quality of Life Index and symptoms. While we found that those with unmet needs at baseline were more likely to have died, this relationship which suggests that unmet need is more prevalent among those with more advanced disease, was relatively weak. Interestingly, the incidence of new unmet needs among survivors is low in general, yet the majority of those with an unmet need at baseline still have one unmet need in that domain at follow-up. Finally, we found that both functional impairment and lack of social support were predictive of having an unmet need at follow-up among survivors.

What has our notion of unmet need contributed to our understanding of quality of life for these cancer patients? First, the notion of not having assistance with necessary daily living tasks that can't be performed independently has a strong measure of face validity as a quality of life indicator. Leaving tasks like light housekeeping undone in our society constitutes a burden that may affect an individual's sense of well-being. While needing assistance in an activity may compromise a patient's sense of independence, leaving that task undone, in some instances with glaring consequences, only serves as a constant reminder to the patient of their inadequacies.

Our data revealed that the presence of unmet need is related to patients' need for assistance and, therefore their health-related quality of life. This is reasonable since the more areas in which patients require assistance, the more likely one of these will be adequately met from available helping sources. Unmet need as a quality-of-life indicator taps a domain of social functioning and support capacity (or the absence thereof) that traditional health-related quality of life measures do not. Traditional quality-of-life measures are related to constructs such as emotional health or social interaction because generally serious functional disability severely limits one's capacity to engage in other spheres of functioning. For example, health-related quality of life is correlated with social interaction because reduced social interaction is due to mobility restrictions arising from impaired function and/or poor health.[21] Social support capacity is generally not adequately captured in social quality of life measures because the authors of such scales were generally interested in the subjective quality of social relations as perceived by the study subject. Since our definition of unmet need is functionally based, persons with need for assistance must have the social support necessary to meet those needs.

Our data reveal that the presence of unmet need is a reflection of both the physical need burden imposed by physiology (and other factors) as well as the individual's social support. This relationship was demonstrated both cross-sectionally and longitudinally. Consequently, a patient's unmet need reflects the interaction of disease and treatment as well as social support factors. It is the social support factor that has traditionally been under-represented conceptually and empirically in previous quality-of-life measures for cancer patients.

The importance of a functionally based approach to defining need cannot be sufficiently stressed. In many respects, one can view unmet needs as tantamount to patients' reported problems as does the CIPS.[12] Patients' reports of problems are likely to be more relativistic than a functionally based approach because a problem for one person is not necessarily seen as a problem for another. Additionally, the reported problem of not being able to cook, for example, may mean the persons' nutrition is compromised because no one cooks for them or it could merely mean that the individual resents being dependent in that activity. Empirically, the number of problems patients' report tends to be strongly related to patients' physiological function, suggesting that respondents tend to interpret problems as functional deficits regardless of whether strategies are in place to solve them.[22] In the CIPS framework, problems are a combination of physical impairment and phenomenological concerns. The unmet need perspective also begins with physical impairment but adds the social support dimension.

While the problem oriented approach to assessing cancer patients' needs is potentially helpful in guiding care planning for doctors, nurses, and social workers, the enumeration of areas of unmet needs offers a mechanism for ranking health and social service interventions in priority order. It also offers a reasonable approach to triaging individuals presenting with a broad range of social problems at medical clinics. Those individuals with several unmet needs are likely to have limited or compromised social support systems suggesting that their needs be addressed first; intervening before a stressed social support network breaks down altogether. Those needing assistance with personal care, the most basic support area, may only be able to tolerate a single unmet personal care need before they move into crisis.

Clearly, there are still many unanswered questions about the meaningfulness of unmet needs as a quality of life indicator. Will such an indicator be sufficiently sensitive to detect the effect introducing formal services might have? Is the functionally based strategy we've adopted likely to underestimate the prevalence of unmet needs because patients tend to minimize the difficulties they experience in performing everyday tasks? Indeed, are patients willing to risk accepting the fact that their family support system is not able to adequately meet their needs? Since some people are reluctant to use formal services, they may refuse to acknowledge the need for assistance if they don't have family members available, or refuse to admit that the help they receive is not adequate. Since the presence of unmet needs can be quite transitory, it may be more interesting in longitudinal analyses to focus on cumulative incidence (i.e., ever having had unmet needs during a given time period) using continuous observation or periodic recall methods. While recall biases may make such an approach difficult, regular observation would make it possible to test whether patients' unmet needs increase as their disease progresses, as in the case with other health related quality of life indicators.

In summary, unmet need appears to hold promise as a quality-of-life indicator on the grounds that it represents the interaction of physical illness and the social support necessary to meet daily living needs. Future research should examine its sensitivity to an intervention, its relationship to more psychological dimensions of stress and burden and its relationship to the interface between receipt of family support and formal agency care.

ACKNOWLEDGMENT

This research is supported in part by National Cancer Institute grants #CA41020, CA46331, and CA36560.

REFERENCES

1. **Bergner, M., Bobbitt, R. A., Carter, W. B., and Gilson, B. S.,** The sickness impact profile: development and final revision of a health status measure, *Med. Care,* 19, 787, 1981.
2. **Kaplan, R. W., Bush, J. W., and Berry, C. C.,** Health status: types of validity and the index of well being, *Health Serv. Res.,* 11, 478, 1976.
3. **Ware, J. E., Brook, R. H., Davies-Avery, A., et al.,** Conceptualization and Measurement of Health for Adults in the Health Insurance Study, Vol. 1, R-1987/HEW, The Rand Corporation, Santa Monica, CA, 1980.
4. **Spitzer, W. O., Dobson, A. H., Hall, J., et al.,** Measuring quality of life in cancer patients: a concise quality of life index for use by physicians, *J. Chronic Dis.,* 34, 585, 1981.
5. **Karnofsky, D. A., Abelmann, W. H., Craver, L. F., and Burchenal, J. H.,** The use of nitrogen mustards in palliative treatment of carcinoma, *Cancer,* 1, 634, 1948.
6. **Shipper, H. et al.,** Measuring the quality of life of cancer patient: the functional living index, cancer patients: development and validation, *J. Clin. Oncol.,* 2, 472, 1984.
7. **Wenger, N. K.,** The concept of quality of life, *Qual. Life Cardiovasc. Care,* 1, 8, 1984.
8. **O'Young, J. and McPeek, B.,** Quality of life variables in surgical trials, *J. Chronic Dis.,* 40, 6, 513, 1987.
9. **Mor, V.,** Cancer patients quality of life over the disease course: lessons from the real world, *J. Chronic Dis.,* 40, 535, 1987.
10. **Mor, V. and Guadagnoli, E.,** Quality of life measurement: a psychometric tower of Babel, *J. Clin. Epidemiol.,* 41, 1105, 1988.

11. **Bergner, M.,** Quality of life, health status and clinical research, *Med. Care,* 27, S148, 1989.
12. **Heinrich, R. L., Schag, C. C., and Ganz, P. A.,** Living with cancer: the cancer inventory of problem situations, *J. Clin. Psychol.,* 40, 972, 1984.
13. **Fillenbaum, G. G.,** *Multidimensional Functional Assessment of Older Adults,* Lawrence Erlbaum, Hillsdale, NJ, 1988.
14. **Steinwachs, D. M.,** Application of health status assessment measures in policy research, *Med. Care,* 27, 512, 1989.
15. **Mor, V., Guadagnoli, E., and Wool, M.,** The role of concrete services in cancer care, in *Psychosocial Aspects of Cancer,* Goldberg, R. J., Ed., S. Karger, Basel, 1988, 102.
16. **Spitzer, W. O.,** State of science, 1986: quality of life and functional status as target variables for research, *J. Chronic Dis.,* 40, 465, 1987.
17. **Mor, V., Guadagnoli, E., and Wool, M.,** An examination of the concrete service needs of advanced cancer patients, *J. Psychosoc. Oncol.,* 5, 1, 1987.
18. **Katz, S., Branch, L. G., Branson, M. H., Papsidero, J. A., Beck, J. C., and Greer, D. S.,** Active life expectancy, *N. Engl. J. Med.,* 209, 1218, 1983.
19. **Spector, W. D., Katz, S., Murphy, J. B., and Fulton, J. P.,** The hierarchical relationship between activities of daily living and instrumental activities of daily living, *J. Chronic Dis.,* 40, 481, 1987.
20. **Mor, V., Laliberte, L., Morris, J. N., and Wiemann, M.,** The Karnofsky Performance Status Scale: an examination of its reliability and validity in a research setting, *Cancer,* 53, 2002, 1984.
21. **Guadagnoli, E. and Mor, V.,** Social Interaction Tests and Scales, in *Quality of Life Assessments in Clinical Trials,* Spilker, B., Ed., Raven Press, New York, in press.
22. **Schagg, C. C., Heinrich, R. L., and Ganz, P. A.,** Cancer inventory of problem situations: an instrument for assessing cancer patients' rehabilitation needs, *J. Psychosoc. Oncol.,* 1, 11, 1983.

Chapter 13

THE SPITZER QUALITY-OF-LIFE INDEX: ITS PERFORMANCE AS A MEASURE

Sharon Wood-Dauphinee and Jack Ivan Williams

TABLE OF CONTENTS

I. INTRODUCTION

Spitzer and colleagues[1] published the Quality of Life (QL) Index in 1981 when much of the medical community was still debating if quality of life should and could be used as an end-point in clinical studies. With the goal of expanding treatment outcome assessments beyond morbidity and mortality, they set out to develop a simple, quantified instrument that would reflect the different dimensions of quality of life. They wanted to provide a measure equivalent to the neonatal Apgar scale,[2] that would be a reliable and valid assessment of an individual's health related quality of life and be responsive to changes in life's quality over time. The measure was to be applicable to patients with cancer as well as to those with other debilitating diseases, and be acceptable to those using the instrument. It was one of the few early scales designated initially as a quality-of-life measure.[3]

The authors largely achieved their objectives. As published, the instrument was brief, reproducible, discriminating, and easy to administer. Since 1981, the QL-Index has been referenced extensively, used as a validating tool and employed as an outcome in clinical studies. In this chapter, we will review the development and original validation of the Index, update information on its measurement properties and describe its application as an outcome variable. Finally, we will discuss the strengths, limitations, and controversies which surround the instrument.

II. METHODS

Primary papers reviewed in this chapter were identified through computerized searches of the Science Citation Index and the Social Science Citation Index. The searches included all journal citations, 115, of the original article by Spitzer and colleagues (to October 1989). Approximately 76% of these articles were editorial comments, letters to the editor, literature reviews, or general notes of comparison in the discussion section of a study. The remaining 28 papers with primary data from the QL-Index form the basis of this chapter as they have provided new psychometric information on the measure or have employed it in an empirically based study assessing the effects of an intervention on quality of life.

III. PSYCHOMETRIC PROPERTIES OF THE MEASURES

A. DEVELOPING THE MEASURES FOR CONTENT VALIDITY

The originators of this Index set out to develop a comprehensive measure that incorporated adequate representation of the different dimensions of quality of life, as perceived by patients, providers, and healthy individuals.[1] After reviewing the existing literature, they created three advisory panels, each made up of 43 individuals divided among patients, their relatives, health professionals, clergy, and ordinary citizens. Using structured and unstructured questionnaires, they determined the factors that comprised quality of life, as well as information on the relative importance of each factor identified. This data was incorporated into two parallel draft indices of seven items each [QL(A) and QL(B)] as well as a linear analog scale (Uniscale) that assessed the global attribute—quality of life.

The two forms and Uniscale were tested on 339 subjects aged 20 to 70 years from hospital clinics, general practices, and a hospice. Each person was assessed by two of the three forms, and the evaluators included eight general practitioners, seven oncologists, nine internists, six nurses, and five social workers. Based on these data, some items were discarded, others were combined to create the five dimensions which made up the QL-Index and the remainder were used to produce Multiscale — a ten-item questionnaire also assessing quality of life.

Score each heading 2, 1 or 0 according to your most recent assessment of the patient.

ACTIVITY   During the last week, the patient
  · has been working or studying full-time, or nearly so, in usual occupation; or managing own household; or participating in unpaid
    or voluntary activities, whether retired or not 2
  · has been working or studying in usual occupation or managing own household or participating in unpaid or voluntary activities;
    but requiring major assistance or a significant reduction in hours worked or a sheltered situation or was on sick leave 1
  · has not been working or studying in any capacity and not managing own household 0

DAILY LIVING   During the last week, the patient
  · has been self-reliant in eating, washing, toiletting and dressing; using public transport or driving own car 2
  · has been requiring assistance (another person or special equipment) for daily activities and transport but performing light tasks 1
  · has not been managing personal care nor light tasks and/or not leaving own home or institution at all 0

HEALTH   During the last week, the patient
  · has been appearing to feel well or reporting feeling "great" most of the time 2
  · has been lacking energy or not feeling entirely "up to par" more than just occasionally 1
  · has been feeling very ill or "lousy", seeming weak and washed out most of the time or was unconscious 0

SUPPORT   During the last week
  · the patient has been having good relationships with others and receiving strong support from at least one family member and/or friend ... 2
  · support received or perceived has been limited from family and friends and/or by the patient's condition 1
  · support from family and friends occurred infrequently or only when absolutely necessary or patient was unconscious 0

OUTLOOK   During the past week the patient
  · has usually been appearing calm and positive in outlook, accepting and in control of personal circumstances, including surroundings 2
  · has sometimes been troubled because not fully in control of personal circumstances or has been having periods of obvious anxiety
    or depression 1
  · has been seriously confused or very frightened or consistently anxious and depressed or unconscious 0

FIGURE 1.   The QL-Index. (From Spitzer, W. O. et al., *J. Chronic Dis.*, 34, 585, 1981. With permission.)

Please mark with an X the appropriate place within the bar to indicate your rating of this person's quality of life during the past week.

Lowest quality applies to someone completely dependent physically on others, seriously impaired mentally, unaware of surroundings and in a hopeless position.

Highest quality applies to someone physically and mentally independent, communicating well with others, able to do most of the things enjoyed, pulling own weight, with a hopeful yet realistic attitude.

LOWEST   HIGHEST

QUALITY   QUALITY

FIGURE 2.   Uniscale. (From Spitzer, W. O. et al., *J. Chronic Dis.*, 34, 585, 1981. With permission.)

The final compositions of the QL-Index and Multiscale were verified by testing to determine if preset criteria for acceptance were met after submission to lay and professional panels. Approximately 70% of each panel agreed completely with all questions relating to relevancy, comprehensiveness, and discriminating ability for the items included in both measures. The QL-Index is presented in Figure 1 and Uniscale in Figure 2. Multiscale has since been employed almost exclusively in validation studies and will be discussed later in the chapter.

The methods of developing the QL-Index were thorough and extensive. The authors carefully pretested, tested, and verified in an effort to ensure content validity. The process has served as a model for others developing clinical measures and the multidimensional outcomes have been confirmed by a number of investigators seeking the determinants of quality of life.[4-9]

Researchers using this instrument have been interested in the usefulness of the individual items as well as in the overall performance of the Index. Slevin et al.[1] tested the instrument using 108 patients with cancer, their doctors, and relatives to assess the contributions of individual items to the total score. In their data, the items assessing activity, daily living, and health each correlated at a 0.8 level with the total score. Collectively, these items accounted for 93% of the variance leaving the other two items, support and outlook, to explain only 7%.

A related issue, the covariation of the items, had been raised in three other investigations. Gough et al.,[4] using the Index in patients with advanced cancer, found that support had a low correlation with the other items and with the Index. As most patients believed they had adequate social support, the responses to the item showed little variation. Similarly, Suissa et al.,[11] in a Canadian study of French and English patients with either cancer or a chronic disease, found low item-to-total correlations for the support item due to lack of variance in raters' scores. They postulated that this was due to the difficulties of an observer rating a subjective phenomena, the probabilty that good support was present and the likelihood that social desirability was influencing the scoring of the item as neither patients nor caregivers like to admit that support is not present.

Using data merged from three studies of cancer patients at different stages in the disease trajectory, Mor[12] found that activity, daily living, and health were the central focus of the measure reflecting physical functioning. However, the remaining items, outlook and support, independently related to external measures of social interaction and psychological state in patients of differing functional capacities. Additionally, the outlook item was strongly related to emotional as well as to physical functioning thereby linking these areas conceptually. On the other hand, responses to the support item were highly skewed, suggesting that cancer patients are generally recipients of strong support from their friends and relatives. This investigator noted that the gradations of response for the support item did not allow differentiation among patients who perceived reasonably good support and suggested modifying the descriptive phrases for scaling the item.

To date, it appears that the Index has been used with medical and surgical conditions where support by family and friends has remained high. However, one group of researchers[13] employed Uniscale to assess quality of life in a group of 50 gay men who were within 3 months of being first diagnosed with autoimmune deficiency syndrome (AIDS), a condition reporting major deterioration of personal support systems.[14] While the group mean for Uniscale was 6.9 (SD = 2.4), 37% of subjects rated their current quality of life as less than 5.0 on the 1—10 visual analog scale. Currently, in Montreal, the QL-Index is being used in another study of patients with AIDS. It will be interesting to observe the behavior of the support item in this population.

Mor[12] also considered the relatively importance of sociodemographic and clinical factors in the three samples of cancer patients to explain responses on the QL-Index. He found that the resulting explanatory regression models were relatively similar across various stages of the disease, and incorporated physical and social functioning, mood, and symptom experience. As noted by Mor, this finding lends support to the idea that the determinants of health-related quality of life are primarily as ascertained by Spitzer and others in the literature.

Other recent evidence in support of content validity has been provided by Parfrey et al.[15] These investigators asked end-stage renal disease patients on dialysis to rank the importance of symptoms prevalent in this disorder. Patients were then requested to score the activity and daily living items of the Spitzer Index and to state how a specific symptom had influenced the score. Additionally, they graded a modified version of Uniscale which was viewed as a more subjective estimation of life's quality. Among the symptoms perceived as being severe, tiredness, cramps, and sleep disturbance affected scores on the Index items and cramps and sleep disturbance negatively influenced their subjective perception of quality of life. Information such as this is helpful in clarifying the relationship between specific symptoms and quality of life.

Morris and colleagues[16] had reservations about the inclusion of the item activity when planning to use the QL-Index in the National Hospice study. They felt that individuals receiving terminal care may give up their previous work roles and focus more strongly on activities of daily living reflecting personal independence. They thus adapted the item by changing the cue from activity to mobility, and wrote descriptors reflecting levels of independence in mobility accordingly.

They included both items so the scores from the adapted measure could be compared with the original QL-Index scores. Starting from the time of death, they looked backward to determine how the scores changed over the last few weeks of life. While the adoption of the mobility item resulted in a change in the average score of about 0.6 points, the shape and distribution of scores were essentially unchanged. Statistically, the form with the mobility rather than the activity item offered no advantages in terms of power or efficiency.

B. SCALING OF THE QL-INDEX

The Index is comprised of five items with three-point responses, each scored on a zero (attribute or activity essentially absent), one (attribute or activity partially present), two (attribute or activity fully present) point scale giving a summated maximum possible score of ten. When developing the measure, the originators also tested a four-point system. The two scoring systems provided similar results but the four-point system took three times as much time for the raters (a median of 3 min compared to 1 min). The three-point system was therefore adopted to minimize the burden on those using the instrument.

The developers choose an equal weighting scheme in the absence of any evidence that any one item was more deserving of extra weight than another. While this result may not in fact reflect reality,[17] it appears to have been an acceptable choice given the limitations of and the difficulties with weighting in clinical scales.[18]

C. RELIABILITY OF THE MEASURES

The reliability of a measure indicates the degree to which its scores are reproducible, thereby reflecting the random error connected to its use. Two basic approaches are employed to establish reliability. Spitzer and colleagues first considered internal consistency or the degree to which the items in a measure relate to each other and to the collection of items as a group. Based on scores for 91 subjects, Cronbach's coefficient alpha[19] gave a value of 0.78. Subsequent work by Mor and associates[12,20] reported consistency coefficients of 0.66 in the National Hospice Study data, and 0.77 and 0.80 in the Concrete Needs Study and the Cancer and Aging Study and 0.61 in the study evaluating day hospital as an alternative to in-patient care. Alpha was also calculated as 0.78 for a sample of 261 chronically ill patients in Canada.[11] A subset of these patients who had cancer gave an alpha of 0.85 when the ratings were made by physicians.

As the measure can be completed by the patient, a significant order, or a health care provider, the level of agreement among raters is an important measure of reliability. In the original testing, inter-physician Spearman Rank correlations ranged between 0.74 and 0.84 and those of patients and physicians between 0.61 and 0.69. In the latter case, it was observed that patients tended to rank themselves one or two points higher than their care-givers. These findings on the reliability among raters and the systematic difference observed when patients rated themselves were replicated in the Canadian study.[11] This latter finding was more striking for Uniscale than for the QL-Index. These investigators also found greater concordance between the ratings of a patient and his friend or relative than between a patient and health professional.

In the Gough study,[4] when cancer patients were rated on four occasions to compare the self administered and professionally rated versions of the Index, Kendall's tau ranged from .51 to .86 giving an overall correlate of 0.72. Recently, McGowan et al.,[21] in a prospective study of palliative laser therapy for inoperable rectal cancer, tested inter-rater reliability between two physicians and found a correlation coefficient of 0.87. Slevin et al.,[10] however, using five raters per patient (usually two doctors and three nurses) noted that they agreed precisely only 45% of the time. When the limits for agreement were expanded to plus or minus one point, this value changed to 70%. This data gave a Kendall's concordance coefficient of 0.54, which while significant was not high.

On the other hand, when patients in the Slevin study rated themselves on the QL-Index five times in one day, their scores agreed completely 78% of the time and were within one point plus or minus, 97% of the time. When these patients rated themselves daily over a 5-day period, these percentages were 80 and 95, respectively, providing evidence for intrarater reliability and stability of the Index.

The stability of the measure was also examined in a study of breast cancer patients.[22] A patient was defined as stable if, during an interview with a nurse, the nurse rated both physical and emotional functioning as unchanged for the last 2-week time period. The QL-Index scores for that interview and the preceding interview were compared, as were the scores for four other measures. The mean change scores were deemed stable by the investigators as they were close to zero. The mean change score for the QL-Index was -0.560 and the standard error was .081, so in fact the change score was statistically significant at the 0.001 level ($t = 6.87$). The mean change score for the Breast Cancer Questionnaire, (BCQ) which the authors developed as a part of the study, was statistically significant (mean change score -0.183, standard error .063, $t = 2.90$, 184 cases) as well even though the other mean change scores for the other four measures were not. Either the QL-Index and the BCQ were picking up changes that did not affect the global self-assessments by the patients, or there were problems with measurement errors.

D. VALIDITY OF THE MEASURES

Validity indicates the degree to which an instrument assesses what it is purported to measure. There are three approaches to validity assessment: content validity which has already been discussed, criterion validity which has been further divided into concurrent and predictive aspects, and construct validity which involves validating the theory behind the measure.

Traditionally, criterion validity has been assessed by comparing the measure under study to a "gold standard" in that area. As there is no gold standard for quality of life, it has become common to choose a variable external to the measure against which the scores can be checked. That variable is then used as a criterion by which to judge the measure. Concurrent criterion validity refers to the ability of a measure to discriminate amoung groups at the time of measurement, whereas predictive criterion validity describes the capacity of the measure to predict future events.

Spitzer[1] assessed concurrent criterion validity by comparing quality-of-life scores in four groups of patients with varying health status. This approach to concurrent validation is termed the "known group technique"[23] and is based on the idea that if one knows that specific groups vary on the characteristic being assessed, the groups can be employed to validate a new measure of it. The Australian samples of healthy individuals, those with chronic disease, cancer patients, and those who were seriously ill, were used. Not only were mean differences discernible among the groups but the within-group scores clustered or spread over the scoring ranges as expected. For example, healthy individuals grouped at the upper levels of the Index while seriously ill people tended to cluster in the lower echelons. On the other hand, patients with various stages of cancer, or those classified as chronically diseased, exhibited a greater spread of scores.

Similarly, in the studies of cancer patients who were recently diagnosed, receiving chemotherapy for progression or recurrence of disease, or in the terminal phase of their illness, QL scores were able to differentiate the groups even though there were overlaps in the distribution of scores.[12] The average score for the recently diagnosed group was 8.1; for those on active treatment it was 7.5 and for the terminally ill patients, it was 3.9.

On the other hand, a study of quality of life in end-stage renal disease had some difficulty differentiating across groups with the Spitzer measures. Churchill and colleagues[24] had patients, their nurses, and nephrologists rate the quality of life of transplant recipients receiving continuous ambulatory peritoneal, home or self, or hospital dialysis. The patients also completed the Rand health status measures, Uniscale, and utility assessments with the time trade-off method (TTO).

In comparing the QL scores, the quality of life was rated the highest for transplant patients, lowest for the patients on hospital hemodialysis, and the patients on continuous ambulatory peritoneal or home dialysis were in between. The utility values followed a different pattern. The absolute values for the TTO were lower than for the QL ratings. More importantly, the utility values for dialysis were clustered together and markedly lower than those for transplant patients.

Uniscale ratings showed far less consistency, either in terms of absolute values or the relative orderings of the mean values, for the four treatment groups across the various raters. The nephrologists gave the lowest ratings and the patients recorded the highest scores. While the scores for the nephrologists were lower for hospital dialysis than the other forms of dialysis, the patients' ratings indicated that they were essentially the same. The nurses' ratings were closer to the nephrologists than the patients'. Overall, Uniscale, as completed by patients, nurses, or nephrologists, ordered the groups as predicted, but the QL-Index complied with prediction only for the patients and nurses. In each case, only small portions of the available range of scores were utilized by the raters making discrimination somewhat difficult.

In a recent study on quality of life in 1981 gastric cancer patients,[25] QL-Index scores were able to discriminate young patients from old and male from female although the data on gender was not standardized for age. In terms of age, this study confirmed work by Mor[12] who noted that older patients reported slightly poorer quality of life. However, gender, in the study, did not appear to be related. Suissa et al.[11] reported that QL scores tended to decrease with age at a faster rate for female than for male cancer patients but that the reverse was true for patients with chronic diseases. In this study, scores from both English and French patients were similar, allowing it to be administered in either language.

In a study comparing intermittent and continuous drug therapy for cancer patients, Coates et al.[26] investigated the predictive ability of the QL-Index and found that changes in scores for individual patients that occurred before 180 days post entry to the trial were significant predictors in the proportional hazards model of survival following that period. In these patients with advanced breast cancer, the QL-Index scores were able to predict survival time. As noted by the authors, this information reinforces the idea that the scores reflect change in the basic disease status.

Quality-of-life measures are often compared to other measures. Hypotheses, stating that the quality of life measure will or will not correlate with related or independent measures, are tested to determine if the instrument will behave as expected. In this manner evidence is accrued concerning the validity of the measure under study and the process is termed construct validation.[27]

The initial approach to construct validation by Spitzer and colleagues was one of positive correlation or convergence. As validating measures, they employed Uniscale and Multiscale. They hypothesized that these measures of quality of life would correlate positively with the QL-Index when tested on sick and healthy groups of individuals using several measurement approaches: self ratings, assessments by physicians and other health professionals and by relatives and friends of the patients. Up to 11 ratings by up to five raters were made per patient. Spearman rank correlations were quite strong for the cancer patients, moderate in magnitude for the chronically diseased and severely ill groups, but low for the healthy individuals. Similar trends appeared across measures and rating approaches and collectively led the researchers to believe that the QL-Index should only be used with people who were definitely diseased.

The QL-Index has been validated against the Karnofsky Performance Status Scale (KPS)[28] in several different settings. The KPS was designed to assess the level of physical activity and medical care requirements in cancer patients and it has been the most widely used indicator to quantify functional performance in these patients. Because of its focus on physical functioning, strong correlations with the QL-Index are to be anticipated. In truth, the results have been variable.

QL-Index and KPS ratings were made in both the National Hospice and the Cancer and Aging studies. Spearman correlations of 0.41 and 0.83 were reported for each sample, respectively.[12] In the Hospice study, Karnofsky ratings were made by a trained interviewer and quality-of-life scores by a family member. In the study of newly diagnosed cancer patients, both ratings were made by the interviewer following a discussion with the patient. Mor postulated that the diverse results were due to the different evaluative procedures.

This investigator also merged the data from the two studies and considered the correlations of each item in the Spitzer Index with the KPS.[12] The results were as follows: activity (r = 0.53), living (r = 0.57), health (r = 0.47), support (r = 0.13) and outlook (r = 0.39). As expected, the functional and health items were more strongly related to the KPS than were the items assessing the psychosocial variables.

Koster et al.[25] compared Karnofsky and Spitzer ratings made by surgeons close to the time of operation in a cohort of 1081 patients with gastric cancer. They used a modified German version of the KPS and achieved a correlation of 0.72. Slevin et al.[10] also considered the degree of similarity of the measures when used with 100 patients with different types and stages of cancer who were undergoing a variety of treatment protocols. They found different correlations dependent upon who made the assessments. For example Kendall's concordance coefficients were 0.65 when the physicians rated, 0.49 when patients rated and 0.66 when the measures were scored by relatives.

Another measurement approach frequently employed to estimate quality of life is the use of visual analog scales (VAS).[29] Gough et al.[4] rated 115 patients with advanced metastatic cancer on four occasions using four measures: a single item VAS concerning "well being"; the QL-Index scored by a social worker, a self-administered QL-Index; and a 21-item linear analog self-assessment questionnaire. All scores were highly and significantly correlated (*p* <0.001) using Kendall's r. When the self-administered version of the QL-Index was tested against the multi-item linear analog questionnaire the coefficients ranged from 0.46 to 0.60 with a combined value of 0.56 and when tested against the single item VAS the coefficients ranged from 0.38 to 0.67 with a combined value of 0.53. Similar results were obtained when the professionally scored versions of this Index were correlated with the two measures using visual analog scales.

This strong association has been replicated in another study. Using a physician-scored QL-Index and a linear analog self assessment on 54 patients with inoperable rectal cancer, McGowan et al.[21] found a correlation coefficient of 0.79 (*p* <.001).

Cancer patients have often stated that certain symptoms such as fatigue, anxiety, depression, nausea, vomiting, and pain were detrimental to the quality of their lives.[4-6] Mor[12] examined the relationships between the QL-Index and depression, pain, and nausea in the Brown University studies of cancer patients at different stages in the disease process. In the investigations involving newly diagnosed or terminal patients, pain was negatively and strongly related to the four items assessing activity, living, health, and outlook but less so to support. The relationships with depression provided a similar pattern. When the total Index was considered, pain and nausea were negatively correlated in the three investigations and this relationship was strongest in the Concrete Needs Study in which patients were receiving treatment. Correlations between depression and the QL-Index in the Hospice Study and the Cancer and Aging Study were all significant but almost three times as great in the newly diagnosed group. The authors felt that this difference was because depression was underestimated in the Hospice study. Forty-eight percent of the terminal patients had been unable to respond to interviews due to being severely ill.

The QL-Index has also been used as a validating tool in several other investigations when instruments with theoretically related constructs were being developed. Wood-Dauphinee and colleagues[30,31] in Montreal designed a Reintegration to Normal Living (RNL) Index to assess global functioning in patients following incapacitating illness or severe trauma. This measure is made up to 11 items, incorporating both objective indicators of reintegration and subjective perceptions of the extent to which patients achieve them.[12,32] As part of the validation proceedings, they hypothesized that patients who were reintegrating well should also perceive themselves as having a higher quality of life than those who were not resuming normal patterns of living. Correlations between the two measures, based on self assessments and on ratings by health professionals were all moderately strong (Pearson's r — .46 to .72), in the expected direction and statistically significant.

Another Montreal team developed a Meaning of Life (ML) Scale which was designed to capture "the sense of purpose, beliefs and faith of patients in hospice and rehabilitative programs".[33] The Scale is composed of 15 statements reflecting diverse beliefs, philosophies, and activities which are scored on a modified visual analog scale. Anchors at each end are provided, but the line is divided into five equal portions. Originally planned as a companion index to the QL-Index, in actual fact the orientations of the two measures are different. While the QL-Index is concerned with physical, psychological, and social functioning, the ML-Scale highlights the spiritual and emotional components of living.[34] This investigative group postulated that different constructs were being measured and the low correlations (r = 0.19 for the terminally ill and r = 0.25 for chronic patients) confirmed this hypothesis and reinforced the divergent construct validity of both measures.

Levine and colleagues[22] have recently published a disease specific quality of life measure for patients in Stage II breast cancer. It was designed to quantify the impact of chemotherapy on physical, emotional, and social function in areas deemed important by the patients. The QL-Index, using ratings by a nurse interviewer, was employed as part of the construct validation process. Based on 346 patients in four settings and a mean of 9.2 assessments per patient, the product-moment correlation was 0.42 ($p < .0001$).

The Spitzer measures were also incorporated in a questionnaire designed to evaluate quality of life in patients with end-stage renal disease.[35] Symptom and affect indices were developed by the authors, included in the overall questionnaire and tested cross-sectionally on two age-matched groups of dialysis and transplantation patients. Based on information available in the literature, the investigators postulated that the group S would differ on symptom scores and "objective" quality of life — the QL-Index, but would score similarly on the affect index and "subjective" quality of life — Uniscale. These hypotheses were confirmed, thereby adding evidence of construct validity for the Uniscale and the QL-Index.

Finally, the QL-Index has been used in the validation of a utility assessment. As discussed previously, Churchill et al.[24] used both the QL-Index and Uniscale as instruments in validating their time trade-off (TTO) method. Four groups representing different treatment approaches in end-stage renal disease were evaluated through self rating and by physicians, nurses, and relatives or friends. The correlation coefficients between the patient TTO values and the Uniscale scores from nephrologists, nurses, and significant others ranged from 0.27 to 0.39. The correlations between the TTO and the QL-Index clustered between 0.38 and 0.40. For the patients, the correlation between TTO and QL Uniscale was 0.22 and for the TTO and QL-Index was 0.43.

These variations in means scores and correlations suggest that while there are some significant covariations in scores, the QL and TTO scores may be tapping separate dimensions. Schuessler[36] suggests that quality-of-life measures yield rankings of states. The utility ratings are designed to indicate the value or worth of health states. In quality-of-life rankings, the scores for dialysis patients were lower than for transplant patients, but not markedly so. However, the utility or worth of life while on dialysis is markedly less than for transplant patients, partly because of the limitations placed on dialysis patients and the uncertainty of their futures as compared to the patients with transplants who lead a near-normal life.

E. RESPONSIVENESS OF THE MEASURES

Responsiveness, or the ability of an instrument to detect changes — especially clinically important changes — over time in individual subjects or groups of subjects, has recently received attention in the health measurement literature.[37] The responsiveness of both the QL-Index and Uniscale was assessed in the National Hospice Study where the family members and professional caregivers of terminally ill cancer patients provided quality-of-life ratings during the final 2 months of the patients' lives.[16] Both measures, whether scored by a relative or a health care provider, demonstrated a deterioration in quality of life as death approached with a fairly acute decline during the last 3 weeks. A similar trend was observed in a sample of terminal cancer patients followed in hospital-based palliative care units in Montreal.[16] Thus, as noted by Mor,[12] these measures are able to capture the physiological process of deterioration. This author expressed concern, however, that if the Index is only a physiological marker, it may not be responsive enough to detect subtle but clinically important changes in patient status. In consequence, its use as an outcome variable might be limited.

This concern has been allayed to some extent by recent findings in a randomized, placebo-controlled trial of congestive heart failure patients by Tandon et al.[38] These investigators employed a nonvalidated Patient Self-Rating Scale and three validated quality-of-life instruments including the Spitzer Index. The patients' Scale and the Index, completed by the physician, demonstrated a significant difference (based on change scores) between the two treatment groups, while the other measures failed to do so. These results support the ability of the Index to respond to fairly small but important changes in the quality of patients' lives as perceived by their caregivers.

IV. SPITZER QUALITY OF LIFE MEASURES AS END-POINTS

This section of the chapter will describe a variety of studies where one or both of the Spitzer measures have been selected as outcome variables expressing quality of life. The National Hospice Study (NHS)[39] has already been referenced extensively in the chapter. To recapitulate, it was a multicentered investigation designed to compare the experiences of terminal cancer patients managed in hospice settings to those receiving a more traditional approach to care. Several outcome variables, felt to indicate the impact of care on both patients and their families were chosen, including the QL-Index and Uniscale. While the results confirmed that patterns of hospice care are distinct from traditional approaches, there were no significant differences in the physical functioning of patients or in the quality of their lives. Results obtained from Spitzer scores were congruent with other measures of similar and related constructs used as outcomes.

Other studies have evaluated diverse approaches to the organization of care for cancer patients. In a randomized trial Mor et al.[20] compared day hospital and in-patient management. These investigators showed day hospital care to be equal to in-patient care in terms of survival, and medical and psychosocial outcomes, at less cost. The performance of the QL-Index conformed with that of the other measures, reinforcing the finding that quality of life was similar in the two groups. Investigators in Boston[40] compared home care services and hospice care for terminally ill patients. QL-Index ratings were made weekly by a research assistant. As the patient approached death, a decline in Index scores was associated with an increased input of services from physicians and nurses. For each point decrease in the score, an average of one and one half extra visits were made. Finally, an Italian study[41] demonstrated the value of a Home Care Program for patients with advanced cancer pain. As measured by the Spitzer Index, quality of life of the patients receiving the program remained unchanged over the final 6 weeks whereas scores in the comparison group demonstrated marked deterioration. Congruently, the Program patients reported less pain, weakness, and anxiety than those cared for by their families.

Studies evaluating specific cancer therapies have also employed the Spitzer instruments. Using a pretest-posttest single group design to assess the palliative effects of laser therapy for inoperable rectal adenocarcinoma in a small group of patients, McGowan et al.[21] were able to demonstrate a consistent and significant improvement in QL-Index scores for several weeks which then changed to a decline as death approached.

Coates and associates[26] conducted a randomized trial of intermittent and continuous chemotherapy in patients with advanced breast disease and employed both self-administered and physician-rated versions of the QL-Index and Uniscale as outcome indicators. Using changes in scores for each patient to make quality of life comparisons between groups, this team unexpectedly found that those receiving continuous therapy demonstrated better quality of life, in line with a longer time to disease progression and a prolonged period of survival.

Levine et al.[9] also used repeated QL-Index assessments in a randomized trial comparing a 12-week regimen of chemotherapy to one given for 36 weeks to patients with Stage II breast cancer. In this study the investigators were unable to demonstrate a difference in the Index scores between the two groups although both a disease-specific quality-of-life measure and the Karnofsky instrument were able to do so.

Similar difficulties with the Index were encountered by a German investigative group[42,43] who presented a preliminary report of a randomized trial of two approaches to surgical reconstructive techniques following total gastrectomy and systematic lymphadenectomy in patients with gastric cancer. The QL-Index scores did not differentiate the groups although differences in survival and in a disease-specific quality-of-life measure created for the study were found. However, in this study the number of patients assessed by the QL-Index was very small and the range of Spitzer scores was extremely restricted in the sample.

The QL-Index and Uniscale also had difficulty distinguishing between "failed" and "successful" transplantation patients following surgery for end-stage renal disease.[44] Of the 82 dialysis patients used in the cross-sectional study reported earlier, 20 had transplants and were interviewed 1 year later. At that time, 5 transplants had failed and the other 15 were successful. For the patients whose transplants failed, the initial QL-Index score was 8.8 and it dropped to 7.8 on the second interview. The initial score for the successful patients was 8.8 and it increased to 9.4. The changes were not statistically significant, presumably because of the small numbers involved.

In addition to the technical difficulties and small sample sizes in the specific studies where responsiveness to clinical change is an issue, the problem may be related to the fact that the QL-Index was designed to reflect the impact of disease and treatment in a global sense over a long follow-up period. As a consequence, the scores are sometimes not as sensitive to short term clinical changes as are the scores in disease-specific measures normally incorporating symptomatology. However, they are better for the long-term response to management.

Quality of life was also evaluated in two matched groups of diabetic patients with severe renal disease who had undergone either a pancreas-kidney transplantation or a kidney transplantation.[45] Physical, mental, and social indicators including the QL-Index were used as outcomes by which to compare the groups. While the groups were too small for statistical analyses, patients with the combined transplantation scored similarly or better than the kidney transplant group on all parameters except the number of days of hospitalization after surgery, due to a more complicated postoperative course. The QL-Index scores were in line with the other measures indicating a better and less restricted quality of life.

Another group of studies has employed the Spitzer measures as end-points in assessing the value of intensive care for critically ill individuals. Sage and associates[46] evaluated 337 mixed medical-surgical ICU patients for severity of illness and chronic health status at admission and assessed "objective" quality of life using the Sickness Impact Profile (SIP)[47] and "subjective" quality of life with Uniscale in survivors 15 to 20 months post discharge.

Quality of life as assessed by both these instruments was inversely related to the severity of illness at admission. The chronic health status measure also predicted Uniscale scores. When the SIP was used, patients over 65 years of age had worse quality of life than younger patients. However when Uniscale data was analyzed, patients who were over 65 years of age had a better quality of life. Based on these findings, this same investigative team specifically considered the outcomes of survivors of intensive care in the elderly[48] and determined with very few exceptions that their quality of life judged either from subjective or objective points of view was similar to that of an age-matched control group.

Also working with ICU patients, Slatyer et al.[49] assessed quality of life retrospectively for the month prior to admission and again 1 month after discharge using the QL-Index. Among survivors the scores were similar at the evaluation points and congruent with interview data obtained in the follow-up period. These investigators noted that the QL-Index was easily administered and a useful tool for outcome assessment.

The Spitzer Index was also used as one of several outcomes in a cross-over trial of elderly homebound patients with arthritis or other orthopedic disabilities that compared a goal-oriented outreach rehabilitation program with standard treatment.[50] These investigators found no clinical or statistically significant differences in functional status, quality of life, contentment, hospitalization, or falls between treatment and control periods. The performance of the Index was concordant with the other measures.

Finally, the QL-Index has been used in investigations focusing on psychiatric problems. It was employed in a clinical study of 20 insomniacs, treated with a multidisciplinary approach directed primarily at an associated personality disorder.[51] Patients reported improvement in nightly sleep congruent with higher scores in the Index, between admission and discharge and at follow-up. In an Australian study,[52] patients who suffered a near miss asthma death were assessed psychiatrically 1 year after the event. Approximately half the patients were judged to have a psychiatric disorder and this group perceived themselves as having a lower quality of life than those without a psychiatric diagnosis. As measured by scores on the QL-Index, this difference was statistically significant.

V. SUMMARY AND CONCLUSIONS

In the Index, quality of life was conceptualized as a construct with several difficult dimensions: day-to-day activity patterns, self care capabilities, general health, outlook on life, and support of family and friends. These dimensions were generated through a comprehensive process involving input from health professionals, patients, their relatives, and other healthy individuals. When completed, it incorporated the concepts presented in the World Health Organization definition, that health is not only the absence of infirmity and disease but also a state of physical, mental, and social well-being.[53] Spitzer and colleagues went on to operationally define the dimensions in terms of how cancer or other chronic diseases and their treatments would impact on the day-to-day lives of patients. Conceptually, this makes sense. Moreoever, the Index has been used successfully to measure quality of life in several studies of cancer and other medical and surgical conditions.

There exists a wealth of information supporting the notion that the Index actually is measuring what it was intended to measure. It is able to distinguish between healthy and sick individuals. In cancer patients it can differentiate among stages of the disease process and it is able to predict survival. The QL-Index correlates substantially with other measures of assessing quality of life including Uniscale and shows the strongest congruency with instruments containing elements of physical performance as opposed to psychosocial functioning. Additionally, the Index has been used as a validating tool by other investigators developing instruments with theoretically related constructs. In most cases, the measure behaved as anticipated.

Extensive evidence has also been assembled over the past few years concerning the reliability of the Index. These studies have used diverse patient populations, varied types of raters in different geographic areas, and have been conducted in both French and English. On balance, the collective documentation from these investigations permits confidence that the Index scores and Uniscale provide data of sufficient reliability for use in a clinical study. None the less, there are two issues which need to be addressed.

The first issue concerns the less than ideal correlations obtained in internal consistency reliability. While there are no hard and fast criteria for acceptable levels of internal consistency, one can agree that a coefficient of 0.80 or greater is desirable, be it Cronbach's alpha, the Kuder-Richardson-20, or other measures.

There are four reasons for not expecting the responses to the items of the QL-Index to have a high level of internal consistency. First of all, items were selected to represent five separate dimensions, and each dimension was represented by one item. The dimensions are sufficiently different that the responses to them could well be statistically independent. Second, items were rejected by design if they had moderate to high levels (rhos of 0.50 or more) of covariation with the preferred items. Third, a coefficient such as Cronbach's alpha reflects the average correlation in the matrix of correlation coefficients as well as the number of items in the scale, and five is a small number of items. Finally, the reponses to the item for social support tend to be univariate and the scores for outlook tend to remain consistently high as well. Items must vary before they can have significant amounts of covariation with other items.

The QL-Index, like the Apgar score,[2] should be thought of as a composite of dissimilar items. If one finds a high level of internal consistency, so much the better, but the lack of an "acceptable" coefficient should not negate the use of the instrument. As the measure can be completed by the patient, a significant other, the attending physician, or other health care provider, the level of inter-rater agreement is a more important measure of reliability than a measure of internal consistency.

In terms of inter-rater agreement, one can raise a question about the objectivity of the QL-Index and Uniscale. If the measures are sufficiently objective for persons other than the patient to observe the phenomena of interest and rate them, scores by proxy raters can be used in place of, or in addition to, the ratings of the patients. If judgments about quality of life are subjective in character, only the patients themselves can give reliable and accurate ratings.

The questions on occupation or principal activity and activities of daily living are sufficiently objective that proxy responses can be used. The questions on health and outlook are more subjective indicators, but persons who know the patients could estimate whether the patients feel better or worse or if their outlook has been altered. In terms of support, one can observe the social interactions around the patients, but those involved may differ as to the degree the interactions are viewed as being supportive.

The lack of strong correlations between the proxy and patient ratings is not surprising. However, they do appear to be stronger the closer the proxy rater is to the patient. Nor is it surprising that the patients tend to give themselves higher ratings than either attending clinicians or significant others. This has been documented with other measures.[54,55]

As the changes in quality of life become more marked, proxy ratings should reflect the patients' status reasonably accurately. Proxy ratings by primary care persons provided the QL scores for the hospice patients in the last weeks of their lives in the National Hospice Study, and they showed the deterioration of quality of life over the last few weeks before death.

Uniscale is a subjective rating of patient status. Consequently the correlations between scores of patients and proxy ratings are less than the correlations for the QL-Index. The response is sufficiently subjective that it probably cannot reliably or accurately be provided by a proxy.

There is a mixed information available on the ability of the Index to respond to clinical change. This may relate to how the Index has been perceived by users. Generally speaking, various investigators testing or using the QL-Index have failed to indicate the conceptual basis for its use as a measure. They have recognized the generic health dimensions covered by the Index, but seldom have gone beyond this in thinking about its purpose.

For example, the QL-Index has been used as an indicator of immediate and short term response to changes in health status or management. Oncologists have used it to measure if it is sensitive to changes in chemotherapy or radiotherapy. Morris and associates[16] used the QL-Index and a variation of it to track weekly changes in health status over the last few weeks of life and investigators in the congestive heart failure trial[38] found that the Index differentiated patients in a placebo group from those receiving standard treatment during a 3-month period.

On the other hand, the measure has been used as indicator of the net effects of disease and management over time. This would suggest that the QL-Index is being used to measure health states that are more stable over time. For example, researchers studying patients with end-stage renal disease have used the measure to compare transplant patients with those on various types of dialysis, or to compare patients whose grafts did and did not fail 1 year after transplantation.

The responses to the questions on health and activities of daily living may fluctuate in response to short-term variations in symptom and treatment effects. The other dimensions, principal activity, support, and outlook, should be less subject to short-term variations in complaints and problems.

There is a case to be made for the use of disease-specific measures of symptoms and response to treatment to gauge short-term responses to variations in management. If there are major short-term effects, the QL-Index could well detect them. However, the measure is more appropriately used to assess changes in quality of health related to health care over longer periods. More specifically, an investigator could use the QL-Index as a pre- and post-measure when assessing an intervention, and use a disease-specific measure to detect specific changes over multiple points during the treatment time.

Several investigators have identified systematic differences in QL scores by gender, age, and disease groupings. In consequence, these variables need to be taken into consideration if the instrument is to be used as an outcome measure. If, for example, in a study that seeks to compare the effectiveness of two approaches to treatment, the interventions are influenced by these variables there is a possibility of misrepresenting the relationship between cause and effect.[11] Methods for remediating this problem through either the design or analysis exist as long as the potential issues have been idenfitied.

In summary, the QL-Index has a great deal of intuitive and practical appeal. It is short and easy to comprehend, administer, and record. It can be scored by professionals, patients, and their family members or friends, thus permitting comparisons among raters. Acceptability among users has been high. As a global measure of quality of life, it has broad applicability across different types of cancer and other chronic diseases. Finally, it has been well validated. Is it a "gold standard"? No, probably not, but there may never be a "gold standard" for assessing quality of life. Perhaps what we have is a standard that could be deemed as "silver" — even sterling silver if used as intended by the developers.

REFERENCES

1. Spitzer, W. O., Dobson, A. J., Hall, J., Chesterman, E., Levi, J., Shepherd, R., Battista, R. N., and Catchlove, B. R., Measuring the quality of life of cancer patients. A concise QL-Index for use by physicians, *J. Chronic Dis.*, 34, 585, 1981.
2. Apgar, V., Proposal for new methods of evaluation of newborn infants, *Anaesth. Analg.*, 32, 260, 1953.
3. Spitzer, W. O., State of science 1986: Quality of life and functional status as target variables for research, *J. Chronic Dis.*, 40, 465, 1987.
4. Gough, I. R., Furnival, C. M., Schilder, L., and Grove, W., Assessment of the quality of life of patients with advanced cancer, *Eur. J. Cancer Clin. Oncol.*, 19, 1161, 1983.
5. Padilla, G. V. and Grant, M. M., Quality of life as a cancer nursing outcome variable, *Adv. Nurs. Sci.*, 8, 45, 1985.
6. Schipper, H., Clinch, J., McMurray, A., and Levitt, M., Measuring the quality of life of cancer patients: the Functional Living Index - Cancer: development and validation, *J. Clin. Oncol.*, 2, 472, 1984.
7. Selby, P. J., Chapman, J.-A. W., Etazadi-Amoli, J., Dalley, D., and Boyd, N. F., The development of a method for assessing the quality of life of cancer patients, *Br. J. Cancer*, 50, 13, 1984.
8. Wenger, N. K., Mattson, M. E., Furberg, C. D., and Elinson, J., Assessment of quality of life in trials of cardiovascular therapies, *Am. J. Cardiol.*, 54, 908, 1984.
9. Levine, S. and Croog, S. H., What constitutes quality of life? A conceptualization of the dimensions of life quality in healthy populations and patients with cardiovascular disease, in *Assessment of Quality of Life in Clinical Trials of Cardiovascular Therapies*, Wenger, N. K., Mattson, M. E., Furberg, C. D., and Elinson, J., Eds., Le Jacq, New York, 1984, 46.
10. Slevin, M. L., Plant, H., Lynch, D., Drinkwater, J., and Gregory, W. M., Who should measure quality of life, the doctor or the patient?, *Br. J. Cancer*, 57, 109, 1988.
11. Suissa, S., Shenker, S. C., and Spitzer, W. O., Measuring the quality of life of cancer and chronically ill patients: cross validation studies of the Quality of Life Index, unpublished data.
12. Mor, V., Cancer patients' quality of life over the disease course: lessons from the real world, *J. Chronic Dis.*, 40, 535, 1987.
13. Wolcott, D. L., Namir, S., Fawzy, F. I., Gottlieb, M. S., and Mitsuyasu, R. T., Illness concerns, attitudes toward homosexuality, and social support in gay men, *Gen. Hosp. Psychiatry*, 8, 395, 1986.
14. Donlou, J. N., Wolcott, D. L., Gottlieb, M. S., and Landsverk, J., Psychosocial aspects of AIDS: a pilot study, *J. Psychosoc. Oncol.*, 3, 39, 1985.
15. Parfrey, P. S., Vavasour, H. M., Henry, S., Bullock, M., and Gault, M. H., Clinical features and severity of nonspecific symptoms in dialysis patients, *Nephron*, 50, 121, 1988.
16. Morris, J. H., Suissa, S., Sherwood, S., Wright, S. M., and Greer, D., Last days: a study of the quality of life of terminally ill cancer patients, *J. Chronic Dis.*, 39, 47, 1986.
17. Clark, A. and Fallowfield, L. J., Quality of life measurements in patients with malignant disease: a review, *J. R. Soc. Med.*, 79, 165, 1986.
18. Selby, P. and Robertson, B., Measurement of quality of life in patients with cancer, *Cancer Surv.*, 6, 521, 1987.
19. Cronbach, L. J., Coefficient alpha and the internal structure of tests, *Psychometrika*, 16, 297, 1951.
20. Mor, V., Stalker, M. Z., Gralla, R., Scher, H. I., Cimma, C., Park, D., Flaherty, A. M., Kiss, M., Nelson, P., Laliberte, L., Schwartz, R., Marks, P. A., and Oettgen, H. F., Day hospital as an alternative to inpatient care for cancer patients: a random assignment trial, *J. Clin. Epidemiol.*, 41, 771, 1988.
21. McGowan, I., Barr, H., and Krasner, N., Palliative laser therapy for inoperable rectal cancer — does it work?, *Cancer*, 63, 967, 1989.
22. Levine, M. N., Guyatt, G. H., Gent, M., De Pauw, S., Goodyear, M. D., Hryniuk, W. M., Arnold, A., Findlay, B., Skillings, J. R., Bramwell, V. H., Levin, L., Bush, H., Abu-Zahra, H., and Kotalik, J., Quality of life in stage II breast cancer: an instrument for clinical trials, *J. Clin. Oncol.*, 6, 1798, 1988.
23. Bohrnstedt, G. W., Measurement, in *Handbook of Survey Research*, Rossi, P. H., Wright, J. D., and Anderson, A. B., Eds., Academic Press, New York, 1983, 69.
24. Churchill, D. N., Torrance, G. W., Taylor, D. W., Barnes, C. C., Ludwin, D., Shimizu, A., and Smith, E. K. M., Measurement of quality of life in end-stage renal disease: the Time Trade Off approach, *Clin. Invest. Med.*, 10, 14, 1987.
25. Köster, R., Gebbensleben, B., Stützer, H., Salzberger, B., Ahrens, P., and Rohde, H., Quality of life in gastric cancer. Karnofsky's scale and Spitzer's index in comparison at the time of surgery in a cohort of 1081 patients, *Scand. J. Gastroenterol.*, 22 (Suppl. 133), 102, 1987.
26. Coates, A. Gebski, V., Bishop, J. F., Jeal, P. N., Woods, R. L., Snyder, R., Tattersall, M. H. N., Byrne, M., Harvey, V., Gill, G., Simpson, J., Drummond, R., Browne, J., van Cooten, R., and Forbes, J. F., Improving the quality of life during chemotherapy for advanced breast cancer, *N. Engl. J. Med.*, 317, 1490, 1987.

27. McDowell, I. and Newell, C., *Measuring Health: A Guide to Rating Scales and Questionnaires*, Oxford University Press, New York, 1987, 12.
28. Karnofsky, D. A. and Burchenal, J. H., The clinical evaluation of chemotherapeutic agents in cancer, in *Evaluation of Chemotherapeutic Agents*, Macleod, C. M., Ed., Columbia University Press, New York, 1949, 191.
29. Bond, A. and Lader, M., The use of analogue scales in rating subjective feelings, *Br. J. Med. Psychol.*, 47, 211, 1974.
30. Wood-Dauphinee, S. and Williams, J. I., Reintegration to normal living as a proxy to quality of life, *J. Chronic Dis.*, 40, 491, 1987.
31. Wood-Dauphinee, S., Opzoomer, M. A., Williams, J. I., Marchand, B., and Spitzer, W. O., Assessment of global function: the Reintegration to Normal Living Index, *Arch. Phys. Med. Rehabil.*, 69, 583, 1988.
32. Mor, V. and Guadagnoli, E., Qualitity of life measurement: a psychometric tower of Babel, *J. Clin. Epidemiol.*, 41, 1055, 1988.
33. Warner, S. C. and Williams, J. I., The Meaning in Life Scale: determining the reliability and validity of a measure, *J. Chronic Dis.*, 40, 503, 1987.
34. Warner, S. C., The Measurement of Subjective Variables in Epidemiology: Development and Validation of an Instrument for Quantifying Self-Perceived Meaning in Life among the Chronically Ill Institutionalized Elderly, Ph.D. Thesis, McGill University, 1986.
35. Parfrey, P. S., Vavasour, H., Bullock, M., Henry, S., Harnett, J. D., and Gault, M. H., Symptoms in end-stage renal disease: dialysis vs transplantation, *Transplant. Proc.*, 19, 3407, 1987.
36. Schuessler, K. F. and Fisher, G. A., Quality of life research and sociology, *Annu. Rev. Sociol.*, 11, 129, 1985.
37. Guyatt, G., Walter, S., and Norman, G., Measuring change over time: assessing the usefulness of evaluative instruments, *J. Chronic Dis.*, 40, 171, 1987.
38. Tandon, P. K., Stander, H., and Schwarz, R. P., Analysis of quality of life data from a randomized, placebo-controlled heart failure trial, *J. Clin. Epidemiol.*, 42, 955, 1989.
39. Greer, D. S., Mor, V., Morris, J. N., Sherwood, S., Kidder, D., and Birnbaum, H., An alternative in terminal care: results of the National Hospice Study, *J. Chronic Dis.*, 39, 9, 1986.
40. Ward, A. W. M., Home care services — an alternative to hospices?, *Community Med.*, 9, 47, 1987.
41. Ventafridda, V., Tamburini, M., Selmi, S., Valera, L., and De Conno, F., The importance of a Home Care Program for patients with advanced cancer, *Tumori*, 71, 449, 1985.
42. Troidl, H., Kusche, J., Vestweber, K.-H., Eypasch, E., and Maul, U., Pouch versus esophagojejunostomy after total gastrectomy, a randomized clinical trial, *World J. Surg.*, 11, 699, 1987.
43. Kusche, J., Vestweber, K.-H., and Troidl, H., Quality of life after total gastrectomy for stomach cancer. Results of three types of quality of life evaluative methods, *Scand. J. Gastroenterol.*, 22 (Suppl. 133), 96, 1987.
44. Parfrey, P. S., Vavasour, H. M., and Gault, M. H., A prospective study of health status in dialysis and transplant patients, *Transplant. Proc.*, 20, 1231, 1988.
45. Nakache, R., Tydén, G., and Groth, C.-G., Quality of life in diabetic patients after combined pancreas-kidney or kidney transplantation, *Diabetes*, 38, 40, 1989.
46. Sage, W. M., Rosenthal, M. H., and Silverman, J. F., Is intensive care worth it? An assessment of input and outcome for the critically ill, *Crit. Care Med.*, 14, 777, 1986.
47. Bergner, M., Bobbitt, R. A., Carter, W. B., and Gilson, B. S., The Sickness Impact Profile: development and final revision of a health status measure, *Med. Care*, 19, 787, 1981.
48. Sage, W. M., Hurst, C. R., Silverman, J. F., and Bortz, W. M., Intensive care for the elderly: outcome of elective and non elective admissions, *J. Am. Geriatr. Soc.*, 35, 312, 1987.
49. Slatyer, M. A., James, O. F., Moore, P. G., and Leeder, S. R., Costs, severity of illness and outcome in intensive care, *Anaesth. Intensive Care*, 14, 381, 1986.
50. Liang, M. H., Partridge, A. J., Larson, M. G., Gall, V., Taylor, J., Berkman, C., Master, R., Feltin, M., and Taylor, J., Evaluation of comprehensive rehabilitation services for elderly homebound patients with arthritis and orthopedic diasbility, *Arthritis Rheum.*, 27, 258, 1984.
51. Tan, T.-L., Kales, J. D., Kales, A., Martin, E. D., Mann, L. D., and Soldatos, C. R., Inpatient multidimensional management of treatment-resistant insomnia, *Psychosomatics*, 28, 266, 1987.
52. Yellowlees, P. M. and Ruffin, R. E., Psychological defenses and coping styles in patients following a life threatening attack of asthma, *Chest*, 95, 1298, 1989.
53. World Health Organization, *The First Ten Years of the World Health Organization*, World Health Organization, Geneva, 1958.
54. Epstein, A. M., Hall, J. A., Tognetti, J., Son, L. H., and Conant, L., Using proxies to evaluate quality of life, *Med. Care*, 27, S91, 1989.
55. Magaziner, J., Simonsick, E. M., Kashner, T. M., and Hebel, J. R., Patient-proxy response comparability on measures of patient health and functional status, *J. Clin. Epidemiol.*, 41, 1065, 1988.

Chapter 14

THE EORTC CORE QUALITY-OF-LIFE QUESTIONNAIRE: INTERIM RESULTS OF AN INTERNATIONAL FIELD STUDY*

Neil K. Aaronson, Sam Ahmedzai, Monika Bullinger, Dirk Crabeels, Jorge Estapè, Antonio Filiberti, Henning Flechtner, Ulrich Frick, Christoph Hürny, Stein Kaasa, Marianne Klee, Miroslav Mastilica, David Osoba, Bettina Pfausler, Darius Razavi, Peter B. C. Rofe, Simon Schraub, Marianne Sullivan, and Fumikazu Takeda for the EORTC Study Group on Quality of Life

TABLE OF CONTENTS

*   EORTC Protocol 15861: Neil K. Aaronson, study coordinator; Dirk Crabeels (formerly of the EORTC Data Center, Brussels, Belgium), data manager; and Ulrich Frick, project statistician. The remaining authors are the national coordinators of the project. The authors are listed in alphabetical order.

I. INTRODUCTION

Traditionally, treatment efficacy in phase III clinical trials in oncology has been assessed in terms of such biomedical outcomes as tumor response, disease-free and overall survival, and level of treatment-related toxicity. In recent years, however, there has been a growing interest in expanding the set of evaluation parameters employed in cancer clinical trials to include an assessment of the impact of treatment on the patients' "quality of life", defined most typically in terms of physical, psychological, and social functioning.[1-3] Indeed, quality-of-life variables have played a salient role in recent prospective, randomized trials in operable[4-7] and advanced[8] breast cancer, and in soft-tissue sarcoma.[9] Nevertheless, such applications remain the exception rather than the rule.[10-12]

Much of the hesitancy in adopting psychosocial research strategies in clinical trials would appear to derive from a basic lack of familiarity of the clinical and social science research communities with one another. On the one hand, clinical researchers are typically untrained in, and perhaps a bit distrustful of, social science research methods. On the other hand, social scientists often fail to familiarize themselves sufficiently with the substantive research questions of interest to clinicians, and can exhibit a lack of sensitivity to the practical constraints operating within clinical trial settings.

In 1980, in an effort to bridge the gap between physicians and behavioral scientists working in the cancer field in Europe, the European Organization for Research and Treatment of Cancer (EORTC) created a Study Group on Quality of Life. A principal function of this group was to serve as a liaison to the various EORTC clinical cooperative groups, providing advice on the design, implementation, and analysis of quality-of-life substudies within selective phase III clinical trials.

An important goal of the Study Group was to achieve consensus on how quality of life should be defined and measured. It was recognized that the lack of such consensus represented a major barrier to the inclusion of quality-of-life evaluations in clinical trial settings. The physician interested in assessing the psychosocial impact of both routine medical care and experimental treatments is confronted with a confusing array of choices. At one end of the spectrum are extensive and time-consuming interview protocols that exceed the practical limits imposed by most clinical trials. At the other end are more concise, patient self-report questionnaires that, while representing a less cumbersome approach to data collection, often leave unanswered the critical questions of instrument reliability and validity.

Much of the early discussion in the EORTC Study Group focused on the relative merits of employing a generic vs. disease-specific approach to quality of life assessment. Quality-of-life measures can be organized along a continuum reflecting their intended spectrum of application: (a) generic instruments designed for use across a wide range of chronic disease populations; (b) disease-specific measures designed for use with cancer patients, in general; (c) diagnosis-specific measures (e.g., intended for use with breast cancer patients only); and (d) *ad hoc*, study-specific measures.

The primary advantage associated with the most generic class of measures is that it allows for comparison of results across studies and, in the long run, can facilitate an ordered, stepwise process of instrument development and validation. Yet, such generic measures, by definition, have not been developed or validated specifically for oncology populations, and thus may not cover adequately topics of particular relevance in evaluating the psychosocial impact of cancer and its treatment. Conversely, while diagnosis-specific and study-specific instruments offer a higher degree of specificity, this is often achieved at the cost of generalizability and instrument standardization.

While a number of cancer-specific questionnaires were available by the mid-1980s, few had yet undergone sufficient field testing to recommend them for more general use. Two instruments that had undergone preliminary psychometric evaluations — the Functional

Living Index-Cancer (FLIC)[13] and the questionnaire developed by Selby and colleagues[14] — were rejected as candidate measures for use in EORTC trials owing to anticipated problems with data reduction and interpretation. The FLIC yields a single, overall score reflecting the sum of the individual items, while the Selby questionnaire treats each item separately. In the former case, the total quality of life score was considered to be too coarse to be of optimal clinical value. In the latter case, there was concern that the absence of subscales summarizing the individual items would lead to information overload.

Given the paucity of well-validated cancer-specific questionnaires, the Study Group elected to embark on the long-term process of instrument development. A subcommittee was formed of physicians, psychologists, psychometricians, and statisticians whose principal tasks were to establish the basic criteria for questionnaire construction, to select and/or generate candidate questionnaire items, and to field test the resulting questionnaire in a cross-cultural context. This chapter presents results of the first phase of this questionnaire development process.

II. METHODOLOGICAL CONSIDERATIONS IN CONSTRUCTING THE QUESTIONNAIRE

The basic measurement strategy that guided the development of the questionnaire reflected a compromise between the generic and disease-specific approaches to quality-of-life assessment. The intent was to generate a *core* questionnaire, composed of a limited number of subscales representing quality of life domains relevant across a wide range of cancer sites and treatment modalities. Additional disease- and treatment-specific questionnaire modules would be developed to complement the core instrument. Adoption of this *modular* assessment strategy could reconcile two principal requirements of a quality of life measure — a sufficient degree of generalizability to allow for cross-study comparisons, and a level of specificity adequate for answering those research questions of particular relevance in a given clinical trial.[15]

Given this general framework, the following specific criteria were employed in constructing the questionnaire:

1. It should be cancer specific.
2. It should be designed for patient self-administration.
3. It should be multidimensional in structure, covering at least three basic quality of life domains — physical functioning (including symptom experience and functional status), emotional functioning, and social functioning.
4. It should be comprised primarily of multi-item scales, with additional single items included only where necessary.
5. It should be relatively short, with an average completion time of approximately 10 to 15 minutes.
6. It should exhibit adequate levels of reliability, validity, and responsiveness to clinical changes in patients' health status.
7. It should be amenable for use across national and cultural boundaries (i.e., should exhibit cross-cultural, as well as statistical validity).

Finally, several technical issues relating to the form and structures of the questionnaire were addressed. First, it was considered essential that the questionnaire employ a specific time frame. In measuring psychosocial outcomes in clinical trials, we may be interested in both the short- and long-term effects of treatment. Particularly in the case of short-term effects (e.g., during or immmediately following a course of chemotherapy or radiotherapy), it is important to provide a relatively short time frame in order to assure that a patient is responding to questions in terms of the relevant period in the treatment cycle. If too long a time frame is employed, or if it is left undefined, the patient may be confused as to which period he or she should report — a treatment period, a rest period, or perhaps both. Even in the case of long-term effects, the use of a relatively short question time frame can be recommended. This will minimize problems associated with memory loss, and will avoid confounding specific symptom experience with a more generalized personality trait characterized by a tendency to complain in either psychological or physical terms.[16] With these considerations in mind, a 1 week time frame was selected for use in the core questionnaire.

Second, a choice has to be made between Likert-type (i.e., categorical) or linear analog response scales. Linear analog scales are purported to be highly sensitive to small changes in symptom levels and to approximate more closely true interval level measurement than do their Likert-type counterparts. However, practical limitations may outweigh these more formal considerations. While a number of investigators report successful use of linear analog methods, others argue that the level of abstraction required by the technique is too great for many patients.[17] Additionally, preparing such data for computer entry (i.e., physically measuring the distance between each response and the scale anchor) can be quite cumbersome, particularly in large scale, multicenter clinical trials. For these reasons, it was decided to employ Likert-type response scales in the core questionnaire.

III. OVERVIEW OF THE CORE QUESTIONNAIRE

The quality-of-life domains selected for inclusion in the core quality-of-life questionnaire are outlined in Table 1. The questionnaire consists of 36 items assessing: (a) physical functioning; (b) role functioning; (c) common physical symptoms of cancer and its treatment; (d) emotional functioning; (e) social functioning; (f) financial impact; and (g) overall perceived health status and global quality of life. A detailed description of the rationale underlying this choice of quality of life domains is provided elsewhere.[15]

An effort was made to include several items to measure each of the quality-of-life domains of interest. To the extent that such multiple items can be combined into summative ratings (i.e., scales or indices) they present a clear advantage over single item measures in terms of reliability, validity and, where necessary, estimation of missing scores.

Additionally, a tumor-specific questionnaire module was developed to provide more detailed information on symptoms of particular relevance to lung cancer patients (the target population for initial psychometric testing of the questionnaire; see below).

In constructing the questionnaire, careful attention was paid to assuring that questions had as close to the same meaning across languages and cultures as possible. Including individuals from a range of countries in the instrument development process was a first, important step toward minimizing cross-cultural problems. Once the choice of items had been made, the questionnaire was submitted to a rigorous "forward-backward" translation process. This entailed translating the questionnaire first from its original language (English) into nine alternative languages, and then translating it back again into English. This was an iterative process, requiring several refinements in question wording before equivalence could be best approximated. Pilot testing of early versions of the questionnaire in various local settings also led to refinements in item content and wording.

IV. METHODS AND PSYCHOMETRIC ANALYSIS PLAN

In order to investigate the psychometric properties and cross-cultural performance of the core questionnaire, a field study was initiated with participants from 15 countries, including most of the Western European countries as well as Australia, Canada, and Japan. The following sections describe the study design and psychometric analysis plan.

TABLE 1

Content and Hypothesized Structure of the EORTC Core
Quality of Life Questionnaire

Content area	No. of items	Type of measure
Physical functioning	7	Guttman scale
Role functioning	2	Guttman scale
Disease symptoms		
Fatigue and malaise	5	Likert scale
Nausea/vomiting	3	Likert scale
Other gastrointestinal	2	Single items
Pain	1	Single item
Dyspnea	1	Single item
Sleep disturbance	1	Single item
Cognitive disturbance	1	Single item
Emotional functioning	8	Likert scale
Social functioning	2	Likert scale
Financial impact	1	Single item
Global health status/quality of life	2	Likert scale

A. THE CHOICE OF THE PATIENT POPULATION FOR STUDY

Although the core questionnaire is intended for use across a range of cancer patient populations, for methodological and practical reasons it was considered desirable to employ initially a study sample that was relatively homogeneous in terms of diagnosis. Nonresectable lung cancer patients were selected for study for the following reasons: (a) the high incidence of the disease would facilitate rapid sample accrual; (b) the palliative nature of available therapies suggested the need for including psychosocial endpoints in treatment evaluations; and (c) there was a paucity of research on the effects of lung cancer and its treatment on patients' quality of life. No further restrictions were placed on patient selection with regard to histological type, age, or performance status.

B. RESEARCH DESIGN AND STUDY PROCEDURES

The study design called for administration of the questionnaire at two points in time: (a) following diagnosis, but prior to the start of treatment (i.e., baseline); and (b) once during the period of treatment (i.e., on the last day of the first course radiotherapy or on the last day of the second cycle of chemotherapy). The current report will focus on data generated from the first, baseline administration of the questionnaire.

Patients were also asked to complete a debriefing form regarding the time required to complete the questionnaire, the need for assistance in its completion, and the presence of questionnaire items that were confusing, difficult to answer, or upsetting. Sociodemographic data included age, sex, marital status, household composition, education, and occupation. Clinical variables included histology, disease stage, weight loss, comorbidity, nature and schedule of treatment, performance status as measured by the ECOG scale,[18] and treatment toxicities (i.e., selective subscales of the WHO Acute and Subacute Toxicity Scales).

C. SCALE CONSTRUCTION AND RELIABILITY ESTIMATION

In order to test whether the individual questionnaire items outlined in Table 1 could be aggregated into a more limited set of scales, either Likert's method of summated ratings[19] or Guttman's Scalogram Analysis[20] was employed. For Likert scaling, items belonging to a hypothesized scale were first summed and then divided by the total number of items in that scale, yielding a total scale score based on the original metric of the individual item responses. Each item of a hypothesized scale was correlated with the total scale score corrected for overlap (i.e., the item score was not included in the total scale score). In order to be retained in the scale, each item should correlate 0.40 or higher with the total scale score.[21]

Principal components factor analysis was used to confirm that only one scale should be constructed from a set of items. A factor is essentially a cluster of items that are highly related to one another. Evidence of scale unidimensionality is provided when the items "load" on (correlate with) a single factor. A factor loading of 0.40 or higher was used as the criterion for retaining an item in a given scale.

Scale reliability (i.e., internal consistency) was assessed by Chronbach's alpha coefficient.[22] Although internal consistency estimates of a magnitude of 0.50 or greater are considered acceptable for group comparisons,[23] values exceeding 0.70 were sought in the current study.

Guttman's Scalogram Analysis is an alternative method for combining items into a single scale score. A Guttman scale can be constructed if a set of items with dichotomous (i.e., "yes" or "no") response choices represent a continuum of increasing levels of intensity, difficulty, or severity. A Guttman scale score is essentially a count of positive responses to such a series of questions. Because of the cumulative nature of the items, a Guttman scale describes rather precisely the logical pattern of responses to all of the items. In the core questionnaire, the physical functioning and role functioning items were hypothesized to form Guttman scales. The two statistics used to evaluate whether these items met the Guttman criteria for scalability were the coefficient of reproducibility (CR) and the coefficient of scalability (CS). Minimal standards of 0.90 for CR and 0.60 for CS were employed as evidence of scale reliability.[21]

D. ASSESSMENT OF CONSTRUCT VALIDITY

Construct validity refers essentially to whether the hypothesized scales are actually measuring the attitudes or behaviors (i.e., the underlying construct) that they are intended to measure and, of equal importance, whether they are *not* measuring some other underlying construct. More formally, construct validation refers to a family of procedures that has as a common denominator the examination of the pattern of correlations within and between various scales. To establish construct validity one looks for evidence of convergence among indicators of the same or similar theoretical constructs, and of divergence between indicators of unrelated or dissimilar constructs.

In the current study, three types of analyses were undertaken to examine the construct validity of the hypothesized questionnaire scales. First, multitrait scaling techniques were employed to test for item-discriminant validity. A matrix of item-scale correlations was created such that each item was correlated with all of the scales being constructed, including the scale to which it was hypothesized to belong (corrected for overlap). According to the discriminant validity criterion, each item should correlate highest with its own scale.

Second, a correlation matrix was constructed of the various quality of life scales. It was expected that those scales that were conceptually related would correlate significantly with one another, whereas those scales with less in common would exhibit low correlations.

Finally, analysis of variance was used to examine whether the quality of life scales were sensitive to differences in the clinical status of the patient sample. The clinical parameters employed included disease stage, ECOG performance status ratings, weight loss and symptom level as recorded by the physician. In general, it was hypothesized that the average scores on the quality-of-life scales would be significantly lower for those subgroups of patients with a poorer clinical status, as defined by this set of variables.

E. ASSESSMENT OF CROSS-CULTURAL VALIDITY

The large majority of available quality of life measures has been developed, validated and subsequently employed in studies based in English-speaking countries. Little attention has been paid to the appropriateness of such instruments for use in other cultural settings. In contrast, the EORTC questionnaire was intended, from the onset, to be used in an international context. Thus, examination of the performance of the questionnaire in a cross-cultural setting represented an essential element of the validation process. Ideally, one would want to replicate the psychometric analyses for each language, culture and/or country of interest. However, practical constraints (i.e., sample size requirements), prohibited the use of this strategy in a single field study. As a more feasible alternative, in the current study the basic psychometric analyses described above were replicated with subsamples formed on the basis of the following three broad categories: (a) English-speaking countries (including Australia, Canada, and Great Britain); (b) northern European countries (including Scandinavia, the Benelux countries, and the German-speaking countries; and (c) southern European countries (including France and French-speaking areas of Belgium and Switzerland, Italy, Spain, and Yugoslavia). As it did not fall logically within one of these categories, Japan formed a fourth, separate subsample. The results of these additional subgroup analyses will be reported only in those cases where they diverge from those based on the analysis of the total study sample.

V. RESULTS

A. CHARACTERISTICS OF THE STUDY SAMPLE

Over an approximate 2-year period, 537 patients were accrued onto the study from 25 institutions located in Western Europe, Australia, Canada, and Japan. Table 2 presents the patient accrual by participating country.

The patients ranged in age between 30 and 87 years, with a mean age of 63 years (standard deviation of 9.6 years). Twenty-one percent of the patients were female and 77% were married. Approximately two thirds of the sample had completed compulsory education only, 28% had received advanced vocational training, and 8% were university graduates.

The clinical characteristics of the sample are presented in Table 3. Sixty-two percent of the patients had non-small cell lung cancer, and 38% small cell lung cancer. In approximately one quarter of the cases the disease was localized, in one third it was locoregional, and in 41% there was evidence of metastasis. Two thirds of the sample had a pretreatment ECOG performance status rating of 0 or 1 (normal or slightly restricted activity level), one quarter had a rating of 2 (ambulatory more than 50% of the time, but unable to work), with the remaining 10% being rated as ECOG level 3 (confined to a bed or chair for more than 50% of waking hours) or 4 (bedridden, unable to carry out self-care activities). Thirty-seven percent of the patients had lost 10% or less of their body weight, and 19% had lost more than 10%. Slightly less than 10% of the sample was asymptomatic, with the remaining patients divided approximately equally between those with local vs. systemic symptoms.

B. ACCEPTABILITY OF THE QUESTIONNAIRE

As the questionnaire was designed for patient self-administration, concerns with ease of completion and acceptability of content were of paramount importance. On average, the questionnaire required slightly less than 15 min to complete (standard deviation of 9 min). Approximately 40% of the sample reported receiving some assistance in completing the questionnaire. In the large majority of cases, however, this involved little more than a brief explanation of the purpose and general content of the questionnaire. Nevertheless, a small number of patients did require help in completing the questionnaire, either due to physical handicap (e.g., poor vision) or very poor physical condition (e.g., extreme fatigue).

Approximately one fifth of the sample reported that one or more of the questionnaire items was confusing or difficult to answer. The majority of these items was concerned with emotional functioning (see below). Less than 5% of the sample found any of the questions to be upsetting.

TABLE 2
Level of Study Participation by Country

Country	N	%
Australia	52	9.7
Austria	18	3.4
Belgium	62	11.5
Canada	57	10.6
Denmark	13	2.4
Federal Republic of Germany	53	9.9
France	31	5.8
Great Britain	21	3.9
Italy	17	3.2
Japan	47	8.7
The Netherlands	24	4.5
Norway	39	7.3
Spain	48	8.9
Sweden	39	7.3
Switzerland	4	0.7
Yugoslavia	12	2.2
Total	537	100.0

TABLE 3
Clinical Characteristics of the Study Sample

Variable	N[a]	Category (%)
Tumor type	518	
Non-small cell		61.6
Small cell		38.4
Disease stage	522	
Local		26.4
Locoregional		32.6
Metastatic		41.0
Performance status[b]	518	
0		18.5
1		47.9
2		23.6
3		8.3
4		1.7
Weight loss	527	
None		43.6
<10%		37.4
>10%		19.0
Symptomatology	524	
Asymptomatic		9.7
Local		46.8
Systemic		43.5

[a]   N varies due to missing data.
[b]   Baseline (pretreatment) ECOG performance status scale.

C. THE SCALING PROPERTIES OF THE QUESTIONNAIRE
1. Physical and Role Functioning

Functional status refers to the performance of (or the capacity to perform) a range of activities that are normal for most people. In the core questionnaire, two scales were employed

TABLE 4
Physical Functioning: Item Frequency Distributions and Scale Summary Statistics

Item	N[a]	%
Can you do hard activities, like moving heavy furniture?	533	26.8
If you wanted to, could you run a short distance?	534	39.7
Do you have any trouble taking a long walk?	535	51.6
Do you have any trouble walking a short distance?	533	20.6
Are you in bed or chair for most of the day?	530	43.0
Do you have to stay indoors most of the day?	533	40.3
Do you need help with eating, dressing, washing yourself, or using the toilet?	534	12.4
Scale[b]	519	
Range: 0—7		
Mean: 3.0		
St. dev.: 1.9		
Reliability:[c] 0.71		

[a] N varies due to missing data.
[b] For scale construction, response categories for questions 1 and 2 were reversed. A higher scale score represents a higher level of dysfunction.
[c] With data in dichotomous form, the Chronbach's alpha coefficient is equal to the reliability coefficient Kuder-Richardson-20 (Hull and Nie, 1981).

to measure physical and role functioning. Physical functioning was assessed with seven items similar to those used previously in healthy populations,[24] in patients with arthritis,[25] and among cancer patients.[26] As these items were hypothesized to form a Guttman scale, the response categories used were a simple "yes" or "no" dichotomy. The item content and score distributions are provided in Table 4. While few patients had difficulties with self-care activities, most were unable to carry out more rigorous forms of activity.

Scalogram analysis indicated that these items did not meet the minimal criteria for a Guttman scale (CR = 0.85; CS = 0.53). Subgroup analyses indicated that this scaling problem could not be attributed to cross-cultural issues, although the Japanese subgroup tended to deviate most strongly from the hypothesized Guttman scale pattern.

As an alternative, these seven items were treated as a less psychometrically demanding Likert-type scale. Scale scores ranged from 0 to 7 (a higher score representing a higher level of dysfunction), with a mean of 3.0. Five of the seven-item-scale correlations were above the 0.40 criterion for additive scales. The reliability of the scale was 0.71.

Two items were included in the questionnaire to assess role functioning, defined in terms of the ability to perform usual work and housework activities. As these two questions were also intended to form a Guttman scale, dichotomous responses categories were used. The item content and score distributions are shown in Table 5. Slightly more than half of the patients reported some limitations in role functioning, with 41% being completely unable to work or to carry out their household jobs.

Scalogram analysis supported the Guttman structure of this two item scale (CR = 0.94; CS = 0.84). Nevertheless, in order to have comparable data across all of the questionnaire scales, these items were further analyzed as a Likert scale. Scale scores ranged from 0 to 2 (a higher score representing a higher level of dysfunction), with a mean of 0.97. The scale reliability was acceptable for group comparisons (alpha coefficient = 0.61).

TABLE 5
Role Functioning: Item Frequency Distributions and Scale Summary Statistics

Item	N[a]	%
Are you limited in any way doing your work or household jobs?	532	56.0
Are you completely unable to work at a job or do household jobs?	530	41.1
Scale[b]	526	

Scale[b]	
Range:	0—2
Mean:	0.97
St. dev.:	0.84
Reliability:[c]	0.61

[a] N varies due to missing data.
[b] A higher scale score represents a higher level of dysfunction.
[c] With data in dichotomous form, the Chronbach's alpha coefficient is equal to the reliability coefficient Kuder-Richardson-20 (Hull and Nie, 1981).

2. Disease Symptoms

Symptoms reported frequently by cancer patients include fatigue and malaise, nausea and vomiting, shortness of breath, pain, constipation, diarrhea, sleeplessness, and cognitive disturbances. In the core questionnaire, these symptoms were assessed with a combination of multiple item scales and single items. All response categories ranged on a four-point Likert-type scale from "not at all" to "very much."

a. Fatigue and Malaise

Five items, similar to those developed by Linssen and colleagues,[27] were employed to assess fatigue and malaise. As can be seen in Table 6, although slightly more than half of the patients reported feeling physically well, a substantial minority reported heightened levels of fatique and malaise.

These five items were combined into a Likert scale, with scores ranging from 1 to 4 (a higher score representing increasing levels of fatigue/malaise). Factor analysis supported the unidimensionality of the scale, with all items loading on a single factor. All item-scale correlations were above the 0.40 criterion for additive scales. The reliability of the scale, as determined by Chronbach's alpha coefficient, was 0.81.

One of the objectives of this study was to determine if the length of the questionnaire could be reduced without sacrificing psychometric performance. The current analysis indicated that a three-item version of the fatigue/malaise scale exhibited better internal consistency (0.85) than the original five-item version. The mean score (2.3) for this truncated scale was identical to that of the five-item version.

b. Nausea and Vomiting

Three of the questionnaire items were hypothesized to form a Likert scale of nausea and vomiting. The item content and score distributions are presented in Table 7. As noted, while one third of the patients reported appetite loss at baseline, few were bothered by symptoms of nausea and vomiting. This was not unexpected, as these latter symptoms are more typically the result of treatment (e.g., chemotherapy) than of the disease process itself.

Factor analysis indicated that the item on appetite loss loaded on a separate factor than the other two items. This was confirmed by the relatively low observed reliability (alpha

TABLE 6
Fatigue: Item Frequency
Distributions and Scale Summary
Statistics

Item	N[a]	%[b]
Did you need to rest?*	534	41.6
Have you felt ill?	535	26.9
Have you felt weak?*	534	36.1
Were you tired?*	535	40.0
Were you physically well?	536	58.0

	5-item scale[c]	3-item scale[d]
N:	520	530
Mean:	2.3	2.3
St. dev.:	0.78	0.86
Reliability:[e]	0.81	0.85

[a] N varies due to missing data.
[b] Response categories included: 1 "not at all", 2 "a little", 3 "quite a bit" and 4 "very much". Percentages reported are for categories 3 and 4 combined.
[c] For scale construction, response categories for question 5 were reversed. The scale was constructed by summing the item scores and dividing by the number of items. A higher score represents a higher fatigue level.
[d] This abbreviated scale is composed of those items marked with an asterisk (*).
[e] Chronbach's alpha coefficient.

coefficient = 0.59) when all three items were combined into a summative scale. A truncated scale, limited to the two questions on nausea and vomiting, yielded significantly improved reliability (alpha coefficient = 0.78).

c. Additional Symptoms

The remaining physical symptom items were treated individually in the analysis. The following baseline levels (moderate to severe) were reported for these symptoms: constipation (18%); diarrhea (4%); dyspnea (38%); pain (30%), difficulty sleeping (36%); and difficulty with memory and concentration (14%).

3. Emotional Functioning

While a range of questionnaires is available for assessing psychological morbidity in general or psychiatric populations, very few have been developed for use with chronic disease patients, in general, or for cancer patients, in particular. Most of these instruments include a number of symptoms (e.g., fatigue, decreased sexual drive, appetite loss, etc.) that, when employed among cancer patients, may reflect the somatic disease process itself, rather than somatic manifestations of psychological distress as intended.

The Hospital Anxiety and Depression Scale (HADS[28]), a 14-item instrument developed for use with physically ill populations, avoids this methodological problem by focusing solely on anxious and depressed affect. Additionally, the wording of the questions avoids allusions to psychopathology, rendering it more appropriate for use with cancer patients

TABLE 7
Nausea and Vomiting: Item
Frequency Distributions and Scale
Summary Statistics

Item	N[a]	%[b]
Did you lack appetite?	536	33.2
Were you nauseated?*	536	9.1
Did you vomit?*	536	4.9

	3-item scale[c]	2-item scale[d]
N:	536	536
Mean:	1.6	1.3
St. dev.:	0.64	0.62
Reliability:[e]	0.59	0.78

[a] One case had missing data on these items.
[b] Response categories included: 1 "not at all",
2 "a little", 3 "quite a bit" and 4 "very much".
Percentages reported are for categories 3 and
4 combined.
[c] The scale was constructed by summing the item
scores and dividing by the number of items. A
higher score represents a higher symptom level.
[d] This abbreviated scale is composed of those
items marked with an asterisk (*).
[e] Chronbach's alpha coefficient.

than other such scales. Despite the relative brevity of the HADS, it was considered too long for inclusion in a multidimensional quality-of-life questionnaire. In consultation with the scale's authors, a subset of eight items was selected that represented a balance between symptoms of depression and anxiety, and between positive and negative question wording. Additionally, the original HADS response categories were adapted to a uniform four-point Likert scale.

The content and score distributions for these eight items are presented in Table 8. Approximately one quarter of the sample exhibited one or more symptoms of anxiety, while about one third reported depressive symptoms. However, the pattern of responses to the individual items suggested that patients may have been confused by the use of both positively and negatively worded questions. A substantial number of "inconsistent" score patterns were detected whereby patients reported both the total absence of symptoms and very severe symptoms within the same hypothesized subscale (i.e., depression or anxiety). While the technique of balancing the direction of question wording is often recommended in order to avoid an "acquiescent response set" (i.e., the tendency to agree with statements, regardless of their content), these findings suggest that it can also lead to mistakes in filling out the questionnaire.

This methodological problem was reflected in the failure to confirm empirically the hypothesized two-dimensional structure of the scale. While two factors emerged from the factor analysis, they reflected the positive vs. negative item wording rather than the substantive distinction between anxiety and depression.

Given the absence of empirical justification for creating separate subscales of anxiety and depression, the 8 HADS items were combined into a single measure of psychological distress. The scale scores ranged from 1 to 4 (a higher score representing a higher distress level), with a mean of 1.9.

TABLE 8
Emotional Functioning: Item Frequency
Distributions and Scale Summary Statistics

Item[a]	N[b]	%[c]
Could you sit at ease and feel relaxed?	526	55.5
Have you lost interest in your appearance?	533	8.6
Have you felt restless as if you had to be on the move?	532	23.1
Did you look forward with enjoyment to things?	524	63.4
Did you get sudden feelings of panic?	535	15.9
Could you enjoy a good book or radio or television program?	534	70.2
Have you felt tense or 'wound up'?	534	25.6
Could you laugh and see the funny side of things?	531	66.9
Scale[d]	511	

Mean:	1.9
St. dev.:	0.54
Reliability:[e]	0.67

[a] These items were selected from the Hospital Anxiety and Depression Scale (Zigmond and Snaith, 1983) in consultation with the scale's authors.

[b] N varies due to missing data.

[c] Response categories included: 1 "not at all", 2 "a little", 3 "quite a bit" and 4 "very much". Percentages reported are for categories 3 and 4 combined.

[d] For scale construction, response categories for questions 1, 4, 6, and 8 were reversed. The scale was constructed by summing the item scores and dividing by the number of items. A higher scale score represents a higher level of dysfunction.

[e] Chronbach's alpha coefficient.

It should be noted that this distress scale was also far from optimal in a psychometric sense. Only four of the eight item-scale correlations surpassed the 0.40 criterion and, given the relatively large number of items, the scale reliability was only fair (alpha coefficient = 0.67). Additionally, the scale exhibited some cross-cultural problems. It performed best with the English-language subsample (alpha coefficient = 0.72), reasonably well with the European subsamples (alpha coefficients of 0.64 for northern Europe and 0.68 for southern Europe), but very poorly with the Japanese subsample (alpha coefficient of 0.34). Replication of the analysis, excluding the Japanese subsample, did not alter significantly the overall results.

4. Social Functioning

Both clinical observations and empirical research point to the importance of social contact and social support in the life of the cancer patient.[29] Yet the physical and emotional condition of the patient may place strains on his or her ability to maintain social contacts, and the reactions of family and friends to the diagnosis of cancer may contribute further to feelings of social isolation.[30]

Assessment of social interaction can be hampered by an underreporting bias, particularly if questions are phrased in terms that imply criticism of family members and friends. By focusing on the behavioral aspects of social contacts rather than on their affective components, such bias may be minimized. In the core questionnaire, two questions were included that assessed the perceived disruption of normal social activities as a result of either the patient's health condition or of the demands of the medical treatment.

TABLE 9
Social Functioning: Item Frequency Distributions and Scale Summary Statistics

Item	N[a]	%[b]
Has your condition interfered with your family or social life?	534	26.8
Has your medical condition interfered with your family or social life?	525	21.9
Scale[c]	525	

Scale[c]

    Mean: 1.8
    St. dev.:   0.93
    Reliability:[d] 0.75

[a] N varies due to missing data.
[b] Response categories included: 1 "not at all", 2 "a little", 3 "quite a bit" and 4 "very much". Percentages reported are for categories 3 and 4 combined.
[c] The scale was constructed by summing the item scores and dividing by the number of items. A higher scale score represents a higher level of dysfunction.
[d] Chronbach's alpha coefficient.

As noted in Table 9, approximately one quarter of the sample reported that their social and family life had been seriously disrupted as a result of their illness. These items were combined into a Likert scale, with scores ranging from 1 to 4 (a higher score representing a greater degree of social disruption). The mean scale score was 1.8. The reliability of the scale, as determined by Chronbach's alpha coefficient, was 0.75.

While not related directly to the issue of social functioning, loss of income due to reduced work levels or altered work schedules can influence adversely the social environment of the patient. An additional single item was included in the questionnaire relating to the impact of the disease and its treatment on the financial situation of the patient. While this question is of more relevance at mid- or posttreatment assessments, it is interesting to note that, at baseline, more than 10% of the patients reported that their illness had already caused them serious financial problems.

5. Global Health Status and Quality of Life

The premise underlying construction of the core questionnaire was that, to be of optimal clinical use, quality of life should be defined and assessed in terms of its component parts. Nevertheless, inclusion of several global questions was considered appropriate in that: (1) they may capture information not covered by the more specific items; (2) they may be useful in assessing the relative value (i.e., weight) attached to specific quality of life components; and (3) they might facilitate incorporating psychosocial variables into formal medical decision-making models (e.g., quality-adjusted life year analysis).[31]

For these reasons, two questions were included in the core questionnaire that assessed, more globally, the patient's sense of well-being. In order to increase score variability, the response scale was expanded to range from 1 ("very poor") to 7 ("excellent"). The specific item content and score distributions are reported in Table 10. While, as expected, the majority of patients rated their physical condition and overall quality of life as fair to poor, a substantial minority of patients (approximately 40%) scored positively on these items.

These two items were combined into a summative scale, with scores ranging from 1 to 7 (a higher score representing a higher level of perceived quality of life). The mean scale value was 4.2. The scale exhibited high internal consistency (alpha coefficient = 0.85).

TABLE 10
Global Quality of Life: Item Frequency Distributions
and Scale Summary Statistics

Item	N[a]	%[b]
How would you rate your overall physical condition during the past week?	533	40.8
How would you rate your overall quality of life during the past week?	532	42.8
Scale[c]	531	

Range: 1—7
Mean: 4.2
St. dev.: 1.4
Reliability:[d] 0.85

[a] N varies due to missing data.
[b] Response categories ranged on a seven-point scale, anchored with 1 "very poor" and 7 "excellent". Percentages reported are for categories 5 through 7 combined.
[c] The scale was constructed by summing the item scores and dividing by the number of items. A higher scale score represents a higher quality of life.
[d] Chronbach's alpha coefficient.

D. CONSTRUCT VALIDITY OF THE QUESTIONNAIRE SCALES

As described earlier, three approaches were taken to assessing the construct validity of the questionnaire scales. First, multitrait scaling techniques were employed to test for item-discriminant validity. A matrix of item-scale correlations was created such that each item in the physical functioning, role functioning, fatigue and malaise, nausea and vomiting, emotional functioning, social functioning, and global quality-of-life scales was correlated with each of the total scales, including its own (corrected for overlap). Across all scales there were 156 such tests of discriminant validity (not presented in tabular form). Using the criteria suggested by Campbell and Fiske,[32] only one definite scaling error was detected (i.e., where the correlation of an item with another scale exceeded the correlation with its own scale by two standard errors), and three probable scaling errors (i.e., where the correlation of an item with another scale was within two standard errors of the correlation with its own scale). The definite scaling error and two of the three probable scaling errors involved items from the physical and role functioning scales. The remaining probable scaling error involved one of the items from the truncated HADS scale. This item exhibited a correlation with the fatigue scale (r = 0.29) similar to that with its own scale (r = 0.32). In general, however, the low number of scaling errors provides fairly strong empirical support for the conceptual distinctiveness of the quality of life domains assessed by these seven scales.

Second, a correlation matrix was constructed that included the seven questionnaire scales. As can be seen in Table 11, all of the inter-scale correlations were statistically significant ($p < .001$). This reflects both the conceptual non-orthogonality of the scales, as well as the effect of a large sample size. Of more importance is the magnitude of the correlations. As expected, the highest correlations were observed between the physical functioning, role functioning, and fatigue scales (ranging from 0.42 to 0.54). The fatigue scale also exhibited a relatively strong (negative) correlation with the global quality of life scale, suggesting that this symptom cluster has a substantial impact on overall sense of well-being. In general, however, the correlations among the seven scales were of only a moderate size, indicating that, although related to one another, these scales are assessing distinct components of the quality of life construct.

TABLE 11
Correlations Among the Core Questionnaire Subscales

Subscale[a]	PF	RF	F	NV	EF	SF	QL
Physical functioning (PF)	(.71)						
Role functioning (RF)	.54	(.61)					
Fatigue (F)	.48	.42	(.85)				
Nausea and vomiting (NV)	.21	.15	.26	(.78)			
Emotional functioning (EF)	.33	.29	.34	.18	(.67)		
Social functioning (SF)	.22	.32	.25	.14	.28	(.75)	
Global quality of life (QL)	− .36	− .31	− .53	− .19	− .37	− .35	(.85)

[a] All correlation coefficients are statistically significant ($p < .001$). Reliability (internal consistency) estimates are given on the diagonal.

Finally, analysis of variance was used to examine the responsiveness of the seven questionnaire scales to differences in the patients' clinical status. Four variables were used to categorize clinical status — disease stage, ECOG performance status, weight loss, and symptom level as rated by the physician. The results of these analyses were very consistent (Table 12). With few exceptions, those patient subgroups classified as having a poor clinical status, however defined, reported significantly lower levels of physical, role, emotional and social functioning, higher levels of fatigue and gastrointestinal symptoms, and lower overall quality of life than did those patient subgroups with a relatively good clinical status. While the strength of association between the clinical variables and the questionnaire scales was modest (see correlations in Table 12), the consistent pattern of results provides additional support for the validity of the questionnaire scales.

VI. SUMMARY

In this paper we have reported interim findings from an on-going, international field study of the EORTC Study Group on Quality of Life concerned with the development and validation of a core quality-of-life questionnaire for use in cancer clinical trials. The questionnaire was designed with an eye toward brevity, ease of administration, comprehensiveness of coverage, psychometric robustness, and cross-cultural applicability. It is composed primarily of multi-item scales tapping the physical, emotional, and social dimensions of quality of life. More specifically, scales are included that assess physical and role functioning, fatigue, nausea and vomiting, emotional functioning, social functioning, and overall quality of life. A number of single items are also included that provide additional information on symptom experience.

The questionnaire appears to be quite acceptable to patients. On average, it requires only about 15 min to complete and, in the majority of cases, can be filled out by the patients themselves with little or no instruction.

When employed with a large sample of lung cancer patients, the questionnaire exhibited satisfactory to excellent psychometric properties. All of the scales met at least minimal criteria for reliability, and were found to have good discriminant validity. Of particular importance is their ability to distinguish between subgroups of patients varying in terms of objective (i.e., clinical) health status.

The single item measures, while difficult to evaluate in a formal psychometric sense, nevertheless represent an important component of the questionnaire. The majority of these items is concerned with common and troublesome physical symptoms such as pain and dyspnea. The fact that most of these items yielded reasonable score variance suggests that they can be useful in providing a more complete symptom profile.

TABLE 12

Analysis of Variance of Questionnaire Subscales by Clinical Criteria

Clinical criterion	Questionnaire subscale						
	PF	RF	F	NV	EF	SF	QL
Disease stage							
Local	2.7[b]	0.8[b]	2.1[b]	1.2	1.8[c]	1.7	4.5[b]
Locoregional	2.8	0.9	2.3	1.3	1.9	1.8	4.2
Systemic	3.3	1.1	2.5	1.3	2.0	1.9	4.0
	(.13)[d]	(.15)	(.15)	—	(.18)	—	(.13)
ECOG performance status							
0—1	2.4[c]	0.8[c]	2.1[c]	1.2[a]	1.8[c]	1.6[c]	4.5[c]
2—4	4.2	1.2	2.8	1.4	2.0	2.0	3.5
	(.42)	(.24)	(.42)	(.09)	(.18)	(.16)	(.36)
Weight loss							
None	2.7[c]	0.8[c]	2.0[c]	1.2[a]	1.9[a]	1.6[c]	4.5[c]
<10%	3.0	1.0	2.4	1.3	1.9	1.9	4.2
>10%	3.7	1.2	2.9	1.4	2.0	2.0	3.6
	(.20)	(.17)	(.35)	(.12)	(.12)	(.15)	(.25)
Symptomatology							
None	2.8[c]	0.8[c]	1.9[c]	1.2	1.8[c]	1.7[c]	4.7[c]
Local	2.6	0.7	2.1	1.3	1.8	1.7	4.5
Systemic	3.4	1.2	2.7	1.4	2.0	2.0	3.8
	(.21)	(.28)	(.36)	—	(.20)	(.16)	(.27)

[a] $p < .05$.
[b] $p < .01$.
[c] $p < .001$.
[d] Figures in parentheses are correlations between the clinical criteria and the questionnaire subscales.

The psychometric characteristics of the questionnaire were found to be quite similar across various languages and cultures. The only exception was the Japanese subsample, where the reliability of several of the questionnaire scales was reduced significantly. It is unclear as to whether this was result of translation problems, or reflects more fundamental cultural differences in symptom perception and illness behavior.

While the overall psychometric results were promising, they also pointed to several areas in which the questionnaire could benefit from further revision. First, the reliability of the physical functioning and emotional functioning scales was judged to be less than optimal, particularly given the fact that both of these scales are comprised of a relatively large number of items. Second, the results indicated that the fatigue scale and the nausea and vomiting scale could be shortened without any loss of reliability or validity. In fact, the truncated versions of these two scales yielded higher reliability coefficients than the original scales. Finally, although not reflected in the psychometric results, patient feedback indicated the need to clarify the wording of several of the individual questionnaire items.

The results reported in this chapter have been limited to those derived from a baseline, pretreatment administration of the questionnaire. It should be noted, however, that the psychometric results based on a cross-sectional analysis of the second, mid-treatment administration of the questionnaire, with only few exceptions, parallel closely those observed for the baseline questionnaire.

Based on these findings, a revised version of the core questionnaire has recently been developed, incorporating the following principal changes: (1) the original physical functioning scale has been reduced to five items, with a slight modification of question wording in order to provide a clearer distinction between scale levels; (2) the 8 HADS items have been replaced by a four item measure of generalized psychological distress employed previously in several EORTC clinical trials; and (3) the single question on memory and concentration has been broken out into two separate items. This 30-item questionnaire is currently undergoing field testing, again in a broad cross-cultural context. It is expected that this revised questionnaire will yield sufficient improvements in psychometric performance to justify its adoption as the standard instrument for the assessment of quality of life in EORTC clinical trials. Continuing efforts will be required to develop a number of additional questionnaire modules that address quality of life issues relevant to specific populations of patients and/or treatment modalities. Combining the core questionnaire with such disease- or treatment-specific modules, will provide a flexible strategy for quality of life assessment in clinical research in oncology.

ACKNOWLEDGMENTS

The authors would like to acknowledge the contribution of the following individuals to this study: Martin Andersson, University of Umeå, Umeå, Sweden; Bengt Bergman, Renstromska Hospital, Göteborg, Sweden; Jürg Bernhard, Medical Division Lory, Bern, Switzerland; J. B. Cookson, Glenfield General Hospital, Leicester, England; Hanneke de Haes, Academic Hospital of the University of Leiden, Leiden, the Netherlands; Alain Depierre, Centre Hospitalier Régional, Besançon, France; Javier García-Conde, University Clinical Hospital, Valencia, Spain; Manfred Heim, Mannheim Clinic Oncological Center, Mannheim, Federal Republic of Germany; F. Kraft, Medical University Clinic, Freiburg, Federal Republic of Germany; Bernard Lebeau, Hospital Saint-Antoine, Paris, France; Antonio Lobo, University Hospital Clinic, Zaragoza, Spain; F. J. F. Madden, Leicester Royal Infirmary, Leicester, England; Enn Nöu, Academic Hospital, Uppsala, Sweden; Luis Salvador, Hospital Clinic, Clinic Hospital of Barcelona, Barcelona, Spain; L. A. Solé-Calvo, Hospital Vall d'Hebrón, Barcelona, Spain; Frits van Dam, the Netherlands Cancer Institute, Amsterdam, the Netherlands; Friederich von Bültzingslöwen, Fachklinik für Erkrankungen der Atmungsorgane, Donaustauf, Federal Republic of Germany; Nina Vranes, Clinical Hospital for Lung Disease, Zagreb, Yugoslavia; David Warr, Princess Margaret Hospital, Toronto, Canada; Kiyokazu Yoshida, Saitama Cancer Center, Saitama, Japan; Robert Zittoun, Hotel-Dieu de Paris, Paris, France.

REFERENCES

1. van Knippenberg, F. C. E. and de Haes, J. C. J. M., Measuring the quality of life of cancer patients: psychometric properties of instruments, *Soc. Sci. Med.*, 41, 1043, 1988.
2. Aaronson, N. K., Quality of life assessment in clinical trials: methodological issues, *Controlled Clin. Trials*, 10, 195s, 1989.
3. McMillen Moinpour, C., Feigl, P., Metch, B., et al., Quality of life endpoints in cancer clinical trials: review and recommendations, *J. Natl. Cancer Inst.*, 81, 485, 1989.
4. Kemeny, M. M., Welisch, D. K., and Schain, W. S., Psychosocial outcome in a randomized surgical trial for treatment of primary breast cancer, *Cancer*, 62, 1231, 1988.
5. de Haes, J. C. J. M., van Oostrom, M. A., and Welvaart, K., The effect of radical and conserving surgery on the quality of life of early breast cancer patients, *Eur. J. Surg. Oncol.*, 12, 337, 1986.
6. Fallowfield, L. J., Baum, M., and Maguire, G. P., Effects of breast conservation on psychological morbidity associated with diagnosis and treatment of early breast cancer, *Br. Med. J.*, 293, 1331, 1986.
7. Gelber, R. D. and Goldhirsch, A., A new endpoint for the assessment of adjuvant therapy in postmenopausal women with operable breast cancer, *J. Clin. Oncol.*, 4, 1772, 1986.
8. Coates, A., Gebski, V., Bishop, J. F., et al., Improving the quality of life during chemotherapy for advanced breast cancer, *N. Engl. J. Med.*, 317, 1490, 1987.
9. Sugarbaker, P. H., Barofsky, I., Rosenberg, S. A., and Gianola, F., Quality of life assessment of patients in extremity sarcoma clinical trials, *Surgery*, 91, 17, 1982.

10. **Bardelli, D. and Saracci, R.**, Measuring the quality of life in cancer clinical trials: a sample survey of published trials, in *Methods and Impact of Controlled Therapeutic Trials in Cancer*, Part I, Armitage, P., Ed., International Union Against Cancer, Geneva, 1978, 75.

11. **O'Young, J. and McPeek, B.**, Quality of life variables in surgical trials, *J. Chronic Dis.*, 11, 513, 1987.

12. **Guyatt, G. H., Veldhuzen van Zanten, S. J. O., Feeny, D. H., and Patrick, D. L.**, Measuring quality of life in clinical trials: a taxonomy and review, *CMAJ*, 140, 1441, 1989.

13. **Schipper, H., Clinch, J., McMurray, A., and Levitt, M.**, Measuring the quality of life of cancer patients: the Functional Living Index - Cancer, *J. Clin. Oncol.*, 2, 472, 1984.

14. **Selby, P. J., Chapman, J. A., Etazadi-Amoli, J., et al.**, The development of a method for assessing the quality of life for cancer patients, *Br. J. Cancer*, 20, 849, 1984.

15. **Aaronson, N. K., Bullinger, M., and Ahmedzai, S.**, A modular approach to quality of life assessment in cancer clinical trials, *Rec. Results Cancer Res.*, 111, 231, 1988.

16. **Huisman, S. J., van Dam, F. S. A. M., Aaronson, N. K., and Hanewald, G.**, On measuring complaints of cancer patients: some remarks on the time span of the question, in *The Quality of Life of Cancer Patients*, Aaronson, N. K. and Beckmann, J., Eds., Raven Press, New York, 1987, 101.

17. **Fayers, P. M. and Jones, S. D. R.**, Measuring and analyzing the quality of life in cancer clinical trials: a review, *Stat. Med.*, 2, 429, 1983.

18. **Zubrod, C. G., Schneidermann, M., Frei, M., et al.**, Appraisal of methods for the study of chemotherapy of cancer in man: comparative therapeutic trial of nitrogen mustard and triethylene thiophosphoramide, *J. Chronic Dis.*, 11, 7, 1960.

19. **Likert, R.**, A technique for the measurement of attitudes, *Arch. Psychol.*, 140, 1, 1932.

20. **Guttman, L. A.**, A basis for scaling qualitative data, *Am. Soc. Rev.*, 9, 139, 1944.

21. **Nie, N. H., Hull, C. H., Jenkins, J. G., et al.**, *Statistical Package for the Social Sciences*, 2nd ed., McGraw-Hill, New York, 1970.

22. **Chronbach, L. J.**, Coefficient alpha and the internal structure of tests, *Psychometrika*, 16, 297, 1951.

23. **Helmstadter, C. G.**, *Principles of Psychological Measurement*, Appleton-Century-Crofts, New York, 1964.

24. **Stewart, A. L., Ware, J. E., and Brooks, R. H.**, *Construction and Scoring of Aggregate Functional Status Measures*, Vol. 1, R-2551-1-HHS, Rand Corporation, Santa Monica, CA, 1984.

25. **Meenan, R. F.**, Measuring health status in arthritis: the arthritis impact measurement scale, *Arthritis Rheum.*, 23, 146, 1980.

26. **Stewart, A. L.**, *Measuring the Ability to Cope with Serious Illness*, N-1907-GRS/RC, Rand Corporation, Santa Monica, CA, 1982.

27. **Linssen, A. C. G., Hanewald, G., Huisman, S., and van Dam, F. S. A. M.**, The development of a "complaint questionnaire" at the Netherlands Cancer Institute, in *Proc. 1st Workshop EORTC Study Group on Quality of Life Workshop*, Amsterdam, 1981.

28. **Zigmond, A. S. and Snaith, R. P.**, The hospital anxiety and depression scale, *Acta Psychiatr. Scand.*, 67, 361, 1983.

29. **Wortman, C. B.**, Social support and the cancer patient: conceptual and methodological issues, *Cancer*, 2217, 1983.

30. **Bury, M.**, Chronic illness as biographical disruption, *Sociol. Health Illness*, 41, 167, 1982.

31. **de Haes, J. C. J. M. and van Knippenberg, F. C. E.**, The quality of life of cancer patients: a review of the literature, *Soc. Sci. Med.*, 20, 809, 1985.

32. **Campbell, D. T. and Fiske, D. W.**, Convergent and discriminant validation by the multitrait-multimethod matrix, *Psychol. Bull.*, 56, 81, 1959.

Chapter 15

QUALITY OF LIFE IN BREAST CANCER

Mark N. Levine

TABLE OF CONTENTS

I. INTRODUCTION

In recent years there have been a number of new exciting developments in the management of patients with breast cancer. Conservative surgery has gained popularity as the definitive surgical procedure for patients with a primary breast malignancy.[1] Adjuvant chemotherapy is now widely used, not only in women with axillary node positive breast cancer, but also in women with node negative disease.[2,3] Patients with metastatic breast cancer are receiving high dose chemotherapy with autologous marrow support or high dose chemotherapy under the protection of hematopoietic growth factors.[4,5] In all of these clinical situations, the therapeutic intervention can have a profound impact on the patient's ability to function in daily living, i.e., on her quality of life. In this chapter, instruments which have been developed specifically for breast cancer will be reviewed, particularly in reference to their use in a particular stage of breast cancer. More generic quality of life instruments which have been developed for cancer patients, but which can be used in the breast cancer patient, will not be described but are discussed in other chapters (see relevant chapters on Spitzer QL-Index and FLIC).

II. ADJUVANT CHEMOTHERAPY FOR OPERABLE BREAST CANCER

Adjuvant chemotherapy decreases recurrence and improves survival in women with axillary node positive breast cancer (Stage II) and is the treatment of choice in premenopausal patients with such disease.[2] Despite the decreased recurrence rate and improved survival, adjuvant chemotherapy can have a profound adverse impact on a patient's quality of life while she is receiving treatment.[6]

Approximately 25% of women who present with breast carcinoma have neither axillary nodal involvement nor metastases at the time of initial surgery and are deemed Stage I. The prognosis of Stage I patients is better than Stage II, with only 10 to 20% of these patients developing recurrence within 5 years of surgery. Recently, results from a number of clinical trials have demonstrated that adjuvant chemotherapy in patients with Stage I breast cancer decreases the recurrence rate by approximately 30% within the first 4 years after initial surgery.[3] However, this has not yet been translated into a survival benefit. The issue of whether to use adjuvant chemotherapy in Stage I breast cancer patients has sparked much discussion and controversy.[7]

III. QUALITY OF LIFE INSTRUMENTS IN STAGE I AND STAGE II BREAST CANCER

A. THE BREAST CANCER CHEMOTHERAPY QUESTIONNAIRE

In 1982, while planning a study to compare two regimens of adjuvant chemotherapy of different duration in women with Stage II breast cancer, it was recognized that quality of life would be an important outcome. Since existing intruments failed to adequately describe the morbidity experienced by Stage II breast cancer patients receiving chemotherapy, a new questionnaire, the Breast Cancer Chemotherapy Questionnaire (BCQ) was developed.[6] It measured the impact of adjuvant chemotherapy on aspects of physical, emotional and social function which were important to such patients. The BCQ consists of 30 questions which focus on loss of attractiveness, fatigue, physical symptoms, inconvenience, emotional distress, and feelings of hope and support from others. The questionnaire is scored on a seven-point categorical scale and initially was evaluated using an interviewer-administered format.

The validity, reproducibility, and responsiveness of the BCQ were evaluated in a randomized trial comparing a 12-week regimen and a 36-week regimen of adjuvant chemo-

TABLE 1
Validity: BCQ vs. other Quality-of-Life Measures

Instrument	Patient no.	Correlation (r)
Global		
Patient physical	232	0.51
Patient emotional	204	0.50
Physician physical	205	0.45
Physician emotional	180	0.41
Karnofsky	213	0.46
Rand physical	212	0.60
Rand emotional	213	0.58
Spitzer QL-Index	346	0.62

TABLE 2
Quality of Life Measures vs. Global Assessments

Instrument	Patient no.	Correlation (r)
Global patient physical vs.		
BCQ	232	0.51
Karnofsky	194	0.26
Rand physical	189	0.29
Rand emotional	200	0.25
Spitzer QL-Index	190	0.40
Global patient emotional vs.		
BCQ	204	0.50
Karnofsky	173	0.24
Rand physical	170	0.21
Rand emotional	182	0.45
Spitzer QL-Index	174	0.40

therapy.[6] The BCQ, other instruments which evaluate quality of life (Spitzer, Karnofsky, and Rand), ECOG toxicity criteria, and patient and physician global assessments were administered serially to 418 patients.

There is no gold standard for quality of life, and therefore, in order to validate the BCQ we adopted the concept of construct validity, i.e., the extent to which the questionnaire was consistent with other established instruments. The correlation coefficients between the BCQ and the other instruments ranged from 0.41 to 0.62 (Table 1). We also used the global rating as an anchor to which to compare the other questionnaires. The global ratings by patient or physician represent changes over a specific 2-week time period. Corresponding differences in the scores of individual quality of life instruments were calculated and the correlations between these and the global ratings were calculated in order to examine the relative validity of the different instruments. It was found that the BCQ correlated more strongly with the ratings of both physical and emotional function by the patient and their physician, than did any of the other instruments (Table 2).

The mean BCQ score changed over time for patients in both treatment groups (Figure 1). The score is presented on a ten-point scale, with ten representing perfect health. A comparison of the quality of life outcomes of patients in the two treatment groups in the period beyond 3 months after initiation of treatment, when one group had completed the treatment course and the other was still on treatment revealed that the BCQ was able to demonstrate differences between the groups (Table 3).

The reproducibility of the BCQ was also determined during the first 2-week period that a patient assessed herself as stable by the global rating. The corresponding change for the

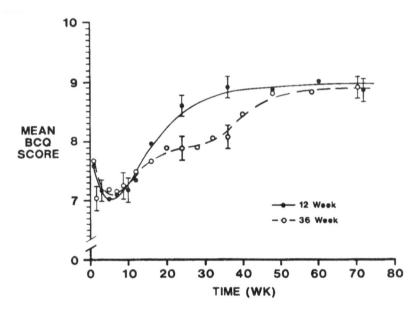

FIGURE 1.   Mean BCQ score over time. Ten represents perfect health.

TABLE 3
Differences between Two Treatment Groups as Measured
by BCQ

	Weeks 1—10	Weeks 10—24
12-week group change score (mean)	−0.53	1.34
36-week group change score (mean)	−0.51	0.59
Difference (mean)	0.02	0.75
p	0.85	<0.001

BCQ was calculated to determine its reproducibility. The mean change score for the BCQ was close to zero which suggested that the instrument was reproducible. However, the assessment of reproducibility in a clinical situation where the patient's health status is constantly changing may be problematic.[8]

Since the original evaluation of the BCQ, a self-administered form of the questionnaire has been evaluated and the agreement with the interviewer-administered form is excellent (Figure 2).

B. THE SELBY AND BOYD QUESTIONNAIRE

Selby and Boyd have developed a questionnaire to measure quality of life in patients with breast cancer.[9,10] This questionnaire consists of 31 items which are assessed by patient self-report using linear analog scales. Two groups of items were used in the development of this instrument. The first group, which are global in nature, were drawn from an existing comprehensive health index, The Sickness Impact Profile (SIP).[11] The 12 categories of the SIP were represented by 18 linear analog scales that inquired about different aspects of general health. In addition, 12 disease-specific items were selected and each was represented by one linear analog scale (Table 4). Finally, an item related to overall quality of life, which was referred to as the Uniscale was included. Each item is on a 10-cm line anchored at each end by descriptive phrases, with the right-hand end corresponding to absence of symptoms and the left, maximum symptoms. The entire instrument was self-administered and took less than 5 min to complete.

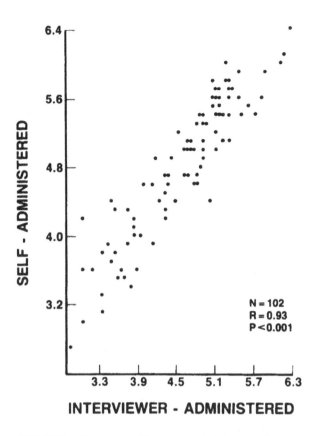

FIGURE 2. Comparison of interviewer-administered and patient self-administered form of BCQ.

TABLE 4
Items of Selby and Boyd Questionnaire

General health items	Disease-related items
Work	Dysuria
Recreation	Sore mouth
Increased eating	Attractiveness
Social life	Breathing
Writing	Pain
Housework	Fatigue
Anger	Information
Reduced eating	Diarrhea
Reduced sleep	Constipation
Physical sleep	Nausea
Concentration	Hair loss
Family relations	Vomiting
Self care	Appearance
Anxiety	Uniscale
Depression	Mobility
Increased Sleep	
Speech	

In the development and evaluation of this instrument, patients with either Stage IV breast cancer or Stage II breast cancer were studied. The patients were asked to consider the previous 24 h or previous 7 days. Reliability was assessed by having the patients complete the instrument on two occasions less than 24 h apart (test/retest reliability). The agreement between the two assessments for most items was high with correlation coefficients greater than 0.7. The validity of the instrument was assessed by several methods. The extent to which scores on individual items correlated with scores on other related items was assessed using factor analysis. This technique examines correlations between scores on all items and creates groups of items whose scores are most strongly correlated with each other. If scores are valid it is expected that the groups created by factor analysis will be comprised of items which are expected, on clinical or other grounds, to be associated with each other. In the analysis for this instrument, five factors were identified.

The scores for the items were also compared with the Sickness Impact Profile and the Karnofsky Index. Validity was also supported by the fact that the instrument was able to distinguish clinically different groups of patients. The scores of patients with metastatic breast cancer were lower than those of patients with Stage II disease. Thus, in summary, through a cross-sectional study of patients with breast cancer, the questionnaire was found to be valid and reproducible. However, further information on the ability of this instrument to measure clinically important change in patients receiving adjuvant chemotherapy is needed.

C. THE TIME WITHOUT SYMPTOMS OF DISEASE AND SUBJECTIVE TOXICITY (TWiST)

There is relatively little information available on how quality of life information obtained from adjuvant breast cancer trials can be used by the patient and physician in clinical decision-making. Quality of life questionnaires are available which measure the effect of treatment on a patients' health status. However, it is important to also consider the negative impact of recurrent breast cancer on quality of life. Based on these considerations, Gelber et al. have recently reported a method for using quality of life as an outcome measurement in trials of adjuvant therapy in women with Stage II breast cancer.[12] They described a new quality-of-life oriented end point, the time without symptoms of disease and subjective toxic effects of treatment (TWiST) which could be used to help determine the optimal adjuvant therapy in postmenopausal patients. Briefly, they discounted from the period of overall survival, the time during which the patient experienced the various toxic effects of treatment or symptoms of disease recurrence. The remaining time, i.e., the time without symptoms and toxicity was then used to calculate actuarial survival curves. Their model indicated that despite the larger initial discount due to subjective toxicity with chemoendocrine therapy, by 5 years postmastectomy the net difference in average TWiST for treated patients compared with no treatment was positive. More recently, Gelber and colleagues have refined their TWiST methodology and reported a way of incorporating a more quantitative assessment of quality of life into their model using a quality-adjusted TWiST.[13]

IV. QUALITY OF LIFE IN STAGE IV BREAST CARCINOMA

Traditionally, chemotherapy has been used to cause tumor regression and thereby palliate symptoms and improve quality of life. More recently, based on the concept of dose intensity, high dose, more intensive chemotherapy regimens have been studied in the research setting. In order to properly evaluate such new therapeutic approaches, physicians and patients must balance improvement in cancer-related symptoms against the morbidity of treatment.

In an early study, Priestman and Baum used a linear analog self-assessment (LASA) technique to measure quality of life in patients with metastatic breast carcinoma.[14] A 10-cm linear analog scale was used in each of ten dimensions; feeling of well-being, mood, level of activity, pain, nausea, appetite, ability to perform housework, social activities, anxiety, and the question, "Is treatment helping?". In the first of three studies, 29 patients with metastatic breast cancer had the assessments repeated 24 h later. There was excellent correlation between the initial and follow-up assessment ($r = 0.7$). Thirteen patients receiving endocrine therapy for advanced breast cancer had the assessment done at baseline and at 3 months. Those patients who had objective tumor response had improvement in the LASA scores. Finally, in a group of 20 women receiving chemotherapy, the LASA scores decreased during the first 3 days of treatment providing preliminary information on the responsiveness of the instrument.

The issue of whether to continue maintenance chemotherapy in patients with metastatic breast cancer who have achieved an initial response to chemotherapy is an important one in the day-to-day practice of oncology. Maintaining control of the tumor and associated symptoms must be balanced against the side effects of chemotherapy. Recently, a clinical trial in which quality of life was a major outcome measure provided important information on this question.[15] Coates et al. randomized 308 patients with metastatic breast cancer to either an approach of continuous chemotherapy until disease progression or intermittent therapy whereby chemotherapy was discontinued after three cycles and then resumed only at disease progression. Besides the traditional outcomes of response and survival, quality of life was also assessed using five linear analog self-assessment scales measuring physical well-being, mood, pain, nausea and vomiting, appetite, and a single uniscale summarizing overall quality of life. In addition, the physician measured quality of life using the Spitzer QL-Index.[16] These assessments were done at baseline and at approximately every 3 months thereafter until disease progression.

Intermittent therapy resulted in a significantly worse response and a significantly shorter time to disease progression. No difference was detected in overall survival. Quality of life improved significantly during the first three cycles when all patients received treatment. Thereafter, intermittent therapy was associated with worse scores for physical well-being, mood, and appetite and for overall quality of life as indicated by the patient and the physician. Thus, in summary, results from this clinical trial suggest that in patients with metastatic breast cancer who have achieved an initial response to chemotherapy, continuing the patient on maintenance chemotherapy and thereby keeping the disease under control is associated with an overall better quality of life of the patient.

Tannock et al. have conducted a trial in patients with metastatic breast carcinoma to evaluate the effect of chemotherapy drug dosage on palliation.[17] In this trial, women with metastatic breast carcinoma were randomized to either high dose cyclophosphamide, methotrexate, 5-fluorouracil (CMF) chemotherapy (66 patients), or lower dose CMF (67 patients). The rate of response to chemotherapy was 30% for patients randomized to the higher dose and 11% for the lower dose ($p = 0.03$). Patients randomized to the higher dose arm had a significantly longer survival, median survival 15.6 months vs. 12.8 months, respectively. A subset of patients in the trial completed a detailed quality of life questionnaire. The questionnaire used was the 34-item linear analog self-assessment scale developed by Selby and Boyd.[9] A subset of 35 patients, 15 receiving lower dose chemotherapy and 20 receiving higher dose, completed one or more LASA scales after the third course of treatment. Only the LASA scale for hair loss was significantly different between the two groups with the higher dose group having a lower score. On the other hand, a number of the scales showed a trend to higher values (i.e., less symptoms) in patients receiving higher dose chemotherapy (pain, mobility, attractiveness, physical activity, recreation, anxiety, social life, and housework). The results from this trial suggest a trend towards better palliation (longer survival without adverse effect on quality of life) from the use of the higher dose of chemotherapy.

Both the study by Coates and the study by Tannock have provided important information for the management of patients with metastatic breast cancer. In addition, they have demonstrated that quality of life measured in a clinical trial can provide results that can be readily incorporated into clinical decision making. On the other hand, it should be pointed out that in both of these trials, compliance with the quality of life assessment was not optimal. In the study by Coates, only 133 of the 305 randomized patients (44%) completed quality of life assessments at both baseline and after three cycles of chemotherapy. Similarly, in the trial by Tannock only 26% of the patients randomized had quality of life assessment studies performed and a much smaller number had serial assessments of quality of life. Clearly, if quality of life measurement is to be incorporated into breast cancer clinical trials, greater attention must be given to ensuring maximum compliance.

V. BREAST CANCER SURGERY

Clinical trials have demonstrated that conservative surgery, i.e., lumpectomy, is an acceptable alternative to a modified radical mastectomy.[1] Studies have shown that women who have undergone modified radical mastectomy have more psychiatric morbidity compared to those with benign breast disease.[18] Despite the ever increasing enthusiasm of patients and physicians for conservative surgery, there is a need for further studies on the effect of conservative surgery on quality of life (see Chapter 16). Although it would appear obvious that breast preservation should be associated with better quality of life than more radical surgery, this does not take into consideration such issues as a lumpectomy patient's fear of local breast recurrence, the impact of a poor cosmetic breast, and the devastation of a local breast recurrence. These issues are supported by the results of a recent study in which women with breast cancer who had undergone conservative surgery were compared with a group who had undergone radical surgery 3 months after the surgery.[19] The women who had conservative surgery had increased psychological morbidity.

There has been recent debate on the need for local breast irradiation in patients who have had lumpectomy. Although the radiation reduces the risk of local breast recurrence, it does not impact on distant disease-free survival and overall survival.[1] This reduced risk for local recurrence must be balanced against the potential negative impact of attending a cancer center daily for at least a month for treatment and the potential effect of breast irradiation on cosmesis. Clearly, information on a patient's quality of life in these clinical situations could help influence clinical decision making.

VI. SUMMARY

In recent years there have been many developments in the therapy of operable and metastatic breast cancer. Such interventions can clearly impact on a patient's quality of life. Instruments are now available that can measure quality of life in the breast cancer patient. Examples already exist which demonstrate that measurement of quality of life as an outcome in breast cancer clinical trials can provide information that can readily be used at the bedside in clinical decision making. Recently, a number of large cooperative clinical trials groups have recognized the importance of measuring quality of life as an outcome measure in breast cancer trials.[20,21] Such policies are welcomed and should ultimately lead to improved care of the breast cancer patient.

REFERENCES

1. Fisher, B., Bauer, M., Margolese, R., et al., Five-year results of a randomized trial comparing total mastectomy and segmental mastectomy with or without radiation in the treatment of breast cancer, *N. Engl. J. Med.*, 312, 665, 1985.
2. Early Breast Cancer Trialists' Collaborative Group, Effects of adjuvant tamoxifen and of cytotoxic therapy on mortality in early breast cancer, *N. Engl. J. Med.*, 320, 527, 1989.
3. De Vita, V. T., Jr., Breast cancer therapy: exercising all our options, *N. Engl. J. Med.*, 320, 527, 1989.
4. Peters, W. P., Shpall, E. J., Jones, R. B., Oslen, G. A., Best, R. C., Gockerman, J. P., and Moore, J. O., High-dose combination alkylating agents with bone marrow support as initial treatment for metastatic breast cancer, *J. Clin. Oncol.*, 6, 1368, 1988.
5. Metcalf, D., Haemopoietic growth factors, *Lancet*, 1, 825, 1989.
6. Levine, M. N., Guyatt, G. H., Gent, M., et al., Quality of life in stage II breast cancer: an instrument for clinical trials, *J. Clin. Oncol.*, 6, 1798, 1988.
7. McGuire, W. L., Adjuvant therapy of node negative breast cancer, *N. Engl. J. Med.*, 320, 525, 1989.
8. Guyatt, G., Walter, S., and Norman, G., Measuring changes over time: assessing the usefulness of evaluative instruments, *J. Chronic Dis.*, 40, 171, 1987.
9. Selby, P. J., Chapman, J. A. W., Etazadi-Amoli, J., Dalley, D., and Boyd, N. F., The development of a method for assessing the quality of life of cancer patients, *Br. J. Cancer*, 50, 13, 1984.
10. Bell, D. R., Tannock, I. F., and Boyd, N. F., Quality of life measurement in breast cancer patients, *Br. J. Cancer*, 51, 577, 1985.
11. Bergner, M., Bobbitt, R. A., and Carter, W. B., The Sickness Impact Profile: development and final revision of a health status measure, *Med. Care*, 19, 788, 1981.
12. Gelber, R. D. and Goldhirsch, A., A new endpoint for the assessment of adjuvant therapy in postmenopausal women with operable breast cancer, *J. Clin. Oncol.*, 4, 1772, 1986.
13. Goldhirsch, A., Gelber, R. D., Simes, R. J., Glasziou, P., and Coates, A. S., Costs and benefits of adjuvant therapy in breast cancer: a quality-adjusted survival analysis, *J. Clin. Oncol.*, 7, 36, 1989.
14. Priestman, T. J. and Baum, M., Evaluation of quality of life in patients receiving treatment for advanced breast cancer, *Lancet*, 1, 899, 1976.
15. Coates, A., Gebski, V., and Stat, M., for the Australian-New Zealand Breast Cancer Trials Group, Improving the quality of life during chemotherapy for advanced breast cancer, *N. Engl. J. Med.*, 317, 1490, 1987.
16. Spitzer, W. O., Dobson, A. J., Hall, J., et al., Measuring the quality of life of cancer patients, *J. Chronic Dis.*, 34, 585, 1981.
17. Tannock, I. F., Boyd, N. F., DeBoer, G., et al., A randomized trial of two dose levels of cyclophosphamide, methotrexate and fluorouracil chemotherapy for patients with metastatic breast cancer, *J. Clin. Oncol.*, 6, 1377, 1988.
18. Morris, T., Greer, H. S., and White, P., Psychological and social adjustment to mastectomy, *Cancer*, 40, 2381, 1977.
19. Levy, S. M., Herberman, R. B., Lee, J. K., Lippman, M. E., and D'Angela, T., Breast conservation versus mastectomy: distress sequelae as a function of choice, *J. Clin. Oncol.*, 7, 367, 1989.
20. Moinpour, C. M., Feigl, P., Metch, P., Hayden, A., Meyskens, F. L., and Crowley, J., Quality of life endpoints in cancer clinical trials: review and recommendations, *J. Natl. Cancer Inst.*, 81, 485, 1989.
21. Skiel, R. T., Quality of life assessment in cancer clinical trials — it's time to catch up, *J. Natl. Cancer Inst.*, 81, 472, 1989.

Chapter 16

WOMEN'S SEXUALITY FOLLOWING BREAST CANCER

Jean-Claude M. Lasry

TABLE OF CONTENTS

I. INTRODUCTION

From the personal experience of a sex therapist[1] to a sexual rehabilitation program of male and female cancer patients,[2] sexual functioning has become a subject of interest for the researchers studying quality of life following cancer treatment. Morris[3] published the first review article on this topic, entitled *Psychological Adjustment to Mastectomy*. In it, she refers to 5 studies (out of 118 cited) that had dealt in some way with the sexuality of the breast cancer patient. The following year, Meyerowitz[4] authored another review article on the same subject, devoting one paragraph to the sexual consequences of mastectomy (in the section "Changes in Life Patterns") in a 24-page essay.

The American Cancer Society, California division, established an Ad Hoc Committee to study the psychosocial aspects of cancer in 1976. In the proceedings of the first scientific session,[5] Mantell[6] devoted a whole chapter to *Sexuality and Cancer*. Yet, the table of contents of a book[7] published 3 years later *Psychosocial Aspects of Early Breast Cancer* seem to ignore the issue of sexuality among the psychosocial consequences of cancer treatment.

Bransfield[8] aptly remarked in the first review of the literature on breast cancer and sexual functioning, with studies ranging from 1953 to 1981, that this field of research is still in its "infancy". As sexual functioning became part of the quality of life assessment, and as some scales became available to measure it,[9] the problem of measuring sexual dysfunction was also raised and addressed.[10-12]

II. LITERATURE REVIEW

In the lines that follow, we will review the literature on female breast cancer treatment and sexual functioning, referring to the main review articles and also to studies that were not analyzed in them (for a review of sexual dysfunctioning in male cancer patients, the reader is referred to the paper of Dobkin and Bradley).[12] We will then present our own study comparing the quality of life of breast cancer patients according to the type of surgery they underwent: radical modified mastectomy or breast conserving procedure.

A. FIRST REVIEW ARTICLE — MORRIS, 1979[3]

In her review of the research assessing the psychological adjustment to mastectomy, Morris mentions five studies that had dealt in some way with the sexuality of the breast cancer patients. The three studies of Morris and colleagues,[13] of Maguire,[14] and of Jamison et al.[15] are well known and deserve some elaboration, while the other two reports[16,17] are rather anecdotal.

Morris et al.[13] followed for 2 years a series of 160 women admitted consecutively to a London hospital for breast tumor biopsy. At operation, 69 patients were diagnosed as having breast cancer. Sexual adjustment was "measured" with two questions. Patients demonstrated a worsening of sexual functioning, over the 2-year period, in the cancer as well as in the benign group. Two years after surgery, about 30% of patients still manifested a deterioration of their sexual functioning.

Maguire[14] interviewed 75 women who had a mastectomy and compared them to a group of 50 matched controls. Two rating scales were used to assess sexual problems and their duration. The follow-up at 1 year revealed one third of the cancer patients (vs. 8% in the control group) experienced moderate or severe sexual problems.

While Jamison et al.[15] used seven questions to examine the sexual functioning of 41 women who had undergone a mastectomy, they only report simple percentages for the alternatives of each question, making it almost impossible to analyze the data. Sexual satisfaction worsened for a quarter of the respondants; about the same percentage found mastectomy made "coital orgasm impossible or more difficult". The authors used the well-known marital adjustment scale of Locke and Wallace[16a] but do not report on it.

B. SECOND REVIEW ARTICLE — BRANSFIELD, 1982[8]

Bransfield[8] reviewed the concomitants of breast cancer treatment on the patients' sexual functioning, in the literature published from 1953 to 1981. She adds only two more studies to those cited by Morris:[3] Silberfarb[18] and Battersby.[19]

Silberfarb and colleagues[18] evaluated the psychosocial functioning of 146 breast cancer patients, at three stages of the disease, with three different groups of patients: primary, recurrent and final. Using a modified version of the *Psychiatric Status Schedule,* they identified disturbance in mate role as the most commonly reported problem (28%), indicating "lack of sexual desire and decreased amount of coitus for all three treatment categories, regardless of age" (p. 452). Bransfield devotes five lines to the other study,[19] stating none of the 30 subjects reported a deterioration of their sexual relationships. We agree with her conclusion that, at the time of her review, no study focused on sexual functioning and breast cancer, while some others reported only incidentally on it.

C. THIRD REVIEW ARTICLE — ANDERSEN, 1986[11]

Since 1983, Andersen has published several papers on the topic of sexual functioning and breast cancer surgery. In a recent book she edited,[20] *Women with Cancer,* Andersen authored a review article[11] on the sexual difficulties women experience following cancer treatment, which includes a section devoted to assessment and another, to intervention. Studies are presented according to cancer sites: breast, gynecologic, and other sites. In addition to the two prospective research already mentioned, of Morris[13] and Maguire,[14] Andersen's breast cancer review includes four studies[21-24] comparing the consequences of two conceptually different surgical procedures: radical modified mastectomy and lumpectomy.

Sanger and Reznikoff[21] were the first to compare the psychological impact of those two types of surgery, with 20 patients matched in each group. They focused on several aspects of body image and marital satisfaction, assessed with the Locke and Wallace scale,[16a] but not on sexual functioning per se. Body satisfaction (adjusted by its covariable, prior body satisfaction) was significantly better with the breast conserving procedure, but there were no differences in marital satisfaction or in social desirability.

Beckmann et al.[22] matched 11 "tumorectomized" patients with another 11 women who had sustained a total mastectomy, and interviewed them 6 to 12 months after the operation. Using a series of ten single questions, the authors demonstrate that body image and sexual functioning are negatively affected by "breast amputation" (total mastectomy). For example, 4 of the 11 mastectomized women (36%) had "lost their libido as a consequence of constant fatigue", vs. only 1 in the tumorectomized group ($p < 0.05$).

Steinberg and team[23] also used a series of questions to assess body image and sexuality in their comparison of psychological outcome of lumpectomy (n = 21) vs. mastectomy (n = 46). Self-image and sexual adjustment were significantly less affected for patients who submitted to the breast conserving procedure. Only one patient in the lumpectomy group (6%) rated a great decrease in her sexual drive compared to six (17%) in the mastectomy group. There were no differences in mood disturbance, depressive symptoms, or an emotional distress factor between the two surgery groups.

It is unfortunate that, for Steinberg as well as for Beckmann, body image and sexuality questions are intermingled with each other and reported on singly. These questions could have been regrouped into specific scales, after reliability analyses had been carried out. As a matter of fact, Steinberg warns the reader of this very limitation in the interpretation of his results.

The fourth study[24] cited by Andersen deals with attribution, psychological control, and cognitive control rather than with sexuality, as expected. The article Andersen refers to, that deals with marital relationships and breast cancer, seems rather to be a paper presented

at the APA convention by Lichtman et al.[25] The authors interviewed 78 patients, of which
26 had undergone a lumpectomy and 29, a radical modified mastectomy. They used the
Locke and Wallace scale[16a] to assess marital relationships, while sexual functioning was
estimated with some questions specifically developed for this purpose. The couple's sexual
relationship was significantly related to the patient's adjustment, and the marital relationship
to the type of surgery. Lumpectomy patients rate marital satisfaction highest, while patients
who underwent a radical modified mastectomy rate it lowest.

D. OTHER STUDIES COMPARING DIFFERENT SURGERIES

We will review two other studies[26,27] comparing the impact of the two surgical procedures
on sexual functioning and body image, which were not mentioned in Andersen's review.[11]
We will also present one study[28] comparing the psychological impact of breast and gynecologic cancer, as well as another one[29] assessing three different types of gynecologic surgery.

Schain and colleagues[26] mailed a questionnaire to 39 women who elected to participate
in a prospective randomized trial comparing mastectomy to lumpectomy. Of the 38 respondants, 20 belonged to the mastectomy group and 18, to the breast "sparing" surgery group.
The type of surgery had no influence on psychosocial symptoms except for a question on
nudity, about which mastectomy patients expressed more negative feelings. Schain reports
a fairly frequent incidence of sexual problems for this type of study, about one in five
patients, in both groups.

Bartelink et al.[27] studied 128 consecutive patients who underwent breast cancer surgery
and compared them to 75 patients who received a mastectomy in the same period. Body
image was measured with six questions that were factor analyzed. The lumpectomy group
exhibited a significantly better body image than the comparison group. The mastectomy
patients manifested a greater degree of dysfunction on a sexual inhibition question, included
in the body image scale.

Andersen and Jochimsen[28] compared the sexual functioning of breast and gynecologic
cancer patients with healthy women, with an extensive sexual inventory.[9] They operationalized the construct of sexual functioning according to sexual behavior and to the sexual
response cycle (desire, excitement, orgasm, resolution). Sexual behavior was significantly
poorer in the two cancer groups ($p < 0.05$), and the subjects' evaluation of their current
sexual life was independent of their current marital adjustment. Gynecologic cancer patients
rated their body image worse than breast cancer patients or healthy women ($p < 0.05$). Lack
of differences could be explained by the very small number of subjects with each condition
($n = 16$).

Only one other study, by Sewell and Edwards,[29] sought to determine the psychological
impact of differing surgeries but on a different cancer site than breast: pelvic genital cancer
(that study is also not reported in Andersen's review). The researchers classified 46 female
patients according to three types of genital surgery: hysterectomy ($n = 16$), vulvectomy ($n
= 15$) and exenterations ($n = 15$). The patients were interviewed at least 6 months post-
surgery with a relationship and sexual adjustment "panel" and some standard scales (for
self-esteem, well-being, and social adjustment). The authors found significant differences
in the predicted direction between the three groups for sexual functioning and body image,
but not for social and psychological well-being.

E. FOURTH REVIEW ARTICLE — HALL AND FALLOWFIELD, 1989[30]

In a very recent paper, Hall and Fallowfield[30] reviewed the studies comparing the
psychological outcomes of mastectomy and breast conserving procedures. Aside from the
previously cited studies, they identified two studies which report some data about sexual
functioning.[31,32] Fallowfield[31] conducted a retrospective research on psychological morbidity
of 101 breast cancer women who had been randomized into either a mastectomy group (n

= 53) or a lumpectomy one (n = 48). Psychiatric symptomatology was assessed with the *Present State Examination* and sexual functioning, with one question from the *Rotterdam Symptom Checklist*. An identical percentage of patients in both groups (38%) expressed loss of sexual interest after their surgical treatment for breast cancer.

Kemeny and colleagues[32] mailed a questionnaire on the psychosocial outcome of three types of breast cancer treatment randomly assigned to 83 women: mastectomy, segmentectomy with or without radiotherapy. The first questionnaire was returned by 62% of the patients, 27 in the mastectomy group and 25 in the segmentectomy one. The second questionnaire, sent 8 months after, was returned by 37 of those 52 patients. Data analysis was fairly simple: *t* tests for each item mean. As the authors point out, the very large number of statistical tests performed augments the probability of finding spurious differences (Type I error). Nevertheless, body image differences, in the expected direction, are the "strongest and most consistent finding". There were no differences in sexual behavior (frequency of intercourse and of orgasm) or in sexual problems.

Another study comparing lumpectomy and mastectomy (with or without breast reconstruction) was published in the same year as Hall and Fallowfield's review. Wellisch and co-workers[33] also sent a questionnaire, similar to the one used by Kemeny,[32] to 103 women who had completed their cancer treatment 1 to 3 years earlier. Fifty patients returned the research materials: 22 in the lumpectomy group, 15 in the mastectomy group with breast reconstruction, and 13 in the one without reconstruction. Of the seven questions assessing body image, four show differences in the expected direction: lumpectomy patients present the best body image, while patients who have undergone a mastectomy with breast reconstruction had scores "midway between the mean scores of the two groups". In terms of sexual functioning, there were no differences between the three groups. The authors underline the fact they used some questions from a previous study[23] in an attempt to replicate some of its findings. The critique we addressed to Steinberg[23] and to Beckmann[22] applies also to the above two studies. Body image and sexuality questions should have been regrouped into scales, after reliability analyses, rather than reported on singly.

We can conclude from this literature review on sexual functioning of breast cancer patients that up to one third of the patients become sexually dysfunctional following surgery (a result found even in studies[32,33] that had a very low return rate of mailed questionnaires). Most studies found that the radical modified mastectomy was followed by a greater percentage of sexual dysfunctions, while the most recent ones tend to find no differences between the two types of surgery.

III. OBJECTIVES AND METHOD OF THE PRESENT STUDY

In the analysis of quality of life following mastectomy or lumpectomy, the issue of how and by whom the type of surgery is decided is of great importance.[30] Of the studies cited above, only those of Schain[26] and of Kemeny[32] compared patients who were randomized into the two types of surgery (in Fallowfield's study,[30] only patients who expressed no preference for either type of intervention were actually randomized). In both cases, the number of patients in each arm is quite small (from 18 to 28).

We decided to take advantage of an on-going multinational trial[34,35] which had randomized hundreds of patients in order to study the efficacy of segmental mastectomy compared to total mastectomy.

Our objective was thus to study the quality of life of the patients entered into this protocol, for randomization would provide a better experimental design than if the surgical procedure was selected by surgeon or by patient, as is mostly the case. In a previous paper,[36] we presented data on depression, body image, and fear of recurrence of the first 123 patients accrued.

The present paper reports on the sexual functioning and the marital relationships of the whole sample of 290 respondents. We hypothesize that patients who submit to a total mastectomy will experience a lower level of quality of life compared to those who receive a breast conserving surgery. They will exhibit a worse body image, more sexual dysfunction, more disturbance in their marital relationships, and a greater number of depressive symptoms than the patients who undergo a lumpectomy.

A. SUBJECTS

The National Surgical Adjuvant Breast Project (NSABP) began, in 1976, a multinational prospective clinical trial (B-06) to compare the efficacy of radical modified mastectomy (total) with partial mastectomy (lumpectomy). Patients were randomly assigned to one of three treatment arms: total mastectomy (TM), lumpectomy (LP), and lumpectomy followed by breast radiation therapy (LPR).

Patients were asked to participate in our quality of life study as they came to one of five cancer clinics for their regular follow-up appointment. Of the 272 patients contacted, 19 refused to answer the questionnaire, while 34 questionnaires were rejected because they contained too many questions or pages left unanswered.

If patients in the B-06 protocol experienced a recurrence of their cancer (or if their margins were not found to be tumor free), a total mastectomy was performed.[34] The protocol required those patients to remain assigned to their initial treatment group, for calculation of survival rates.

This classification was necessary to assess the effectiveness of the surgical procedures, but it was not deemed appropriate for quality-of-life assessment. In the case of recurrence, patients experienced a heightened threat of cancer and death, and also had to face the psychological consequences of a total mastectomy. To offset this methodological difficulty, we created a fourth type of treatment group, the multiple surgery group (MUL).

Figure 1 presents the original random assignment of patients from the B-06 protocol to the three surgery groups. A total of 219 questionnaires had been retained for data analysis, answered by 93 patients from the total mastectomy group (TM), 62 from the lumpectomy group (LP), and 64 from the lumpectomy with radiotherapy group (LPR). Dissection of the axillary nodes had proven positive for 80 patients, who had then received adjuvant chemotherapy. They numbered 37 in the TM group, 19 in the LP group, and 24 in the LPR group.

For comparison purposes, a control group (BIO) of 63 patients was established the following year, composed of women who had undergone a biopsy for a tumor that revealed itself as benign. For most of the control group patients, the only contact they had with the oncology center was for their biopsy. Since tracking down these biopsy patients, after several years and several address changes, became extremely difficult, we had to limit the time period since biopsy to a duration of 5 years.

B. INSTRUMENTS

To assess the impact of breast cancer on body image, we have elaborated a set of ten questions based on the studies of Polivy[37] and Steinberg.[23] A reliability analysis reduced the scale to seven items, for a Cronbach alpha of 0.81. Details of this *Body Image Index* were reported in our previous paper.[36]

Scales previously used to assess sexual functioning were found to be inappropriate for our purposes, since they are either extremely lengthy or their aim is to measure sexual dysfunction in order to plan for treatment. A *Sexual Functioning Scale* of 17 items was constructed from questions used in cancer studies[23,38,39] or from general sexual scales.[40,41] A reliability analysis led us to eliminate two questions, reducing it to 15 items, to obtain a Cronbach alpha of 0.84. Details of the scale (frequencies for each alternative and mean score for each question) are to be found in the Appendix.

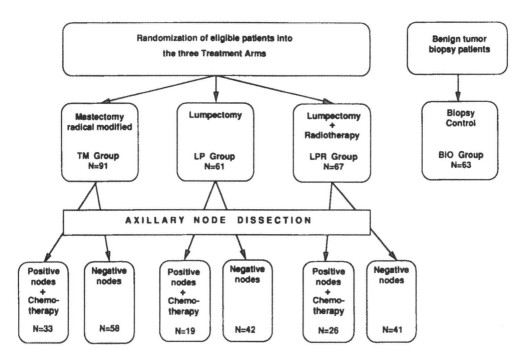

FIGURE 1. Number of patients initially assigned to the three Treatment Arms and to the Biopsy Control group.

Marital Adjustment was measured with the Locke and Wallace[16a] scale, as several of the reviewed studies did. Kimmel and Van Der Veen[42] have identified one general Marital Adjustment factor, after factor analyzing the scale. The 21-item test includes three questions about sexual relations (which showed an alpha of 0.83 when we regrouped them as a subscale). The reliability of the total scale in our study is quite high (Chronbach alpha of 0.92).

Psychological distress is measured with the *CES-Depression* scale, a 20-item checklist developed by Radloff,[43] at the National Institute of Mental Health's Center for Epidemiologic Studies, to measure depressive symptomatology in a general population. Of the 20 questions, 4 are destined to evidence the presence of positive affect. Answers are of the Likert type, ranging from 0 to 3, yielding a global score of 0 to 60. Radloff has established the population average to be around 8, and the psychiatric cut-off point, at 15. The reliability of this scale, in our study, is 0.88.

IV. RESULTS

The results reported previously[36] presented data of the first 123 patients accrued, classified according to the B-06 protocol: 43 in the TM group (total mastectomy), 44 in the LP group (lumpectomy), and 36 in the LPR group (lumpectomy followed by breast radiation therapy). For the subsequent analyses, the subjects were reclassified according to the creation of the fourth treatment category. For the complete sample of 219 cancer patients, the MUL group (multiple interventions) regrouped 42 patients.

Table 1 presents the basic characteristics of the four surgery groups as well as those of the biopsy control group. Time since operation is significantly shorter for the biopsy group than for the four treatment groups, respectively, a little less than $2\frac{1}{2}$ years compared to $3\frac{1}{2}$ to 4 years (F = 5.32, $p < 0.001$). The biopsy patients are also slightly younger than the patients who underwent surgical treatment for cancer. There are no differences between the five groups in terms of marital or occupational status: about two thirds of the whole

TABLE 1
Characteristics of the Four Treatment Groups and of the Biopsy Control Group

	Treatment groups[*]				Biopsy group	
	(LP)	(LPR)	(TM)	(MUL)	(BIO)	p <
Time since operation (in months)	43.6	41.8	43.3	47.8	27.7	0.001[a]
Age (in months)	55.3	54.1	55.1	53.0	51.1	0.14[a]
Education (in years)	11.3	11.4	11.2	11.3	12.5	0.18[a]
Married (in %)	74	61	68	74	60	0.55[b]
Employed (in %)	42	48	42	48	51	0.83[b]
n	58	60	59	42	63	

Note: [*] TM = total mastectomy group, LP = lumpectomy group, LPR = lumpectomy with radiotherapy group, MUL = multiple surgery group.

[a] Based on one-way Anovas, among the five groups.
[b] Based on chi-square since variables are nominal.

sample is married and half, gainfully employed. The biopsy control group is thus quite similar to the surgery groups, but for time interval since operation, which we had to limit for practical reasons to a period of 5 years.

Table 2 presents four dependent variables that the literature has shown to be influenced by breast cancer surgery. The type of mastectomy significantly impacts on the patients' body image (F = 12.27, p <0.000). Results on the whole sample confirm what has already been reported in our previous paper. The breast conserving intervention (LP and LPR groups) yields a better body image than radical modified mastectomy (TM and MUL groups). The patient who undergoes a lumpectomy experiences a body image similar to that of the patient who did not require cancer surgery but a simple biopsy.

Whatever the type of surgery, be it total or partial, it significantly influences, in a negative way, the sexual functioning of the patient (F = 5.23, p <0.001). Compared to the biopsy control group, the four surgery groups manifest a higher level of sexual dysfunction (F = 22.93, p <0.000).

The global Marital Adjustment score is not affected by surgery. There are no differences among the four types of surgery, as well as no difference between the biopsy control group and the surgery groups. Yet, when the three items dealing with sexual relations are grouped as a subscale, differences appear, similar to those evidenced with the Sexual Functioning scale. Surgery impacts negatively on sexual relations: the biopsy control group exhibits better sexual functioning than the other four treatment groups (F = 4.78, p <0.01).

Contrary to our expectations, women who were subjected to a total mastectomy do not express more depressive symptoms than those who received a lumpectomy. And those who had a simple biopsy manifest a depressive level equivalent to that of the breast cancer surgery patients who were subjected to either a total or a partial mastectomy.

V. DISCUSSION

The lumpectomy, a breast conserving procedure for treatment of breast cancer, had been resisted by surgeons who feared the less extensive resection would lead to higher mortality rates. The recently published data from the 5- and 10-year follow-up studies of Fisher and colleagues[34,35] demonstrated the breast conserving procedure and the more radical intervention were not different in terms of long-term survival rates nor in terms of incidence of metastases.

The literature on quality of life following breast cancer treatment has shown body image differences, in favor of the lesser surgery, are the most frequent finding.[21-23,27,32-34] Our

TABLE 2
Body Image, Sexual Functioning, Marital Adjustment and Depressive Symptoms, According to the Four Treatment and the Biopsy Control Groups

	No. of items	Alpha (α)	Treatment groups				Biopsy group (BIO)	F	$p <$	LP, LPR vs. TM, MUL $p <$	LP, LPR, TM, MUL vs. BIO $p <$
			(LP)	(LPR)	(TM)	(MUL)					
Body image	7	81	31.5	31.3	27.4	26.7	31.9	12.27	0.000	0.000	0.001
Sexual functioning[a]	15	84	28.6	31.1	30.7	32.0	24.9	5.23	0.001	0.26	0.000
Marital adjustment[a]	21	92	39.8	38.7	39.8	38.1	37.1	0.32	0.86	0.89	0.39
Depressive symptoms[a]	20	88	14.3	12.2	13.1	15.7	12.8	0.97	0.42	0.39	0.50

[a] The lower the score, the better the functioning.

results are consistent with the literature: the breast conserving operation exerts a significant influence on the patient's body image. The patients who submitted to a total (radical modified) mastectomy are not as satisfied with their body appearance as are the ones who had the less extensive surgery. In the latter case, the impact of a lumpectomy is not different from that of a simple biopsy. This result demonstrates the validity of the appellation "breast conserving procedure" attributed to the lumpectomy.

Contrary to our hypothesis, this breast conserving procedure does not influence the sexual functioning, the marital adjustment nor the depressive symptomatology of the patients, when compared to total mastectomy. Data from the biopsy control group shows sexual functioning is disrupted by cancer surgery, be it a mastectomy or a lumpectomy. The breast conserving intervention thus does not shield patients from sexual difficulties associated with breast surgery. On the other hand, cancer surgery, whether minimal or extensive, does not affect the patients' marital adjustment. The breast conserving procedure then has also no significant influence on the couples' marital harmony. An absence of difference in results was also found in recent studies of sexual functioning[28,31-44] and of marital adjustment.[13,21]

Results from the whole sample confirm the preliminary data we found previously about depressive symptoms. Contrary to our hypothesis, lumpectomy patients are not less subject to depression than mastectomy patients. Whether the patient had her whole breast removed or only the cancerous part, does not affect her level of depressive symptomatology. Recent studies[23,32,33,46] failed also to obtain differences between the two surgical procedures.

While there were no differences among the four surgery groups, the biopsy control group also was not any different from them in terms of depressive symptoms. So, having experienced cancer and the effect of its surgery or only the threat of cancer (in the biopsy group), is linked to a similar level of depression. We should underline that the level of depression in the five groups is almost double that of a normal population. Our results are consistent with the findings from the very first studies on the quality of life of cancer patients,[4,13-15,45] which established depression as an almost "normal" reaction to cancer surgery.

To conclude, total mastectomy does alter the patients' body image, while the breast conserving intervention does not affect it. Unfortunately, this lack of impact on the self concept is not reflected at the psychological level: depressive symptoms in the lesser surgery patients are as high as in the "disfiguring" surgery group, and problems in sexual functioning arise following cancer surgery, as much with the breast conserving operation as with a total mastectomy.

APPENDIX
Lasry Sexual Functioning Scale
for Breast Cancer Patients

	Frequencies (N_{max} = 180)	$\bar{X}$
1. How would you describe your mate's sexual drive, since your surgery?		1.71
(1)* Very high (1) High	80	
(2) Moderate	78	
(3) Low	7	
(4) Absent	11	
2. How would you describe your own sexual drive, since surgery?		2.02
(1) Very high (1) High	49	
(2) Moderate	88	
(3) Low	33	
(4) Absent	10	

* Indicates the weight attributed to each response.

APPENDIX (continued)
Lasry Sexual Functioning Scale
for Breast Cancer Patients

	Frequencies ($N_{max} = 180$)	$\overline{X}$
3. What was the time interval between surgery and the first time you had sexual relations with your mate? *(open ended question)*		1.47
(1) 1—4 weeks	120	
(2) 5—11 weeks	24	
(3) 12—78 weeks	12	
(4) Not resumed yet	10	
4. What is the approximate frequency of your sexual relations, at present?		2.02
(1) Once/day (1) 3—4/week (1) Twice/week	54	
(2) Once/week (2) Once/2 weeks	75	
(3) Once/month (3) Less than once/month	31	
(4) Not resumed yet	13	
5. When you think of having sexual relations, how anxious do you feel?		1.92
(1) Not at all anxious	87	
(2) A little anxious	29	
(3) Moderately anxious	37	
(4) Very anxious	18	
6. How often do you see your mate completely undressed?		1.73
(1) Very often	95	
(2) Often	41	
(3) Sometimes	34	
(4) Never	7	
7. How often does your mate see you completely undressed?		1.98
(1) Very often	75	
(2) Often	41	
(3) Sometimes	49	
(4) Never	11	
8. During lovemaking, do you keep some sort of clothing (nightgown, T-shirt...) on you?		1.72
(1) No	94	
(2) Sometimes	46	
(3) Usually	23	
(4) Nearly always	11	
9. How satisfied are you presently with your sex life?		1.84
(1) Very satisfied (1) Quite satisfied	85	
(2) Rather satisfied	50	
(3) Rather dissatisfied	23	
(4) Quite dissatisfied (4) Very dissatisfied	17	
10. Since surgery, have you felt the need to have a professional discuss sexual issues with you and/or your mate?		1.25
(1) No need at all	150	
(2) A little need	10	
(3) A moderate need	9	
(4) A great need	5	
Since you had breast surgery, has there been any change in the following behaviors?		
11. In your mate's sexual drive		2.18
(1) Increase	3	
(2) Same	153	
(4) Decrease	17	
12. In your own sexual drive		2.46
(1) Increase	8	
(2) Same	121	
(4) Decrease	44	

APPENDIX (continued)
Lasry Sexual Functioning Scale
for Breast Cancer Patients

	Frequencies (N$_{max}$ = 180)	$\overline{X}$
13. In the frequency of your sexual relations		2.43
(1) Increase	6	
(2) Same	126	
(4) Decrease	40	
14. In your degree of satisfaction with your sexual relations		2.40
(1) Increase	4	
(2) Same	136	
(4) Decrease	34	
15. In how frequently you appear undressed in front of your mate		2.38
(1) Increase	5	
(2) Same	133	
(4) Decrease	35	

REFERENCES

1. Witkin, M. H., Sex therapy and mastectomy, *J. Sex Marital Ther.*, 1, 290, 1975.
2. Schover, L. R., Evans, R. B., and VonEschenbach, A. C., Sexual rehabilitation in a cancer center: diagnosis and outcome in 384 consultations, *Arch. Sex. Behav.*, 16, 445, 1987.
3. Morris, T., Psychological adjustment to mastectomy, *Cancer Treat. Rev.*, 4, 41, 1979.
4. Meyerowitz, B. E., Psychosocial correlates of breast cancer and its treatments, *Psychol. Bull.*, 87, 108, 1980.
5. Cohen, J., Cullen, J. W., and Martin, L. R., Eds., *Psychosocial Aspects of Cancer*, Raven Press, New York, 1982.
6. Mantell, J. E., Sexuality and cancer, in *Psychosocial Aspects of Cancer*, Cohen, J., Cullen, J. W., and Martin, L. R., Eds., Raven Press, New York, 1982, chap. 20.
8. Bransfield, D. D., Breast cancer and sexual functioning: a review of the literature and implications for future research, *Int. J. Psychiatry Med.*, 12, 197, 1982.
9. Derogatis, L. R. and Melisaratos, N., The DSFI: a multidimensional measure of sexual functioning, *J. Sex Marital Ther.*, 5, 244, 1979.
10. Greenberg, D. B., The measurement of sexual dysfunction in cancer patients, *Cancer*, 53, 2281, 1984.
11. Andersen, B. L., Sexual difficulties for women following cancer treatment, in *Woman With Cancer*, Andersen, B., Ed., Springer-Verlag, New York, 1986, chap. 8.
12. Dobkin, P. L. and Bradley, I., Assessment of sexual dysfunction in oncology patients: review, critique and suggestions, *J. Psychosoc. Oncol.*, in press.
13. Morris, T., Greer, S. H., and White, P., Psychological and social adjustment to mastectomy: a two-year follow-up study, *Cancer*, 40, 2381, 1977.
14. Maguire, P., Psychiatric problems after mastectomy, in *Cancer — Psychosocial Aspects of Early Detection and Treatment*, Brand, P. C. and VanKeeps, P. A., Eds., University Park Press, Baltimore, 1978, chap. 6.
15. Jamison, K. R., Wellisch, D. K., and Pasnau, R. O., Psychosocial aspects of mastectomy: the woman's perspective, *Am. J. Psychiatry*, 135, 432, 1978.
16. Torrie, A., Like a bird with broken wings, *World Med.*, 7, 36, 1970.
16a. Locke, H. J. and Wallace, K. M., Short marital adjustment and prediction tests: their reliability and validity, *Marriage Fam. Living*, 21, 251, 1959.
17. Lyon, J. S., Management of psychological problems in breast cancer, in *Breast Cancer Management — Early and Late*, Stoll, B. A., Ed., Heinemann Medical, London, 1977, 225.
18. Silberfarb, P. M., Maurer, H., and Crouthamel, C. S., Psychosocial aspects of neoplastic disease. I. Functional status of breast cancer patients during different treatment regimens, *Am. J. Psychiatry*, 137, 450, 1980.

19. Battersby, C., Armstrong, J., and Abrahams, M., Mastectomy in a large public hospital, *Austr. N. Z. J. Surg.*, 48, 401, 1978.

20. Anderson, B. L., Ed., *Women with Cancer: Psychological Perspectives*, Springer-Verlag, New York, 1986.

21. Sanger, C. K. and Reznikoff, M., A comparison of the psychological effects of breast-saving procedures with the modified radical mastectomy, *Cancer*, 48, 2341, 1981.

22. Beckmann, J., Johansen, L., Richardt, C., and Blichert-Toft, M., Psychological reactions in younger women operated on for breast cancer, *Dan. Med. J.*, 30, 10, 1983.

23. Steinberg, M. D., Juliano, M. A., and Wise, L., Psychological outcome of lumpectomy vs. mastectomy in the treatment of breast cancer, *Am. J. Psychiatry*, 142, 34, 1985.

24. Taylor, S. E., Lichtman, R. R., and Wood, J. V., Attribution beliefs about control and adjustment to breast cancer, *J. Pers. Soc. Psychol.*, 46, 489, 1984.

25. Lichtman, R. R., Wood, J., and Taylor, S. E., Close relationships after breast cancer, presented at the annual meeting of the American Psychological Association, Washington, D. C., 1982.

26. Schain, W., Edwards, B. K., Gorell, C. R., DeMoss, E. V., et al., Psychosocial and physical outcomes of primary breast cancer therapy: mastectomy vs excisional biopsy and irradiation, *Breast Cancer Res. Treat.*, 3, 377, 1983.

27. Bartelink, H., Van Dam, F., and Van Dongen, J., Psychological effects of breast conserving therapy in comparison with radical mastectomy, *Int. J. Radiat. Oncol. Biol. Phys.*, 11, 391, 1985.

28. Andersen, B. L. and Jochimsen, P. R., Sexual functioning among breast cancer, gynecologic cancer, and healthy women, *J. Consult. Clin. Psychol.*, 53, 25, 1985.

29. Sewell, H. H. and Edwards, D. W., Pelvic genital cancer: body image and sexuality, *Front. Radiat. Ther. Oncol.*, 14, 35, 1980.

30. Hall, A. and Fallowfield, L., Psychological outcome of treatment for early breast cancer: a review, *Stress Med.*, 5, 167, 1989.

31. Fallowfield, L. J., Baum, M., and Maguire, G. P., Effects of breast conservation on psychological morbidity associated with diagnosis and treatment of early breast cancer, *Br. Med. J.*, 293, 1331, 1986.

32. Kemeny, M. M., Wellisch, D. K., and Schain, W. S., Psychosocial outcome in a randomized surgical trial for treatment of primary breast cancer, *Cancer*, 62, 1231, 1988.

33. Wellisch, D. K., DiMatteo, R., Silverstein, M., et al., Psychosocial outcomes of breast cancer therapies: lumpectomy vs mastectomy, *Psychosomatics*, 30, 365, 1989.

34. Fischer, B., Bauer, M., Margolese, R., Poisson, R., et al., Five-year results of randomized clinical trial comparing total mastectomy and segmental mastectomy with or without radiation in the treatment of breast cancer, *N. Engl. J. Med.*, 312, 665, 1985.

35. Fischer, B., Redmond, C., Fischer, E., and Bauer, M., et al., Ten-year results of a randomized clinical trial comparing radical mastectomy and total mastectomy with or without radiation, *N. Engl. J. Med.*, 312, 674, 1985.

36. Lasry, J. C., Margolese, R. G., Poisson, R., Shibata, H., et al., Depression and body image following mastectomy and lumpectomy, *J. Chronic Dis.*, 40, 529, 1987.

37. Polivy, J., Psychological effects of mastectomy on a woman's feminine self-concept, *J. Nerv. Ment. Dis.*, 164, 77, 1977.

37. Ray, C. and Baum, M., *Psychological Aspects of Early Breast Cancer*, Springer-Verlag, New York, 1985.

38. Wellisch, D. K., Jamison, K. R., and Pasnau, R. O., Psychosocial aspects of mastectomy. II. The man's perspective, *Am. J. Psychiatry*, 135, 543, 1978.

39. Grandstaff, N. W., The impact of breast cancer on the family, *Front. Radiat. Ther. Oncol.*, 11, 146, 1976.

40. Nowinsky, J. K. and Lopicollo, J., Assessing sexual behavior in couples, *J. Sex. Marit. Ther.*, 5, 225, 1979.

41. Harbison, J. M., Graham, P. J., Queen, N. J. T., Mcallister, H., and Woodward, R., A questionnaire measure of sexual interest, *Arch. Sex. Behav.*, 3, 357, 1974.

42. Kimmell, D. and Van Der Veen, F., Factors of marital adjustment in Locke's Marital Adjustment Test, *J. Marr. Fam.*, 36, 57, 1974.

43. Radloff, L. S., The CES-D scale: a self-report depression scale for research in the general population, *Appl. Psychol. Measur.*, 1, 385, 1977.

44. DeHaes, J. C. J. M. and Welvaart, T. K., Quality of life after breast cancer surgery, *J. Surg. Oncol.*, 28, 123, 1985.

45. Ray, C., Adjustment to mastectomy: the psychological impact of disfigurement, in *Breast Cancer — Psychosocial Aspects of Early Detection and Treatment*, Brand, P. C. and Van Keeps, P. A., Eds., University Park Press, Baltimore, 1978, chap. 5.

46. DeHaes, J. C. J. M., Van Oostrom, M. A., and Welvaart, K., The effect of radical and conserving surgery on the quality of life of early breast cancer patients, *Eur. J. Surg. Oncol.*, 12, 337, 1986.

Chapter 17

METHODOLOGICAL ISSUES IN ANTIEMETIC STUDIES

Andrew R. Willan, David Warr, Joseph L. Pater, Martin Levitt,
Charles Erlichman, and David Osoba

TABLE OF CONTENTS

I. INTRODUCTION

One of the major ways in which chemotherapy may exert an adverse effect on quality of life is through the induction of nausea and vomiting.[1,2] Controlled trials have established that high dose metoclopramide[3] and glucocorticoids[4,5] are effective antiemetics but a substantial proportion of patients will still experience acute or delayed upset.

The ability to identify new treatments that will provide better protection requires a sound methodologic approach. Previous reviews of antiemetic methodology have identified the potential for erroneous conclusions when the trial design is flawed.[6-8] An example is the initial failure to explore the dose-response relationship of metoclopramide in phase II chemotherapy-based studies before evaluation in a phase III setting. The use of an inappropriately low dose led to a conclusion that this drug was ineffective for upset induced by cytotoxic agents.[9] A later study by Gralla using much higher doses demonstrated potent antiemetic activity that made metoclopramide the treatment of choice.[3] If such pitfalls are to be avoided in the future, studies will have to adhere to clinical trial design strategies that are quite similar to those used in the development of antineoplastic agents.[10]

The purpose of this chapter is to review several methodologic aspects in the conduct of antiemetic studies. The emphasis will be on randomized studies but the earlier steps in drug evaluation will be briefly reviewed. The nomenclature for these studies is identical to that employed for cytotoxic trials, i.e., phase I, II, and III.[10] Parallels will be drawn between studies of cytotoxic agents and antiemetics and several important differences will be discussed. The lessons learned from antiemetic studies over the past decade will be used to suggest designs for future antiemetic studies.

II. PHASE I AND II CLINICAL TRIALS

Phase I studies are carried out to define pharmacokinetics and dose-limiting toxicities. Unlike phase I trials of cytotoxic agents, the earliest studies of antiemetics may include normal volunteers. Because of the lesser co-intervention and co-morbidity in these subjects as compared to patients with cancer, it is easier to attribute adverse effects to the experimental drug. It is important, though, to realize that toxicities that are considered dose-limiting for the general population may nonetheless be considered tolerable in the setting of chemotherapy if the benefits are substantial and the period of administration is brief. Examples are the doses of metoclopramide and lorazepam recommended for use as antiemetics[11] which are far above the amount that would be considered reasonable for other indications. It is possible that the pharmacokinetics or toxicity profile of a drug in patients will differ from normal volunteers because of drug interaction or co-morbidity. Phase I studies are therefore also conducted in patients who are receiving chemotherapy.

After the dose-limiting toxicities and pharmacokinetics have been documented, a decision must be made about whether or not the new treatment has sufficient antiemetic activity to warrant large scale trials against standard therapy. In the case of cytotoxic agents, this assessment would be made by conducting a separate phase II study. The reason for a separate study is that patients in phase I trials are often heavily pretreated and heterogeneous in tumor type with the result that responses are infrequent even with agents that are subsequently judged to be active.[12] Proper evaluation for efficacy therefore requires assessment in a different patient population.

In contrast, an antiemetic trial may be both phase I and II in intent. Patients entered into these early studies often have had no prior therapy and thus would have a reasonable chance of responding to an effective new therapy. Examples include phase I studies of metoclopramide and selective 5-HT$_3$ receptor antagonists where protection from emesis occurred in a substantial proportion of cases.[13-16] Since there is no control group, statements about effectiveness in this type of study are meaningful only if the emetic stimulus would be expected to produce vomiting in virtually 100% of patients (e.g., high-dose cisplatin[3]) and the patients have not had extensive prior chemotherapy (in which case the probability of response to any antiemetic agent is greatly diminished[17,18]). These protocols require entry of only three to five patients per dose level[10] which means that the confidence limits on results will be extremely wide. For example, even if one pools the results of four or five dose levels, a 50% response rate in 20 patients still has a 95% confidence interval of 27 to 73%. With such a wide range it is not possible to make definitive statements about optimal antiemetic dose in these combined phase I/II studies. Precise estimates of efficacy require entry of more patients at the dose of drug which will be selected for phase III investigations.

Decisions regarding optimum dose and schedule (single bolus, continuous infusion, q 2 h vs. q 6 h etc.) can only be properly addressed in separate phase II studies that are large enough to detect differences of moderate size, e.g., an absolute 20% increase or decrease in protection from emesis. In practice, however, these trials are often so small that there is a considerable potential for false negative conclusions.[19-23] The principles regarding selection of patients, assessment of outcome, and analysis for such studies are similar to those used in phase III trials and are discussed below.

III. PHASE III STUDIES

A. OBJECTIVE

The intent of a phase III study is usually to demonstrate superior efficacy.[10] Alternatively, the objective may be to demonstrate lesser toxicity[24] or more convenient scheduling with equivalent antiemetic effect.[25] The requirement for comparison with a standard therapy imposes constraints on the design that differ from phase I and phase II studies. The principle design elements are discussed below.

B. RANDOMIZATION

It could be argued that the initial studies with high dose metoclopramide did not require a control group because 100% of patients would be expected to vomit with antiemetics available at that time. The predictability of emesis, however, may be challenged by three studies. Kahn[26] reported that a single oral dose of metoclopramide 20 mg (a dose documented in controlled studies to be ineffective) prevented emesis in 17/24 patients (71%) who received cisplatin in a dose of 100 mg/m². In a study by D'Olimpio, 7/32 patients (22%) in the placebo group did not vomit.[27] Using patients deemed refractory to standard antiemetics, Sallan reported that 10 mg of oral prochlorperazine (a standard antiemetic) produced a complete response in 16/78 (21%) of subjects.[28] Thus the absence of emesis does not necessarily indicate a response to therapy.

With current antiemetic therapy it is possible to prevent vomiting in up to 60% of patients receiving the most highly emetogenic therapy.[24] Further improvements of the magnitude seen with the introduction of high-dose metoclopramide are unlikely to occur; yet even a 15% decrease in the proportion of patients with emesis should be considered worthwhile.

Given the number of variables that may influence the probability of emesis (see below), it is impossible to be certain that any differences between the experimental treatment and control treatment (whether concurrent or historical) is not due to patient selection. Predictive models that might help with assessing comparability to nonrandomized controls are being developed[29,30] but they have not been validated and it is not clear how much of the variance is left to be explained by other (unknown) factors. Randomization should be regarded as a necessary aspect of phase III studies. Information from nonrandomized studies should rarely change clinical practice.

C. BLINDING

The double-blind technique is frequently (but not universally) used in comparative antiemetic trials. There are several reasons why blinding is occasionally not employed. First, patients may be ill at ease when they do not know which treatment has been administered. In one study 25% of patients refused further participation because of the uncertainty associated with blinding.[31] Second, investigators may be reluctant to randomize patients because they will not know whether or not the drug administered is an experimental agent with a less certain profile of adverse effects than the standard therapy. Third, it is also cumbersome when blinding necessitates the manufacture of special tablets or capsules which must be identical, from the patient's perspective, to the active treatment and which must (if they contain active ingredients) be approved by regulatory bodies.

Despite these concerns, it is desirable to maintain blinding whenever possible. Unlike tumor response in chemotherapy studies, the outcome in antiemetic trials is sometimes highly subjective (nausea severity). Though more *objective*, the number of emetic episodes is not data that is available for independent review unless the entire study period has been recorded on videotape.[32] Cognitive-behavioral intervention studies demonstrate that pre- and post-chemotherapy upset can be modified by training[33,34] and one must assume that beliefs regarding a new treatment may influence the results. Patient expectations may also influence the frequency with which adverse effects are recorded, e.g., *highs* were experienced with prochlorperazine in a double-blind study also involving a cannabinoid.[31]

Single-blind technique is not an acceptable alternative to double-blind design for several reasons. Although most studies use data from patient self-report, there may be unintended communication of expectations regarding efficacy and adverse effects from the (unblinded) investigator to the patient. As stated above, this may influence the outcome. Another issue is the potential for bias in the search for adverse effects (more adverse effects are recorded when there is direct questioning[35]). A third problem is the subjective nature of the decision whether or not to attribute an adverse event to a treatment. In antiemetic studies, a large number of the recorded adverse events may be due to the underlying cancer or its treatment. If a decision is made to abbreviate the list of events to those that are felt to be drug related, investigator expectations may then influence the adverse effect profile.

When drugs such as lorazepam or cannabinoids are used, blinding is difficult to maintain because of adverse effects.[8] It has been stated that in studies where a new agent is associated with sedation a sedative could be added to the alternative arm to maintaining blinding.[7] This recommendation is unacceptable for two reasons. First, the addition of a sedative to a standard arm might alter the antiemetic efficacy of the standard *therapy* (as has been documented with lorazepam[36]). Second, the sedation would certainly alter the adverse effect profile of that group (increased sedation and possibly decreased akathisia[24] if dopamine-blocking agents are used) making it difficult to compare treatments in terms of toxicity. In these situations, double-blind technique should still be used because a proportion of patients receiving cannabinoids, lorazepam, etc. will experience little or no sedation[35,36] and even patients on placebo may report sedation.[35] In a cross-over study of prochlorperazine vs. tetrahydrocannabinol over one third of patients were unable to identify the correct identify of the antiemetic despite the fact that there was prior exposure to prochlorperazine and marijuana in 71 and 40.5%, of subjects, respectively.[31] Of the 19 patients who reported a *high*, 6 were receiving prochlorperazine. Some degree of unblinding will invariably occur when the antiemetic agents differ substantially in adverse effects and particularly when crossover design is used. Failure to use double-blind technique, however, will only increase the potential that the differences measured in efficacy or adverse effects are due to patient/investigator expectations as opposed to a true drug effect.

D. SELECTION OF A CONTROL (STANDARD THERAPY) ARM

Since the objective of a phase III study is usually to assess whether or not the new treatment is superior to conventional therapy, the choice of the standard arm is crucial. In the initial studies of high-dose metoclopramide and dexamethasone, placebo was sometimes used.[3,4,27] Since there are now treatments that have been shown to be effective for cisplatin and noncisplatin chemotherapy, it has been argued that a placebo control group is unethical.[7] Apart from ethical concerns there is another reason why placebo is unacceptable in phase III trials. The study objective is to compare a new treatment with standard therapy, and that standard can no longer be regarded as placebo.

There is no single therapy that can be regarded as the standard but reasonable alternatives are stated in reviews of antiemetics.[11] For high-dose cisplatin, an appropriate control arm would be a combination of high-dose metoclopramide, a steroid, and lorazepam. While this combination may be widely used outside of clinical trials, it poses two problems if selected as a control group. First, unless the new agent were sedating it would be difficult to maintain blinding because of the lorazepam in the standard arm. Second, one might overlook new agents that are inferior to the combination but have the potential to add to the effectiveness of standard therapy. For this reason, investigators may opt to use high-dose metoclopramide alone as the control arm, particularly if the experimental agent shares a mechanism of action, e.g., selective $5-HT_3$ receptor antagonists.[37] It should be recognized however that such studies do not involve a comparison with a standard therapy. While they establish that there is potent antiemetic activity, further studies involving combinations are required.

E. PATIENT SELECTION
1. Inclusion/Exclusion Criteria

Although in phase III studies one would like to have results that apply to a large cross-section of the chemotherapy population, there are practical and ethical reasons for excluding certain individuals. A necessary reason for exclusion from study is that one or more of the drugs to be administered is contraindicated because of co-morbidity. Examples would be brittle diabetes in a study involving high dose steroids or drug allergy to a benzamide in a study of metoclopramide. One should also not enter those patients who are deemed unlikely to benefit from the new treatment. The nausea due to bowel obstruction, brain metastases, morphine (due to prior exposure to cytotoxics) may well be unaffected by an antiemetic that is very effective for chemotherapy-induced upset. For example, in animal models the $5-HT_3$ receptor antagonists are ineffective against emesis induced by xylazine or motion, yet are very potent inhibitors of upset due to cisplatin.[38] Since patients with other causes for upset are a heterogeneous group, there is little to be learned by their inclusion and they are unlikely to benefit from treatment.

Many studies have excluded any individual with prior exposure to chemotherapy.[3,24,35,36,39] The rationale is that these patients do not respond as well to subsequent antiemetic therapy[17,18] either because of a conditioning effect or simply the fact that they are poorer responders to antiemetic therapy in general (good responders are unlikely to volunteer for such studies). Exclusion of these patients does not greatly compromise the applicability of the results. Inclusion of these individuals, however, may decrease the change of detecting a positive overall result.

TABLE 1
Patient Characteristics Associated with
Favorable Antiemetic Response

Characteristic	Ref.
Increasing age	29, 30, 39, 40
Male	29, 30, 39
Alcohol intake	22, 41, 42
Not susceptible to motion sickness	43
Poor performance status	29
Inpatient	30, 39
No prior chemotherapy	17, 18

False positive results are less likely but may arise because of co-intervention. Glucocorticoids may be a component of the treatment for diseases such as breast cancer or lymphomas and should not be allowed during the study period because of their potent antiemetic effect. Supportive therapy such as sedatives, anxiolytics, or antidepressants may also have antiemetic effects.[40,41] Unfortunately the list of potential co-interventions is so large than an attempt to exclude all such patients may impair accrual and lead to the selection of a population that does not reflect clinical practice. It is reasonable to prohibit the use of drugs with well-documented antiemetic activity, e.g., steroids and cannabinoids, but compromises such as allowing the use of the patient's usual nighttime sedative may be required. A record should be kept of all medications taken shortly prior to and during the study period. This allows investigators to identify potentially important co-interventions that should lead to exclusion from the analysis and lesser co-interventions can be checked to see that there is no major imbalance between groups.

2. Patient Characteristics Affecting Response

Even after the exclusion of many individuals because of co-intervention and co-morbidity there is still substantial patient-to-patient variability in outcome (see above) some of which is predictable (see Table 1). There are discrepancies between studies with respect to the variables identified as important. This may be related to size (smaller studies are less likely to detect significant differences in subgroups) or perhaps the chemotherapy/antiemetic that is administered. While alcohol intake is a powerful factor in univariate analysis there is confounding with age and sex (alcoholics tend to be older males) and the independent role of alcohol is unclear.[29] Performance status has generally not been found to influence the probability of emesis,[17,39,44] but one study suggested that poorer status was associated with improved tolerance.[29] Prior exposure to chemotherapy has a major impact on antiemetic efficacy even in the absence of anticipatory symptoms.[17,18]

It is not possible to stratify for more than a few of these variables but a tabulation of the balance between groups should be provided for age, sex, and alcohol intake and adjustment should be made in the analysis for significant covariates. An alternative would be to devise a predictive model[29,30] and stratify treatment allocation based upon risk but the validity of this approach has not been tested.

Another aspect of selection is the variability in the frequency of adverse effects of the antiemetic agent. Young patients are at greater risk of developing extrapyramidal reactions following high-dose metoclopramide[47,48] or intermediate doses for maintenance therapy. Older patients may demonstrate poorer tolerance for the adverse effects of cannabinoids.[8] Awareness of these differences may allow investigators to select an appropriate group of individuals in which to test the hypotheses and to explain apparent discrepancies with other studies.

F. EMETIC STIMULUS

It is clear that there are major differences between the emetogenic potential of various chemotherapy agents.[11] Cisplatin is regarded as the most emetogenic agent but the effect has been shown to vary with dose,[27,39,49] rate of infusion,[50] time of administration,[51] co-administration of other cytotoxics,[42,52] and whether the drug is administered as an in-patient or out-patient.[30,39] The rate of infusion also appears to be important for doxorubicin.[53] If the study population includes a wide variation in dose or prolonged infusions are used then this should be clearly stated and the distribution between study groups should be indicated with adjustment of results if these are significant covariates.

The ability to demonstrate antiemetic activity may be affected by the type of chemotherapy against which the drug is tested. In animal models the mechanism of antiemetic effect appears to differ for the various cytotoxic agents.[54] It would not be surprising if some antiemetics were useful only for selected antineoplastic agents. For example, the cannabinoids are useful for moderately emetogenic therapy but their efficacy for high-dose cisplatin is limited.[55] Similarly, dexamethasone was readily established as an effective agent for noncisplatin chemotherapy[4,5] but was comparable to placebo as a single agent in patients receiving high-dose cisplatin.[27,56] The highly emetogenic nature of cisplatin and its widespread use account for the fact that it is commonly the cytotoxic drug administered in antiemetic studies. Phase III evaluations of any new antinauseant should be regarded as incomplete unless there is information regarding efficacy in patients who receive anthracyclines or cyclophosphamide.

G. ANTIEMETIC ADMINISTRATION

1. Dose-Response Relationships

A dose-response relationship has not been investigated for most antiemetics. This issue, however, was important in establishing the efficacy of metoclopramide[13] and may also be relevant to prochlorperazine.[57] For cannabinoids[31,35] and lorazepam[36,40] dose-limiting toxicities have been reached and the only question is whether lower doses might achieve equivalent results. On the other hand, conventional antiemetic doses of steroids are well tolerated and are largely based upon results achieved with arbitrarily selected doses rather than dose-response information. One controlled study showed no difference in efficacy between two dose levels of methylprednisolone.[58] A small study of dexamethasone reported in abstract form suggested that efficacy increased with higher doses.[59] Although further trials of steroids are warranted to define optimal therapy, at present a wide range of steroid dose is considered acceptable.[11]

2. Influence of Schedule

One would anticipate that drug schedule would be most important when the antiemetic possesses a relatively short terminal half-life (e.g., 6 h for metoclopramide[60]) and the cytotoxic agent causes prolonged upset (e.g., cisplatin). A study of high-dose metoclopramide has suggested that a bolus plus continuous infusion may be more effective than the schedule of intermittent injections originally described by Gralla et al.[61] Other trials have not shown differences between infusions and bolus administration[19,21,62] and even a single dose of metoclopramide has been reported to give favorable results.[63] Although no controlled trials have directly compared the five dose (intravenous) regimen to two doses, a recent study is suggestive that an abbreviated regimen may indeed be more effective[30] and current practice would indicate that two or three doses is an acceptable standard for phase III studies.

There are no studies that have addressed whether repeated doses of steroids in the first 24 h are more beneficial than a single dose. In one study sustained-release methylprednisolone failed to improve the results achieved with a single intravenous dose of the same drug.[64] A single dose for antiemetic control over the first 24 h is considered acceptable.

A related issue is the value of continuing antiemetics beyond the first 24 h especially for cisplatin. For patients receiving high-dose cisplatin, maintenance with dexamethasone and metoclopramide appears to be useful in decreasing the proportion of patients with delayed onset upset.[65] The relative value of dexamethasone vs. metoclopramide for this problem is not clear. The use of maintenance antiemetics for chemotherapy other than cisplatin has not been evaluated.

3. Route of Administration

Another source of variation in results may be route of antiemetic administration as noted in the following examples:

1. Interpatient variation in the absorption of tetrahydrocannabinol may account for some of the inconsistency in reports of efficacy.[8]
2. Oral dosing with steroids[66] (or possibly any other agent) immediately prior to the intravenous administration of chemotherapy may produce suboptimal results because of inadequate blood levels.
3. Metoclopramide may cause more adverse effects when given by mouth as opposed to intravenously.[67]

Because of the large number of ways in which an antiemetic may be given and the uncertain influence of these changes, investigators should administer these drugs in ways that have been demonstrated to be effective by controlled trials.

H. OUTCOME ASSESSMENT
1. What Should We Measure?
a. Nausea, Retching, and Emesis

Table 2 lists some of the outcomes that have been assessed in phase III studies. Because of the large number of potential end-points it is possible that in any given study where there is a true treatment difference that only some of these will be associated with statistically significant results. This is due to differences in sensitivity of the outcome measures, random variation and possibly due to true differences in the drug effect on various outcomes. It is important to select one or at most two outcomes to be the ones upon which sample size calculations and post-study decisions will be made. In most studies, both nausea and emesis are assessed.

Some studies do not count several successive emeses unless they occur outside of a specified time limit.[22,32] This appears to have been introduced because of some limitations of time-lapse videotaping.[32] There is no rationale for this alternative definition in studies not using videotape to assess response. Because of the potential for confusion, the term 'frequency' of emesis rather than 'episode' is preferable.

Although there is a neurological basis for distinguishing retching from emesis,[70] this is rarely done.[68] Several studies indicate that retching is included in the evaluation.[14,22,25,31,32,68,71] In some studies, episodes of retching have been regarded as equivalent to one episode of emesis if they occur within a 5-min period.[22,25] The reason for this time requirement is unclear and this is not a practical definition for patient self-assessment. Since retching is very troublesome to the patients it should be recorded and either reported separately[68] or grouped with emesis.[22,31,32,71]

Volume of emesis will be dependent upon the amount of food/liquid ingested and the gastric emptying properties of the antiemetic. It is not a practical outcome measure for outpatient studies and its contribution to decision making about efficacy is doubtful.

Some studies have combined nausea and emesis into one scale assuming that nausea and emesis are on a continuum.[27,31,52] While most studies report that a higher percentage of

TABLE 2
Antiemetic Outcomes and Method of Assessment

Outcome	Assessment method	Ref.
Nausea severity	Visual analog scale	23, 36, 64
	Categorical scale	4, 58, 68
Nausea duration	Hours	4, 36, 55
Emesis frequency	Number of episodes	3, 55, 57
Emesis severity	Visual analog scale	36, 65
Emesis volume	Mililiters	3, 55, 69
Retching	Number of episodes	68
Nausea/emesis	Combined categorical scale	27, 52, 31
Preference	Choice	17, 28, 36
Appetite	Categorical	4, 5, 68

patients experience nausea than emesis[5,39,58,68,71] there are studies where the reverse is true.[27,30] The results from the latter studies indicate that there are patients who may experience emesis but no nausea and thus a single scale would be inappropriate.

b. Patient Preference

Preference is an outcome that has been used in several antiemetic trials of cross-over design.[17,28,36,52,54] Its strength lies in the fact that choice of one therapy implies that the difference is clinically significant, i.e., appreciable to the patient. This in contrast to the assumption that 'x' mm on a visual analog scale or a specified percent difference in the likelihood of emesis is clinically significant. In addition, the preference reflects any trade-offs that must be made because of toxicity. This end-point may be used to establish the validity of other end-points (see Section III.H.4).

2. Who Should Measure the Outcome?

Observers have been used in some antiemetic studies to quantify the outcomes of interest.[3,56,57,69,72] It is conceivable that patients may be so distressed by their discomfort or so sedated by the treatment that they may not accurately record the number of episodes of vomiting. In one study in which videotaping was used, the reviewer's scores showed a statistically significant difference between two treatments but there was no significant difference in the patient's scores.[73]

There are several disadvantages to using observers.[72] It would be inappropriate to use them to record nausea since this is a totally subjective phenomenon. They may intrude on the patient's privacy. They are not practical for out-patient therapy or monitoring for periods of 24 h or longer and even with shorter periods, it is not reasonable to expect that one individual will be in constant attendance. Despite theoretical concerns about the validity of patient data, studies reporting both observer and patient data show similar results.[19,20,72] It is appropriate to reserve observers for phase I studies where frequent monitoring of vital signs and sampling of blood for pharmacokinetics necessitates the constant presence of an individual.

3. Period of Observation

The intensity of post-chemotherapy emesis is greatest in the initial 24 h.[70] The vast majority of studies have not been extended beyond this period although there are exceptions.[35,65,68] With the introduction of high-dose metoclopramide it became evident that approximately two thirds of patients who receive high dose cisplatin and are free of emesis in the first 24 h will vomit later with the most troublesome period being 48 to 72 h.[74] It is not clear to what degree this delayed onset upset occurs with noncisplatin chemotherapy. Since patient self-assessment is now frequently used, all phase III antiemetic studies should record nausea and vomiting for a minimum of 5 days.

There has also been attention directed toward anticipatory upset although this is virtually never reported as part of phase III studies because of their limited duration, e.g., one course.[65] This problem occurs after several courses of chemotherapy following which there has been marked upset. There are methodological issues which are particularly relevant to this problem but it is beyond the scope of this chapter to review the potential problems in detail. Examples are the definition of *anticipatory* (does this include nausea that occurs while the chemotherapy is being infused?), distinguishing anticipatory symptoms from upset due to multiple other etiologies, the inability to blind behavioral intervention studies, greater difficulty in specifying the exact nature of the intervention in nonpharmacologic studies, and the decision to include only those patients who are already experiencing symptoms vs. a prophylactic study.

A final consideration is the number of courses over which the therapy is evaluated. The efficacy of therapy may decline over time[58,76] although in other cases it is said to be maintained.[46,77] In the case of cannabinoids, it has been speculated that loss of efficacy may be due to drug tolerance.[76] An alternative explanation relates to conditioning. Those patients who experienced nausea but no emesis may, with repeated exposure (especially if they are in a hospital bed beside someone who is vomiting), start to vomit. Individuals with one or two emetic episodes after one course, i.e., partial responders, may also experience less satisfactory results for the same reason. In any event, information from observation of patients over several courses is useful because the requirement for good antiemetic control extends throughout the entire course of treatment. The dropout rate due to tumor progression, refusal, etc., however, means that this information will be primarily descriptive in nature and the decision-making analysis will be based upon the data obtained at the time of the first course.

4. Validation of Visual Analog Scales for Measuring Nausea

As discussed in a previous section, there are several potential outcome measures for antiemetic studies. The most common is emesis. Its validity is somewhat self-evident, although the validity of self-reported emesis could be verified using an independent clinical observer. The validity of patient preference in crossover trials is also self-evident, although preference is a measure of treatment comparison with respect to all outcomes that affect patient perception including adverse effects. The validation of measures of nausea is also possible despite it not being an observable entity. Typically nausea is measured on a four- or five-point ordered categorical scale or using a visual analog scale (VAS).

The use of the VAS has been assessed as a valid measure of pain in several studies comprising of over 2000 patients.[78,79] Although commonly employed,[64,72,88-91] validation of its use as a measure of nausea is less extensive. Fetting et al.[72] investigated the reliability of the VAS for nausea in 18 patients, achieving a test-retest correlation of 0.83. They also studied the validity of the VAS for nausea and of the self-reporting of vomiting in 20 patients by making a comparison with the assessment with a single clinical observer. There were statistically significant associations between the patient self-reports and those of the clinical observer. The authors conclude that the "visual analog scale may provide information about nausea not obtained by the more frequently employed categorical verbal rating scales." In 28 patients, Kris et al.[74] observed high correlations between patient VAS ratings and an observer rating scale of delayed (post 24 h) nausea and vomiting, Pearson correlations ranged from 0.50 to 0.71. Melzack et al.[92] used the data from 25 patients undergoing cancer chemotherapy to examine the correlation coefficients between three measures of nausea: the Nausea Rating Index (NRI), a modification of the McGill Pain Questionnaire; the Overall Nausea Intensity (ONI), a five-point scale (0—no nausea, 1—mild, 2—discomforting, 3—distressing, 4—horrible, 5—excruciating); and, the 10-cm VAS. The strongest correlation between the ONI and VAS ($r = 0.75$, $p < 0.001$). There was also a strong correlation between VAS and the *affective* subset of the NRI ($r = 0.61$, $p < 0.001$). The patient scores on these three scales were also correlated with physician and nurse estimates of the nausea intensity of the chemotherapy regimens. The ONI and VAS were mostly highly correlated with these estimates ($r = 0.55$ to 0.63). Of all the scales VAS discriminated best between patients receiving cisplatin or 5-fluorouracil. The remainder of this section uses data from an antiemetic trial to illustrate the validation of the VAS for measuring nausea.

The study was a randomized, double-blind, cross-over trial, comparing the efficacy of methylprednisolone sodium succinate (MSS) and low-dose metoclopramide (MTC) in controlling the nausea and vomiting induced by a variety of moderately emetogenic chemotherapy regimens, and was a joint venture of the National Cancer Institute of Canada (NCIC) and the Upjohn Company of Canada. The therapeutic results of the study are reported elsewhere.[64] The study medications were administered intravenously immediately prior to each of the first two cycles of identical chemotherapy given 3 or 4 weeks apart. Supplemental antiemetic treatment with prochlorperazine was permitted, but the study medications were only to be administered once.

The major outcome of the trial was designed to be the patient's preference between the study medications as assessed 7 to 10 days after the second chemotherapy treatment. Patients were asked in a telephone interview to state which antiemetic they preferred overall, and which they preferred with respect to nausea and vomiting separately. Also, patients rated their nausea on a 100-mm horizontal VAS for each of the four 6-h intervals following chemotherapy. The VAS had the words *never* on the left-hand side and *constantly* on the right-hand side. Severity of nausea was measured as the number of mm from the left-hand side to where the patient had marked the scale. There were 115 evaluable patients for analysis, 70 females (61%) and 45 males (39%). The age range was 24 to 81 with a median of 62.

For both treatment periods the average of the four 6-hourly measurements on the VAS was calculated for each patient. The difference of the average score on MSS minus the average score on MTC was determined. If the VAS is valid we would expect patients who preferred MSS to have negative differences and patients who preferred MTC to have positive differences. The distribution of these treatment differences by patient preference with respect to nausea is displayed in Figure 1. Of the 57 patients who preferred MSS with respect to nausea, only 5 had positive differences. Similarly, only 5 of the 21 patients who preferred MTC with respect to nausea, 17 had negative differences and 12 positive. The average treatment difference of patients preferring MSS is -23.8, while the means for patients with no preference and for patients preferring MTC are -7.00 and 9.41, respectively. The means are significantly different at the 0.0001 level. The weight of this evidence leads us to conclude that the VAS for measuring nausea is valid because of its high association with patient preference.

Patient preference was used here as the standard by which to assess the validity of the VAS because modification of patient perception is the most important clinical objective in treating nausea and vomiting induced by chemotherapy, and thus the most relevant in treatment comparisons. Because nausea is a subjective experience, scales to measure it should be able to differentiate between experiences as expressed by patient preferences. The use of an independent clinical observer as a standard for validation for such a subjective measurement seems questionable at best. This argument for the use of patient preference as a standard by which to assess scales for nausea holds, of course, only in circumstances, such as in the above trial, where preference between treatments can only be influenced by their relative antiemetic effects. This method of validation would not apply, for example, when the treatments being studied have additional effects which might influence preference.

5. What Constitutes a Response?

Although results could be expressed solely in terms of means or medians, it is conventional to break the findings into categories that will give an idea of the percentage of patients

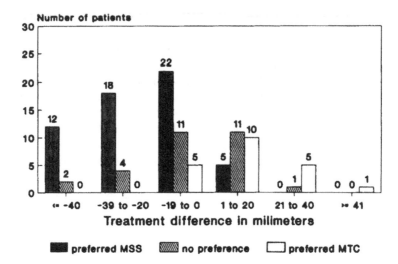

FIGURE 1.   Distribution of treatment differences by preference with respect to nausea.

for whom the antiemetic produced an acceptable result. To a large extent antiemetic studies have adopted the same terminology used for assessing antitumor response. A complete response may indicate the total absence of emesis or it may also mean that there has been no nausea or emesis. A partial or major emetic response most frequently means that there have been 2 or less episodes of vomiting[14,17,18,25,39,55] but alternative definitions exist.[5,29,42,69] The term minor response has been used to signify three to four[17] episodes but this is difficult to defend as a desirable response. We recommend that all investigators report the complete emetic response rate. For patients who receive cisplatin, the major response rate should be routinely reported with the latter defined as ≤two episodes of vomiting.

I. SAMPLE SIZE AND POWER

1. Introduction

Previous reviews have noted the small sample size of many antiemetic studies, and cautioned that this may lead to false negative conclusions.[6,7] As an example, there are eleven studies cited in this chapter which purport to show equivalence, and in only three instances was the sample size greater than 100 patients. In the two articles in which there was a statement about statistical power, the clinical difference that could be detected was an absolute difference in efficacy of 44% in one study[62] and 50% in the other.[19] The effectiveness of standard therapy for all types of chemotherapy is sufficiently great that a difference of this magnitude is unattainable. We recommend that all reports of randomized studies include information about the power of the study to detect specified differences in efficacy.

Parameter estimates from the cross-over trial used in the Validation section, and from two randomized, double-blind, parallel trials are used in this section to provide calculations of sample size requirements for antiemetic trials. The two parallel trials, which are yet to be reported, were joint ventures of the NCIC and Beecham Clinical Pharmacology (Canada). One was a comparison of Beecham's 5-HT$_3$ antagonist, granisetron (80 μg/kg, single dose i.v.), vs. high dose metoclopramide (2 mg/kg, i.v., every 2 h for five doses) plus dexamethasone (10 mg i.v. single dose) in patients receiving at least 50 mg/m^2 of cisplatin. The other was granisetron (80 μg/kg, single dose i.v.) vs. dexamethasone (10 mg single dose i.v.) plus prochlorperazine (10 mg single dose i.v.) in patients receiving moderately emetogenic chemotherapy (mainly doxorubicin and cyclophosphamide-containing regimens). In both trials patients scored their nausea on a VAS every 6 h for the first 24 h and every 24 h for the next 48 h. The scale was anchored on the left by *no nausea* and on the right by *extremely severe nausea*. They also reported the vomiting/retching on a five-point scale (none, 1 to 2 episodes, 3 to 5 episodes, 6 to 10 episodes, and 11 or more episodes) at the same time points. Each trial had approximately 150 evaluable patients.

The issue of which end-point should be used to determine the sample size arises. For cross-over trials the use of patient preference provides a measure which should encompass nausea, vomiting, and side effects, and therefore would seem the most appropriate. For parallel trials there appears to be some preference to base the sample size on comparing treatments with respect to proportion of patients vomiting. However for less emetogenic chemotherapy with very low rates of vomiting, treatment comparisons of nausea on VAS may be more sensitive.

2. Patient Preference

For a one-sided, level alpha test of significance to have a power of $1 - $ beta when the proportion of patients preferring one treatment to another is p, the sample size required is approximated by $(Z_{alpha} + Z_{beta})^2/[2(p - 0.5)]^2$ where Z_{alpha} and Z_{beta} are the upper normal cut-off points corresponding to a level of alpha and a power of $1 - $ beta, i.e., $Z_{0.05} = 1.65$ and $Z_{0.20} = 0.84$. Alpha should be halved for a two-sided test. From the literature,[64,88] whether there is a treatment difference or not, approximately 25% of patients have no preference, and are not included in the analysis. Consequently, the sample size from the above equation should be inflated by about 33%. An additional inflation factor should be used to account for dropouts between treatment courses. Twenty-five percent should be adequate to account for a dropout rate of 20%.[64] A trial which is designed to use one-sided test of significance at the 5% level and achieve an 80% power if patients have a 65% probability of preferring the study treatment over the standard (i.e., a 2:1 ratio) should, allowing for 25% no preference and a 20% dropout rate, enter 115 patients.

3. Vomiting

The proportion of patients reporting some vomiting in the first 24 h in the best arm is 50% for the high-dose cisplatin trial and 30% for the moderately emetogenic trial. Using these figures to provide a range of baseline rates for the control arm, and tables from Cassagrande et al.,[93] total sample sizes for various significant levels, power and treatment differences for parallel designs are displayed in Table 3. These are the same sample sizes one would use for comparing response rates in antineoplastic trials.

4. Nausea

Estimates of the standard deviations of the VAS for nausea from all three NCIC trials are 30 mm for each 6-h measurement and 20 mm for the average score over 24 h. (For the cross-over trial only the first period data was included). The sample size equation[94] $4(Z_{alpha} + Z_{beta})^2(s/d)^2$ can be used to calculate the total number of patients required for various significance levels (one-sided), power and treatment differences, where s is the appropriate standard deviation and d is the smallest clinically relevant difference. The mean of the average score of 24 h ranges between 10 and 20 mm depending on the emetogenicity of the chemotherapy regimen. It seems reasonable to choose d between 5 and 10 mm, since this represents a 25 to 50% difference between treatments.

5. Parallel vs. Cross-Over

The existence of validated scales for measuring nausea implies that the use of cross-over trials to generate preference data is no longer a necessity and that investigators are freer to choose between parallel or cross-over designs in antiemetic trials. The much cited reason for preferring cross-over designs is that because patients are used as their own control; there is no between-patient variability in the treatment comparison. This reduction in variance

TABLE 3
Total Sample Size Based on Vomiting, Parallel
Design, One-Sided Test

Reduction in rate in study arm	Rate of vomiting in the first 24 h in the control arm				
	0.20	0.30	0.40	0.50	0.60
0.10	346	498	604	642	642
	464	676	818	890	890
	428	622	750	808	808
	562	820	992	1066	1066
0.15	134	212	264	286	288
	178	284	356	400	404
	164	262	328	366	366
	212	344	432	484	488

Note: First figure: 5% level, 80% power. Second figure: 5% level, 90% power. Third figure: 2.5% level, 80% power. Fourth figure: 2.5% level, 90% power.

reduces the sample size required by the factor $(1 - rho)/2$, where rho, usually positive, is the intra-patient correlation coefficient. One would conclude then, that the cross-over design is more efficient in terms of the number of patients required and the time required to complete patient accrual. However, this conclusion fails to take into account the problems of residual carryover, patient dropouts between treatment periods and the requirement that cross-over trials be restricted to patients receiving two consecutive identical courses of chemotherapy.

Psychological carryover is often present in antiemetic cross-over trials, especially in those using previously untreated patients. This results because patients are conditioned by their experience in the first treatment period to have more nausea and vomiting in the second. Patients on the inferior antiemetic in the first treatment period will be conditioned to a greater extent than patients receiving the superior antiemetic first. The result is that the difference in efficacy between the two antiemetics is diminished during the second treatment period. This treatment by period interaction (residual carryover) reduces the power of the crossover design. The amount by which the treatment difference is diminished in the second period is referred to as the residual carryover, and is defined as the difference between treatments in the first period minus the difference between treatments in the second period. Using the average over intervals, the means of the VAS from the crossover trial referred to above[64] are presented by period and treatment in Figure 2. Residual carryover can be seen since the difference between antiemetics is considerably smaller during the second treatment period. In addition, patients who fail to enter the second treatment period cannot be used in the crossover analysis, further reducing the power.

A simple adjustment accounting for dropouts to the results found in Willan and Pater[95] yields the result that a cross-over design is more powerful (i.e., more likely to reject the null hypothesis when its false) than a parallel design with the same number of patients if, and only if, the residual carryover, expressed as a proportion of treatment effect, is less than

$$2 - \text{square root}\{2(1 - rho)/(1 - rate)\}$$

where *rate* is the between-treatment dropout rate. As *rho* increases and *rate* decreases, the relative power of the cross-over design increases.

In the cross-over trial[64] mentioned previously the dropout rate is 0.19. Using the average over intervals, *rho* is 0.45, and the residual carryover becomes 0.83. This carryover, ex-

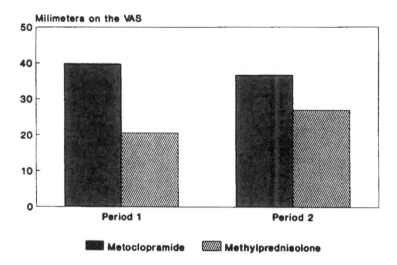

FIGURE 2. Average nausea by treatment and period.

pressed as a proportion of treatment effect, is 0.51. Thus we can conclude we have evidence that our choice of a cross-over design is justified. Readers may find it surprising that even though the residual carryover was sufficient to reduce the difference in antiemetics in the second treatment period by 51% and the dropout rate was 19%, the cross-over design provides more statistical power. In fact, even with a 19% dropout rate, residual carryover has to be sufficient to reduce the difference in antiemetics in the second treatment period by more than 80% before the parallel design is more powerful.

Although the above investigation implies that, in spite of the presence of residual carryover and dropouts, a cross-over trial may require fewer patients, it is possible that the corresponding parallel trial, which in fact needs more patients, could have a shorter accrual time. Many chemotherapy patients are on alternating regimens or are taking other treatments (steroids, radiotherapy) between chemotherapy cycles and would not ordinarily be eligible for cross-over trials. The inclusion of these patients in antiemetic trials in a parallel design may well shorten accrual time and would broaden the range of chemotherapy regimens included and strengthen the generalizability of the results. Furthermore, parallel designs allow investigators to compare antiemetics over several courses of chemotherapy, thereby permitting an examination of whether treatment differences diminish or increase in subsequent courses of chemotherapy. Another argument against cross-over designs is that the U.S. Food and Drug Administration[96] discredits the evidence they provide. For all the same reasons multiperiod cross-overs should be avoided, since the problems of dropouts and conditioning would be further compounded.

J. STATISTICAL ANALYSIS
1. Vomiting
a. Parallel Designs
Many investigators are interested in comparing treatment groups for statistical significance with respect to the proportion of patients who vomit within a certain period of time from chemotherapy, usually 24 h, but more frequently with more emetogenic chemotherapy, 48 or 72 h. This is achieved easily using a Fisher exact test[97] or for larger treatment groups (25 patients or more) with contingency chi-square for 2 by 2 tables.[97] Treatment comparisons should be controlled for discrete prognostic factors using the Mantel-Haenszel[98] procedure and for both continuous and discrete prognostic factors using logistic regression.[99] Logistic regression for prognostic factor adjustment should be considered valid for larger treatment groups only, perhaps as many as 50 patients per treatment group.

b. Cross-Over Designs

Treatment comparison for statistical significance in cross-over designs with respect to proportions can be done with an application of the common McNemar chi-square test.[100] If A is the number of patients who vomit on treatment 1 but not on treatment 2, and B the number of patients who vomit on treatment 2 but not on treatment 1, then the McNemar test statistic is $(A - B)^2/(A + B)$. In the absence of a treatment effect this test statistic is distributed as a one degree of free chi-square. This test is considered valid only if $A + B$ is 25 or more. For smaller values of $A + B$ a continuity correction can be applied, $(|A - B| - 1)^2/(A + B)$, or an exact binomial test can be used.[97] Since treatment comparisons are made within patients for the cross-over design, prognostic factor adjustment is not ordinarily an issue.

2. Nausea Measured on a VAS

a. Parallel Designs

Comparing treatment groups for statistical significance with respect to mean nausea can be done using a simple two-sample t-test. Adjustment for prognostic factors can be provided using the analysis of covariance. Skewness is often present in observations taken on a VAS. It is advisable to examine the data for skewness, and if necessary take the natural logarithm or the square root of each observation prior to performing tests of significance.

b. Cross-Over Designs

Treatment comparison for statistical significance in cross-over designs with respect to means, in the absence of period and residual carryover effect, is performed using a paired t-test. Unfortunately, a period effect is almost always present, since patients tend to have more nausea during the second treatment period, having been conditioned from their experience in the first. A valid test for treatment effect, in the presence of a period effect, requires what amounts to a simple adjustment of the paired t-test.[95] A more difficult problem arises when the treatment difference diminishes the second treatment period due to conditioning (see Section III.I). Since this treatment by period interaction (residual carryover) can only occur when the treatments differ, a valid test using data from both treatment periods can be performed.[101] Two significance levels are calculated; one using the parallel design analysis on the first period data and the other using the cross-over analysis of both periods of data. The null hypothesis is rejected if the smaller of these is less than some significance level cut-off which is adjusted to account for the multiplicity (having taken the smaller of to significance levels) to maintain the nominal level. The adjusted significance level cut-off depends on the value of rho, the intrapatient correlation coefficient, but is fairly insensitive for values in the 0.4 to 0.6 range observed in cross-over trials.[64-68] For values of rho in this range, the adjusted significance level cut-off for a nominal level of 0.05 is 0.028, for a nominal level of 0.025, 0.014, and for a nominal level of 0.01, 0.0053. It is conceivable that residual carryover could occur for reasons other than conditioning. If the time between treatment periods is short compared to treatment half-lives, one treatment may still be active in the second period, adding to the efficacy of the second treatment. This type of residual carryover invalidates the crossover design. Consequently, cross-over trials should be avoided unless treatment half-lives are considerably shorter than the time between treatment periods. As discussed in the previous section, transformation may be required to remove skewness.

c. Repeated Measurements

In the NCIC trials, patients were asked to score the VAS for nausea every 6 h for the first 24 h and, in parallel design trials, every 24 h for the next 48 h. The primary nausea outcome in parallel trials was the average of the first four scores, partly because of simplicity and partly because the average exhibited far less skewness. In addition, the reason patients were asked to score every 6 h was not so much because of an interest in the time profile but because of a desire to record the patients experience while it is most fresh in their minds. Nonetheless, repeated measures analysis of variance[102] can be performed on the individual scores which provide for a possible increase in power and allows for an examination of whether treatment differences diminish or increase over time. Such observations may be crucial to understanding the need for redosing.

IV. CONCLUSIONS

In this chapter, the current status of antiemetic study methodology has been reviewed. Although there are some unique challenges in the design and execution of these studies, the underlying principles should be familiar to those who have participated in phase I—III studies in other fields. There are valid ways of assessing even *soft* outcomes such as nausea or indeed using this end-point as a means of determining sample size.

The ability to determine the most effective treatments and the subgroups most benefitted by them will require even larger controlled studies than has been generally the case in the past when standard therapy was less effective than it is now.

REFERENCES

1. **Coates, A., Fischer-Dillenbeck, C., McNeil, D. R., Kaye, S. B., Sims, K., Fox, R. M., Woods, R. C., Milton, G. W., Solomons, J., and Tattersall, M. H. N.**, On the receiving end. II. Linear analogue self-assessment (LASA) in evaluation of the quality of life of cancer patients receiving therapy, *Eur. J. Cancer Clin. Oncol.*, 19, 1633, 1983.
2. **Palmer, B. V., Walsh, G. A., McKinna, J. A., and Greening, W. P.**, Adjuvant chemotherapy for breast cancer: side effects and quality of life, *Br. J. Med.*, 281, 1594, 1980.
3. **Gralla, R. J., Itri, L. M., Pisko, S. E., Squillante, A. E., Kelsen, D. P., Braun, D. W., Jr., Borden, L. A., Braun, T. J., and Young, C. W.**, Antiemetic efficacy of high-dose metoclopramide: randomized trials with placebo and prochlorperazine in patients with chemotherapy-induced nausea and vomiting, *N. Engl. J. Med.*, 305, 905, 1981.
4. **Cassileth, P. A., Lusk, E. J., Torri, S., DiNubile, N., and Gerson, S. L.**, Antiemetic efficacy of dexamethasone therapy in patients receiving cancer chemotherapy, *Arch. Intern. Med.*, 143, 1347, 1983.
5. **Markman, M., Sheidler, V., Ettinger, D. S., Quaskey, S. A., and Mellits, E. D.**, Antiemetic efficacy of dexamethasone. Randomized, double-blind, crossover study with prochlorperazine in patients receiving cancer chemotherapy, *N. Engl. J. Med.*, 311, 549, 1984.
6. **Pater, J. L. and Willan, A. R.**, Methodologic issues in trials of antiemetics, *J. Clin. Oncol.*, 2, 1984.
7. **Olver, N., Simon, R. M., and Aisner, J.**, Antiemetic studies: a methodological discussion, *Cancer Treat. Rep.*, 70, 555, 1986.
8. **Carey, M. P., Burish, T. G., and Brenner, D. E.**, Delta-9-tetrahydrocannabinol in cancer chemotherapy: research problems and issues, *Ann. Intern. Med.*, 99, 106, 1983.
9. **Moertel, C. G. and Reitemeier, R. J.**, Controlled clinical studies of orally administered antiemetic drugs, *Gastroenterology*, 57, 262, 1969.
10. **Simon, R. M.**, Design and conduct of clinical trials, in *Cancer: Principles and Practice of Oncology*, Vol. 1, 3rd ed., De Vita, V. T., Hellman, S., and Rosenberg, S., Eds., J. B. Lippincott, Philadelphia, 1989, 396.
11. **Gralla, R. J.**, Nausea and vomiting, in *Cancer: Principles and Practice of Oncology*, Vol. 2, 3rd ed., De Vita, V. T., Hellman, S., and Rosenberg, S., Eds., J. B. Lippincott, Philadelphia, 1989, 2137.
12. **Estey, E., Hoth, D., Simon, R., Marsoni, S., Leyland-Jones, B., and Wittes, R.**, Therapeutic response in phase I trials of antineoplastic agents, *Cancer Treat. Rep.*, 70, 1105, 1986.
13. **Gralla, R. J., Braun, T. J., Squillante, A., Steele, N., Kelsen, D. P., and Young, C. W.**, Metoclopramide, in *The Treatment of Nausea and Vomiting Induced by Cancer Chemotherapy*, Poster, D., Ed., Masson, New York, 1981, 167.
14. **Grunberg, S. M., Stevenson, L. L., Russell, C. A., and McDermed, J. E.**, Dose ranging phase I study of the serotonin antagonist GR38032F for prevention of cisplatin-induced nausea and vomiting, *J. Clin. Oncol.*, 7, 1137, 1989.

15. Tyson, L. R., Gralla, R. J., Kris, M. G., and Clark, R. A., Phase I antiemetic study of the serotonin antagonist ICS 205-930, *Proc. Am. Soc. Clin. Oncol.*, 8, 331, 1989.

16. Sartiano, G. P., Early, W., Early, J., Fairchild, C. J., Crenshaw, R. R., and Schwartz, S. E., BMY-25801-01: a non-antidopaminergic agent to prevent cisplatin-induced nausea and vomiting, *Proc. Am. Soc. Clin. Oncol.*, 6, 272, 1987.

17. Strum, S. B., McDermed, J. E., and Liponi, D. F., High-dose intravenous metoclopramide versus combination high-dose metoclopramide and intravenous dexamethasone in preventing cisplatin-induced nausea and emesis: a single-blind crossover comparison of antiemetic efficacy, *J. Clin. Oncol.*, 3, 245, 1985.

18. Strum, S. B., McDermed, J. E., Streng, B. R., and McDermott, N. M., Combination metoclopramide and dexamethasone: an effective antiemetic regimen in outpatients receiving non-cisplatin chemotherapy, *J. Clin. Oncol.*, 2, 1057, 1984.

19. Dana, B. W., McDermott, M., Everts, E., and Abdulhay, G., A randomized trial of high dose metoclopramide versus low dose continuous infusion metoclopramide in the prevention of cisplatin-induced emesis, *Am. J. Clin. Oncol.*, 10, 253, 1987.

20. Onsrud, M., Moxnes, A., Sollien, A., Grande, T., and Solesvik, O., High-dose versus low-dose metoclopramide in the prevention of cisplatin-induced emesis. A randomized crossover study in patients with ovarian cancer, *Cancer*, 61, 2429, 1988.

21. Presant, C. A., Wiseman, C., Gala, K., Kennedy, P., Bouzaglou, A., Blayney, D., Schindler, J., Rigas, M., Melville, J., Dolan, J., and Jund, L., Antiemetic effects of metoclopramide (m) continuous infusion (ci): safety, efficacy, patient preference, and cost reduction, in *Advances in Cancer Control: The War on Cancer — 15 Years of Progress*, Engstrom, P., Mortensen, L., and Anderson, P., Eds., Alan R. Liss, New York, 1987, 299.

22. Hesketh, P. J., Murphy, W. K., Lester, E. P., Gandara, D. R., Khojasteh, A., Tapazoglou, E., Sartiano, G. P., White, D. R., Werner, K., and Chubb, J. M., GR 38032F (GR-C507/75): a novel compound effective in the prevention of acute cisplatin-induced emesis, *J. Clin. Oncol.*, 7, 700, 1989.

23. Abad-Esteve, A., Rosell, R., Moreno, I., Serichol, M., Moya, L., and Ribas-Mundo, M., Antiemetic efficacy of escalating doses of alizapride against chemotherapy-induced emesis, *Oncology*, 46, 235, 1989.

24. Kris, M. G., Gralla, R. J., Clark, R. A., Tyson, L., and Groshen, S., Antiemetic control and prevention of side-effects of anticancer therapy with lorazepam or diphenhydramine when used in combination with metoclopramide plus dexamethasone: a double-blind, randomized trial, *Cancer*, 60, 2816, 1987.

25. Kris, M. G., Gralla, R. J., Tyson, L. B., Clark, R. A., Kelsen, D. P., Reilly, L. D., Groshen, S., Bosl, G. J., and Kalman, L. A., Improved control of cisplatin-induced emesis with high-dose metoclopramide and combinations of metoclopramide, dexamethasone, and diphenhydramine: results of consecutive trials in 255 patients, *Cancer*, 55, 527, 1985.

26. Kahn, T., Elias, E. G., and Mason, G. R., A single dose of metoclopramide in the control of vomiting from cis-dichlorodiammineplatinum (II) in man, *Cancer Treat. Rep.*, 62, 1106, 1978.

27. D'Olimpio, J. T., Camacho, F., Chandra, P., Lesser, M., Maldonado, M., Wollner, D., and Wiernik, P. H., Antiemetic efficacy of high-dose dexamethasone versus placebo in patients receiving cisplatin-based chemotherapy: a randomized, double-blind controlled clinical trial, *J. Clin. Oncol.*, 3, 1133, 1985.

28. Sallan, S. E., Cronin, C., Zelen, M., and Zinberg, N. E., Antiemetics in patients receiving chemotherapy for cancer. A randomized comparison of delta-9-tetrahydrocannabinol and prochlorperazine, *N. Engl. J. Med.*, 302, 135, 1980.

29. Pollera, C. F. and Giannarelli, D., Prognostic factors influencing cisplatin-induced emesis. Definition and validation of a predictive logistic model, *Cancer*, 64, 1117, 1989.

30. Roila, F., Tonato, M., Basurto, C., Picciafuoco, M., Bracarda, S., Donati, D., Malacarne, P., Monici, L., Di Costanzo, F., Patoia, L., Ballatori, E., Tognoni, G., and Del Favero, A., Protection from nausea and vomiting in cisplatin-treated patients: high-dose metoclopramide combined with methylprednisolone versus metoclopramide combined with dexamethasone and diphenhydramine: a study of the Italian Oncology Group for Clinical Research, *J. Clin. Oncol.*, 7, 1693, 1989.

31. Ungerleider, J. T., Andrysiak, T., Fairbanks, L., Goodnight, J., Sarna, G., and Jamison, K., Cannabis and cancer chemotherapy: a comparison of oral delta-9-THC and proclorperazine, *Cancer*, 50, 636, 1982.

32. Triplett, W. C., Schroeder, J. E., Minnick, D. J., Dugan, W. M., and Berry, J. A., Reliability of videotape technology in assessing the efficacy of anti-emetic drugs, *Advances in Cancer Control: Health Care Financing and Research*, 1986, 377.

33. Zeltzer, L., LeBaron, S., and Zeltzer, P. M., The effectiveness of behavioral intervention for reduction of nausea and vomiting in children and adolescents receiving chemotherapy, *J. Clin. Oncol.*, 2, 683, 1984.

34. Lyles, J. N., Burish, T. G., Krozely, M. G., and Oldham, R. K., Efficacy of relaxation training and guided imagery in reducing the aversiveness of cancer chemotherapy, *J. Consult. Clin. Psychol.*, 50, 509, 1982.

247

35. Frytak, S., Moertel, C. G., O'Fallon, J. R., Rubin, J., Creagan, E. T., O'Connell, M. J., Schutt, A. J., and Schwartau, N. W., Delta-9-tetrahydrocannabinol as an antiemetic for patients receiving cancer chemotherapy. A comparison with prochlorperazine and placebo, *Ann. Intern. Med.*, 91, 825, 1979.

36. Kearsley, J. H., Williams, A. M., and Fiumara, A., Antiemetic superiority of lorazepam over oxazepam and methylprednisolone as premedicants for patients receiving cisplatin-containing chemotherapy, *Cancer*, 64, 1595, 1989.

37. de Mulder, P. H. M., Seynaeve, C., Van Liessum, P. A., Verweij, J., Vermorken, J., and Lane-Allman, E., A multicentre double blind comparison of ondansetron (GR38032F) and metoclopramide in the prophylaxis of acute emesis induced by cisplatin, presented at ECCO 5, London, September 3, 1989 (#0-0501).

38. Lucot, J. B., Blockade of 5-hydroxytryptamine3 receptors prevents cisplatin-induced but not motion- or xylazine-induced emesis in the cat, *Pharmacol. Biochem. Behav.*, 32, 207, 1989.

39. Roila, F., Tonato, M., Basurto, C., Bella, M., Passalacqua, R., Morsia, D., DiCostanzo, F., Donati, D., Ballatori, E., Tognoni, G., Franzosi, M. G., and Del Favero, A., Antiemetic activity of high doses of metoclopramide combined with methylprednisolone versus metoclopramide alone in cisplatin-treated cancer patients: a randomized double-blind trial of the Italian Oncology Group for Clinical Research, *J. Clin. Oncol.*, 5, 141, 1987.

40. Laszlo, J., Clark, R. A., Hanson, D. C., Tyson, L., Crumpler, L., and Gralla, R., Lorazepam in cancer patients treated with cisplatin: a drug having antiemetic, amnesic and anxiolytic effects, *J. Clin. Oncol.*, 3, 864, 1985.

41. Morran, C., Smith, D. C., Anderson, D. A., and McArdle, C. S., Incidence of nausea and vomiting with cytotoxic chemotherapy: a prospective randomized trial of antiemetics, *Br. Med. J.*, 1, 1324, 1979.

42. Parikh, P. M., Charak, B. S., Banavali, S. D., Koppikar, S. B., Giri, N., Nadkarni, P., Saikia, T. K., Gopal, R., and Advani, S. H., A prospective, randomized double-blind trial comparing metoclopramide alone with metoclopramide plus dexamethasone in preventing emesis induced by high-dose cisplatin, *Cancer*, 62, 2263, 1988.

43. D'Acquisto, R. W., Tyson, L. B., Gralla, R. J., Clark, R. A., Kris, M. G., and von Witte, D. M., The influence of a chronic high alcohol intake on chemotherapy-induced nausea and vomiting, *Proc. Am. Soc. Clin. Oncol.*, 5, 257, 1986.

44. Sullivan, J. R., Leyden, M. J., and Bell, R., Decreased cisplatin induced nausea and vomiting with alcohol ingestion, *N. Engl. J. Med.*, 309, 796, 1983.

45. Morrow, G. R., The effect of a susceptibility to motion sickness on the side effects of cancer chemotherapy, *Cancer*, 55, 2766, 1985.

46. Sridhar, K. S. and Donnelly, E., Combination antiemetics for cisplatin chemotherapy, *Cancer*, 61, 1508, 1988.

47. Kris, M. G., Gralla, R. J., and Allen, J. C., Extrapyramidal reactions with high dose metoclopramide, *N. Engl. J. Med.*, 309, 433, 1983.

48. Grunberg, S. M., Aler, E., McDremed, J. E., and Akerley, W. L., Oral metoclopramide with or without diphenhydramine: potential for prevention of late nausea and vomiting induced cisplatin, *J. Natl. Cancer Inst.*, 80, 864, 1988.

49. Ell, Ch., Konig, H. J., Brockmann, P., Domschke, S., and Domschke, W., Antiemetic efficacy of moderately high-dose metoclopramide in patients receiving varying doses of cisplatin, *Oncology*, 42, 354, 1985.

50. Jordan, N. S., Schauer, P. K., Schauer, A., Nightingale, C., Golub, G., Martin, R. S., and Williams, H. M., The effect of administration rate on cisplatin-induced emesis, *J. Clin. Oncol.*, 3, 559, 1985.

51. Hrushesky, W., Vukelich, M., Halberg, F., Levi, F., Langevin, T., Kennedy, B. J., Gergen, J., Goetz, F., and Theologides, A., Optimal circadian treatment time reduces cis-diamminedichloroplatinum-induced vomiting, *Int. J. Chronobiol.*, 64, 257, 1981.

52. Frustaci, S., Grattoni, E., Tumolo, S., Crivellari, D., Figoli, F., Galligioni, E., Veronesi, A., Tirelli, U., and Grigoletto, E., Randomized crossover antiemetic study in cisplatin-treated patients, *Cancer Chemother. Pharmacol.*, 17, 75, 1986.

53. Benjamin, R. S., Chawla, S. P., Hortobagyi, G. N., Ewer, M. S., Mackay, B., Legha, S. S., Carrasco, C. H., and Wallace, S., Continuous infusion adriamycin, in *Clinical Applications of Continuous-Infusion Chemotherapy and Concomitant Radiation Therapy*, Rosenthal, C. I. and Rotman, M., Eds., Plenum Press, New York, 1986, 19.

54. Siegel, L. S. and Longo, D. L., The control of chemotherapy-induced emesis, *Ann. Intern. Med.*, 95, 352, 1981.

55. Gralla, R. J., Tyson, L. B., Bordin, L. A., Clark, R. A., Kelsen, D. P., Dris, M. G., Kalman, L. B., and Groshen, S., Antiemetic therapy: a review of recent studies and report of a random assignment trial comparing metoclopramide with delta-9-tetrahydrocannabinol, *Cancer Treat. Rep.*, 68, 163, 1984.

56. Dana, B. W., Everts, E. C., and Dickinson, D., Dexamethasone vs. placebo for cisplatin-induced emesis. A randomized cross-over trial, *Am. J. Clin. Oncol.*, 8, 426, 1985.

57. Carr, B. I., Bertrand, M., Browning, S., Doroshow, J. H., Presant, C., Pulone, B., and Hill, L. R., A comparison of the antiemetic efficacy of prochlorperazine and metoclopramide for the treatment of cisplatin-induced emesis: a prospective, randomized, double-blind study, *J. Clin. Oncol.*, 3, 1127, 1985.

58. Chiara, S., Campora, E., Lionetto, R., Bruzzi, P., and Rosso, R., Methylprednisolone for the control of CMF-induced emesis, *Am. J. Clin. Oncol.*, 10, 264, 1987.

59. Drapkin, R., McAloon, E., Sokol, G., Paladine, W., and Marks, R., The antiemetic effect of dexamethasone in patients receiving cis-platinum, *Proc. Am. Assoc. Cancer Res./Am. Soc. Clin. Oncol.*, 22, 419, 1981.

60. Taylor, W. B., Simpson, J. M., and Bateman, D. N., High dose metoclopramide by infusion: a double-blind study of plasma concentration-effect relationships in patients receiving cancer chemotherapy, *Eur. J. Clin. Pharmacol.*, 33, 161, 1987.

61. Warrington, P. S., Allan, S. G., Cornbleet, M. A., MacPherson, J. S., Smyth, J. F., and Leonard, R. C. F., Optimizing antiemesis in cancer chemotherapy: efficacy of continuous versus intermittent infusion of high dose metoclopramide in emesis induced by cisplatin, *Br. Med. J.*, 293, 1334, 1986.

62. Agostinucci, W. A., Gannon, R. H., Golub, G. R., Martin, R. S., Schauer, P. K., and Dinonno, E. B., Continuous i.v. infusion versus multiple bolus doses of metoclopramide for prevention of cisplatin-induced emesis, *Clin. Pharm.*, 7, 454, 1988.

63. Clark, R. A., Gralla, R. J., Kris, M. G., and Tyson, L. B., Exploring very high doses of metoclopramide (4—6 mg/kg): preservation of efficacy and safety with only a single dose in a combination antiemetic regimen, *Proc. Am. Soc. Clin. Oncol.*, 8, 330, 1989.

64. Osoba, D., Erlichman, C., Willan, A. R., Levitt, M., and Pater, J. L., Superiority of methylprednisolone sodium succinate over low dose metoclopramide hydrochloride in the prevention of nausea and vomiting produced by cancer chemotherapy, *Clin. Invest. Med.*, 9, 225, 1986.

65. Kris, M. G., Gralla, R. J., Tyson, L. B., Clark, R. A., Cirrincione, C., and Groshen, S., Controlling delayed vomiting: double-blind, randomized trial comparing placebo, dexamethasone alone, and metoclopramide plus dexamethasone in patients receiving cisplatin, *J. Clin. Oncol.*, 7, 108, 1989.

66. Williams, C. J., Davies, C., Raval, M., Middleton, J., Luken, J., and Stone, B., Comparison of starting antiemetic treatment 24 hours before or concurrently with cytotoxic chemotherapy, *Br. Med. J.*, 298, 430, 1989.

67. Tyson, L., Gralla, R. J., Clark, R. A., Kris, M. G., Bosl, G. J., Reich, L. M., and Young, C. W., High dose oral metoclopramide: dose-finding, efficacy, and preliminary pharmacokinetic evaluation, *Proc. Am. Soc. Med. Oncol.*, 3, 102, 1984.

68. Cunningham, D., Evans, C., Gazet, J., Ford, H., Pople, A., Dearling, J., Chappell, D., and Coombes, C., Comparison of antiemetic efficacy of domperidone, metoclopramide, and dexamethasone in patients receiving outpatient chemotherapy regimens, *Br. Med. J.*, 295, 250, 1987.

69. Pollera, C. F. and Calabresi, F., Effective control of moderate-dose cisplatin by a short-course regimen including metoclopramide, chlorpromazine and hydrocortisone: results of a randomized trial with metoclopramide alone, *Oncology*, 46, 238, 1989.

70. Borison, H. L. and McCarthy, L. E., Neuropharmacology of chemotherapy-induced emesis, *Drugs*, 25, 8, 1983.

71. Allan, S. G., Cornbleet, M. A., Warrington, P. S., Gollard, I. M., Leonard, R. C. F., and Smyth, J. F., Dexamethasone and high-dose metoclopramide: efficacy in controlling cisplatin induced nausea and vomiting, *Br. J. Med.*, 289, 878, 1984.

72. Fetting, J. H., Grochow, L. B., Folstein, M. F., Ettinger, D. S., and Calvin, M., The course of nausea and vomiting after high-dose cyclophosphamide, *Cancer Treat. Rep.*, 66, 1487, 1982.

73. Rhinehart, S. N., Dugan, W. M., Parashos, P. J., Triplett, W. C., Minnick, D. J., and Fry, M. W., The value of dexamethasone when added to combination drug therapy in the prevention of cisplatin-induced nausea and vomiting, evaluated by time-lapse video technology, in *Progress in Clinical and Biological Research*, Vol. 216, Alan R. Liss, New York, 1986, 407.

74. Kris, M. G., Gralla, R. J., Clark, R. A., Tyson, L. B., O'Connell, J. P., Wertheim, M. S., and Kelsen, D. P., Incidence, course, and severity of delayed onset nausea and vomiting following the administration of high-dose cisplatin, *J. Clin. Oncol.*, 3, 1379, 1985.

75. Morrow, G. R., The assessment of nausea and vomiting. Past problems, current issues, and suggestions for future research, *Cancer*, 53, 2267, 1984.

76. Chang, A. E., Shiling, D. J., Stillman, R. C., Goldberg, N. H., Seipp, C. A., Barofsky, I., Simon, R. M., and Rosenberg, S. A., Delta-9-tetrahydrocannabinol as an antiemetic in cancer patients receiving high-dose methotrexate: a prospective, randomized evaluation, *Ann. Intern. Med.*, 91, 819, 1979.

77. Cognetti, F., Carlini, P., Pinnaro, P., Ruggeri, E. M., and Caporali, C., Maintenance of antiemetic effect of a metoclopramide-dexamethasone combination during subsequent cisplatin courses, *Oncology*, 43, 292, 1986.

78. Joyce, C. R. B., Zutshi, D. W., Hrubes, V., and Mason, R. M., Comparison of fixed interval and visual analogue scales for rating chronic pain, *Eur. J. Clin. Pharmacol.*, 8, 415, 1975.

79. Elton, D., Burrows, G. D., and Stanley, G. V., Clinical measure of pain, *Med. J. Aust.*, 1, 109, 1979.
80. Kremer, E., Atkinson, J. H., and Ignelzi, R. J., Measurement of pain: patient preference does not confound pain measurement, *Pain*, 10, 241, 1981.
81. Woodforde, J. M. and Merskey, H., Some relationships between subjective measures of pain, *J. Psychosom. Res.*, 16, 173, 1972.
82. Scott, J. and Huskisson, E. C., Graphic representation of pain, *Pain*, 2, 175, 1976.
83. Downie, W. W., Leatham, P. A., Rhind, V. M., Wright, V., Branco, J. A., and Anderson, J. A., Studies with pain rating scales, *Ann. Rheum. Dis.*, 37, 378, 1978.
84. Carlsson, A. M., Assessment of chronic pain. I. Aspects of the reliability and validity of the visual analogue scale, *Pain*, 16, 87, 1983.
85. Sriwatanakel, K., Kelvie, W., Lasagna, L., Calimlim, J. K., Weis, O. F., and Mehta, G., Studies with different types of visual analog scales for measurement of pain, *Clin. Pharmacol. Ther.*, 34, 234, 1983.
86. Ohnhaus, E. E. and Adler, R., Methodologic problems in the measurement of pain: a comparison between verbal rating scales and the visual analogue scale, *Pain*, 1, 379, 1975.
87. Littman, G. S., Walker, B. R., and Schneider, B. E., Reassessment of verbal and visual analog ratings in analgesic studies, *Clin. Pharmacol. Ther.*, 38, 16, 1985.
88. Osoba, D., Erlichman, C., Willan, A. R., Brigden, M. L., Geggie, P., Pater, J. L., Rusthoven, J. J., and Wilson, K. S., Failure of methylprednisolone acetate to prolong the antinauseant effect of intravenous methylprednisolone sodium succinate in patients receiving chemotherapy, *Clin. Invest. Med.*, 11, 377, 1988.
89. Hurley, J. D. and Eshelman, F. N., Trimethobenzamide HCL in the treatment of nausea and vomiting associated with antineoplastic chemotherapy, *J. Clin. Pharmacol.*, 21, 86S, 1980.
90. Kaan, S. K. and Eshelman, F. N., The antiemetic effects of Trimethobenzamide during chemotherapy: a controlled trial, *Curr. Ther. Res.*, 26, 210, 1979.
91. Redd, W. H., Andresen, G. V., and Minagawa, R. Y., Hypnotic control of anticipatory emesis in patients receiving cancer chemotherapy, *J. Consult. Clin. Psychol.*, 50, 14, 1982.
92. Melzack, R., Rosberger, Z., Hollingsworth, M. L., and Thirlwell, M., New approaches to measuring nausea, *Can. Med. Assoc. J.*, 133, 755, 1985.
93. Cassagrande, J. T., Pike, M. C., and Smith, P. G., The power function of the "exact" test for comparing two binomial distributions, *Appl. Stat.*, 27, 176, 1978.
94. Lachin, J. M., Introduction to sample size determination and power analysis for clinical trials, *Controlled Clin. Trials*, 2, 93, 1981.
95. Willan, A. R. and Pater, J. L., Carryover and the two-period crossover clinical trial, *Biometrics*, 42, 593, 1986.
96. O'Neill, R. T. and Cornfield, J., A report on the two-period crossover design and its applicability in trials of clinical effectiveness, Biometric and Epidemiological Methodology Advisory Committee, Bureau of Drugs, U. S. Food and Drug Administration, Washington, D.C., 1977.
97. Siegel, S., *Nonparametric Statistics for the Behavioral Sciences*, McGraw-Hill, New York, 1956.
98. Mantel, N. and Haenszel, W., Statistical aspects of the analysis of data from retrospective studies of disease, *J. Natl. Cancer Inst.*, 22, 719, 1959.
99. Cox, D. R., *Analysis of Binary Data*, Chapman and Hall, London, 1970.
100. McNemar, Q., Note on the sampling error of the differences between correlated proportions or percentages, *Psychometrika*, 12, 153, 1947.
101. Willan, A. R., Using the maximum test statistic in the two period crossover clinical trial, *Biometrics*, 44, 211, 1988.
102. Winer, B. J., *Statistical Principles in Experimental Design*, 2nd ed., McGraw-Hill, New York, 1971.

Chapter 18

ANTICIPATORY NAUSEA AND VOMITING SIDE EFFECTS EXPERIENCED BY CANCER PATIENTS UNDERGOING CHEMOTHERAPY TREATMENT

Gary R. Morrow and Peter M. Black

TABLE OF CONTENTS

I. INTRODUCTION

The most common side effects of cancer treatment by chemotherapy are nausea and vomiting. Cancer patients may develop as much apprehension and dread about treatment, and the side effects of treatment, as they do about their disease. If not adequately controlled, these side effects can lead to further complications such as anorexia and metabolite imbalance, along with contributing to a general deterioration of the cancer patient's psychological and physical condition. Many cancer patients treated with chemotherapy drugs request dosage reductions or even stop potentially curative treatment prematurely due to inadequately controlled nausea and vomiting.[1,2] The impact of inadequately controlled nausea/vomiting on patient's quality of life is substantial.

In addition to becoming nauseous and/or vomiting following chemotherapy treatment, cancer patients can begin to experience these aversive side effects *prior to* a treatment session.[3-5] This is referred to as anticipatory nausea and vomiting (ANV). It is a side effect that appears to link psychological, neurological, and physiological systems and may provide an unusual opportunity to study the natural occurrence of what appears to be a form of aversive learning in humans.[6] This chapter examines the prevalence, etiology, and treatment of anticipatory nausea and vomiting. The principal models of treatment presented are behavioral; there are recent reviews of pharmacologic treatment of posttreatment nausea/vomiting.[7]

II. PREVALENCE OF ANTICIPATORY NAUSEA AND VOMITING

The prevalence of anticipatory nausea and vomiting in adult and pediatric cancer chemotherapy patients has been reported in a number of studies (summarized in Table 1). On the lower end of estimates, 18% of 71 patients examined by Nicholas[8] reported anticipatory side effects while Cella et al.[9] reported that over half of 60 patients previously treated for Hodgkin's Disease developed ANV.

Several factors have been proposed to account for variation in prevalence rates.[4,7,10,12-14] These reviews develop one or more of the following explanations for differences in prevalence rates of anticipatory nausea. (1) Nausea and vomiting side effects occur *during* chemotherapy treatment with some drugs. While this may represent anticipatory phenomenon it is more likely a largely physiological response. (2) Some researchers have studied anticipatory nausea and vomiting symptoms independently of each other, whereas other researchers combined them and viewed the symptoms as one phenomenon. (3) Prevalence rates may be influenced by the type of chemotherapy drugs administered to cancer patients since posttreatment side effects vary across different treatment regimens. (4) The time frame in which ANV symptoms were studied has differed across studies. For example, Morrow et al.[4] assessed patients prior to their fourth chemotherapy cycle whereas Wilcox et al.[15] did so prior to the tenth chemotherapy cycle. (5) A portion of the variation in prevalence rates may be due to different measurement methodology. A variety of self-report measures have been used to assess ANV across studies.[13] Some studies involved interviewing patients by asking retrospective questions[16] whereas others used patient-completed logs during and following treatment.[6]

As a means of approximating how much variation in prevalence rates may be due to the factors mentioned above, data from a series of consecutive chemotherapy patients of ours[17] can be compared with the rates cited in Table 1. By aggregating the data from Table 1, it appears that the overall prevalence rate of anticipatory nausea is about 33%. From our data, collected on 1480 patients from a single cancer center, assessed with the same scale (Morrow Assessment of Nausea and Emesis), at a standard time (prior to the fourth chemotherapy cycle), it appears that the overall prevalence rate is 23%. Thus, perhaps about 10% of the variability in prevalence rates may be due to the factors mentioned above.

TABLE 1
Prevalence of Anticipatory Side Effects in Cancer Chemotherapy Patients

Ref.	Number studied	Anticipatory nausea (%)	Anticipatory vomiting (%)	Anticipatory nausea and/or vomiting (%)
Andrykowski[38]	78	33	—	—
Andrykowski[40]	71	37	—	—
Andrykowski[38]	77	57	—	—
Cella et al.[9]	60	63	—	—
Cohen[25]	149	42	27	—
Dobkin et al.[16]	125	32	12	—
Dolgan et al.[41]	80	29	20	—
Fdez-Arguelles et al.[81]	72	—	—	31
Fetting et al.[26]	123	14	—	31
Hursti et al.[90]	39	67	0	—
Jacobsen et al.[91]	27	57	—	—
Ingle et al.[27]	60	—	—	25
Love et al.[19]	126	38	—	38
Morrow[21]	406	24	9	—
Morrow et al.[18]	225	—	—	21
Morrow and Dobkin[21]	736*	26	8	—
Nesse et al.[31]	18	44	—	—
Nerenz et al.[82]	61	24	—	—
Nicholas[83]	71	—	—	18
Nicholas[84]	50	42	—	—
Olafsdottir et al.[20]	50	40	14	—
Palmer et al.[85]	24	22	9	—
Schultz[37]	68	—	—	31
Scogna and Smalley[86]	41	—	—	37
van Komen and Redd[28]	100	33	11	—
Weddington[87]	17	53	12	—
Weddington et al.[88]	50	—	—	38
Wilcox et al.[15]	52	—	33	—
Wilson[29]	66	20	8	—
Total	2,452	18	10	9
Median	80	33	12	
Range	17—736	14—63	9—27	18—38

* These patients were part of a consecutive series; therefore, the patients reported in Morrow (1982) and Morrow (in press) are part of the n = 736 in Morrow and Dobkin (1985).

III. ETIOLOGY OF ANTICIPATORY NAUSEA AND VOMITING

Several potential correlates of anticipatory nausea and vomiting have been studied. This section begins with a detailed examination of how available data support a model of ANV development based on learning principles. Studies exploring associations among demographic, clinical and psychological variables of ANV are then presented and discussed, followed by a critique of three conceptual models of how ANV develops.

A. LEARNED ETIOLOGY MODEL

The development of anticipatory side effects closely follows the principles of learning. While potential differences between them are often complex and controversial, there are basically two principal models of learning: operant and classical.

An operant model suggests that behavior develops and continues because it is reinforced. Such a view of the development of anticipatory side effects would state that the patient

The First Few Chemotherapy Treatments

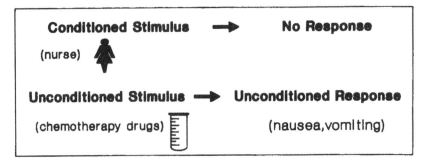

After Several Chemotherapy Treatments

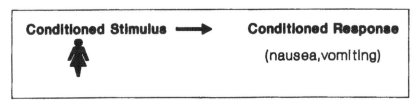

FIGURE 1.   Conditioning explanation of how anticipatory side effects develop.

received some reward for nausea and vomiting behavior. While it is certainly the case that nausea and vomiting side effects are attended to by treating staff and others, it stretches credibility that someone would continue these behaviors for the rather meager reinforcement being provided. The high prevalence of ANV casts further doubt on the validity of this potential explanation.

A classical conditioning explanation of how ANV might develop is outlined below. The conditioning process proposed involves the elements in the top part of the model of Figure 1 which was modified from Burish and Carey.[6] An unconditioned reponse (posttreatment nausea and vomiting) which follows an unconditioned stimulus (the chemotherapy drugs administered) in the context of potentially conditionable stimuli (sensations, thoughts, images of the clinic and/or nurse) will, after a number of repeated trials (chemotherapy treatments), give rise to a conditioned stimulus (such as the chemotherapy nurse) eliciting a conditioned response of anticipatory nausea and vomiting. A number of indirect lines of evidence support such a model.

B. PARAMETERS OF CLASSICAL CONDITIONING WHICH SUPPORT THE VIEW THAT ANV IS LEARNED

Course of development — Anticipatory nausea and vomiting develops only after a number of administrations of chemotherapeutic agents have been given.[18,19] Clinical reports, along with clinical studies support the notion that anticipatory nausea and vomiting is virtually never seen before a number of administrations of chemotherapeutic agents have been given. The percent of patients who develop anticipatory nausea and vomiting increases with the number of courses of chemotherapy given.[4,20,21] Figure 2 combines data from several studies and suggests that the development of anticipatory symptoms is a function of the number of treatment cycles administered. The observation is consistent with the development of a learned reponse where the strength of that response increases with the number of conditioning trials given. In a clinical situation, each administration of chemotherapy agents would correspond to a conditioning trial.

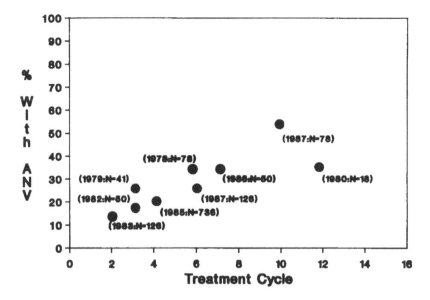

FIGURE 2. Percent of patients developing anticipatory side effects by number of chemotherapy treatments.

Stimulus generalization — The learning phenomenon of a stimulus generalization, where a response may be elicited by a stimulus similar to the original conditioned stimulus, fits the available clinical data. Patients' anticipatory side effects may be elicited by an increasing constellation for stimuli and situations as treatment continues. It is not uncommon, for example, for patients to report nausea when they see *the clinic nurse* who administers their drugs, and then report, after a few more chemotherapy treatments, that the sight of *any clinic nurse* elicits nausea.[22]

Correspondence between unconditioned and conditioned responses — Several investigations have shown a relationship between the occurrence of posttreatment nausea/vomiting and the likelihood of an individual patient developing anticipatory nausea and vomiting. There has not been a study that reported the presence of anticipatory nausea/vomiting in the absence of posttreatment nausea/vomiting. The fact that anticipatory nausea and vomiting so closely resemble the posttreatment nausea and vomiting fits a traditional Pavlovian or classical conditioning model, in which the posttreatment nausea and vomiting is an unconditioned response and the anticipatory nausea and vomiting is a conditioned response.

Intensity of unconditioned response — The intensity of an unconditioned response has been shown to affect the development of a conditioned response.[23,24] When applied to ANV, this finding from classical conditioning would hypothesize that the severity of *posttreatment* nausea/vomiting (intensity of unconditioned response) would be related to the development of anticipatory nausea/vomiting (the conditioned response). All studies (summarized in Table 3) which have examined severity of posttreatment nausea/vomiting have found it significantly associated with the development of ANV; the greater the severity of posttreatment nausea/vomiting, the higher the incidence of anticipatory nausea/vomiting.

C. UNIVARIATE CORRELATES OF ANTICIPATORY NAUSEA AND VOMITING

A number of characteristics have been examined for their possible role in how anticipatory side effects develop. They fit loosely in categories of demographic, clinical and psychological characteristics.

TABLE 2
Demographic Variables Associated with Anticipatory Nausea and Vomiting

Ref.	n	Gender	Age	Race
Andrykowski et al.[40]	71	—	x	—
Cohen[25]	149	x	Younger	—
Dolgan et al.[41]	80	x	x	x
Fetting et al.[26]	123	Female	Younger	x
Ingle et al.[27]	60	x	Younger	x
Love et al.[19]	126	—	Younger	x
Morrow[4]	225	x	Younger	x
Morrow et al.[7]	530	x	Younger	—
Nesse et al.[31]	18	x	x	—
Schultz[37]	68	x	x	—
van Komen and Redd[28]	100	x	Younger	—
Weddington et al.[87]	17	x	x	—
Weddington et al.[88]	50	x	x	x
Wilson[29]	66	Female	Younger	x

Note: x indicates that the factor was investigated and was not found to correlate with ANV. — indicates that the factor was not investigated.

Demographic variables — Table 2 summarizes the types of demographic variables examined for a correlation with anticipatory side effects. Every investigator who has included it[4,25-28] has found an association between age (that is, being younger than 50 years old) and experiencing ANV. Only two of the eleven studies investigating gender[26,29] found it to be associated with ANV symptomatology. None of six studies including data on ethnicity[4,26-28,30] has reported a relationship between race and anticipatory side effects. Education level and socioeconomic and marital status do not appear to be critical factors for the development of ANV symptoms.[4,26,30] Overall, with the marked exception of age, there appears to be little association between patient demographic characteristics and the development of anticipatory side effects. The effect of age has been found independent of other factors such as amount and type of chemotherapy drug given. Younger patients have also been found to experience greater nausea/vomiting as a result of anesthesia. Whether or not some common mechanism is responsible for both findings is a topic for further research.

Clinical variables — Table 3 summarizes results of clinical variables examined for their association to ANV. Nesse et al.[31] reported that cancer patients with anticipatory nausea, when compared to those cancer patients without anticipatory nausea, had been treated for a significantly longer period of time (M = 9.3 months vs. M = 4.2 months, respectively). We[4,32] have noted that, compared to patients who did not report ANV symptoms, ANV patients experienced more postchemotherapy nausea and vomiting, of longer duration and greater severity.

All three studies that examined a potential relationship between how much nausea and vomiting a chemotherapy drug typically caused after treatment (its emetic potential) and ANV reported a significant relationship. Seven out of seven studies, and seven out of nine studies reported a relationship between postchemotherapy nausea and vomiting, respectively, and ANV symptoms. The neural pathway between the vomiting center (an area in the dorsolateral reticular formation of the medulla) and the vestibular system has been implicated in motion induced nausea and vomiting as well as vomiting from poisons given to animals.[33] Thus, a possible relationship between motion sickness susceptibility and chemotherapy nausea/vomiting has been studied. Using a case control methodology, we have shown that cancer patients who self-report a susceptibility to motion sickness (compared to patients

TABLE 3
Clinical Variables Associated with Anticipatory Nausea and Vomiting

Ref.	n	No. of Rx	Emetic potential	Post Rx nausea		Post Rx vomiting	
				S	D	S	D
Andrykowski et al.[40]	71	a	—	*	—	*	—
Andrykowski et al.[38]	77	*	—	*	—	—	—
Cohen[25]	149	x	—	—	—	—	b*
Dobkin et al.[16]	125	—	—	—	b*	—	b*
Dolgan et al.[41]	80	x	*	*	—	*	x
Fetting et al.[26]	123	—	—	—	*	—	*
Ingle et al.[27]	58	x	—	*	—	—	—
Morrow[4]	225	—	*	*	*	*	*
Morrow[32]	176	—	—	*	—	*	—
Nesse et al.[31]	18	*	—	*	*	*	*
Nerenz et al.[82]	61	—	—	—	x	—	x
Nicholas[84]	71	*	—	—	*	—	*
van Komen and Redd[28]	100	*	—	*	—	*	—
Weddington et al.[87]	17	*	—	—	—	—	—
Weddington et al.[88]	50	*	—	—	bx	—	bx
Wilcox et al.[15]	52	—	*	*	—	*	—

Note: x indicates that the factor was studied and was not found to correlate with ANV. — indicates that the factor was not studied. * indicates that the factor was found to correlate significantly with ANV. Rx = chemotherapy regimen; S = severity; D = duration.

a Indicates length of infusion.
b Indicates frequency (rather than duration).

without susceptibility) had (a) significantly more side effects from chemotherapy drugs[34]; (b) significantly more posttreatment nausea and vomiting[35]; (c) significantly more anticipatory nausea and vomiting.[36]

Psychological variables — Consistent with a view that emotions and cognitions may contribute to the development of ANV[28,37] anxiety, depression, hostility, and coping styles in cancer chemotherapy patients have been studied.

As shown in Table 4, 10 out of 11 investigations found that state anxiety levels were significantly elevated in patients with ANV compared to patients without ANV. Two out of three investigations found trait anxiety related to ANV. Love et al.,[19] using a prospective research design, studied 126 cancer patients being treated with chemotherapy for breast cancer (n = 94) and malignant lymphoma (n = 32). Patients were interviewed repeatedly during their initial 6 months of chemotherapy. Thirty-eight percent of the patients developed ANV, with patients who experienced anxiety during injections significantly more likely to develop anticipatory nausea than nonanxious patients. Interestingly, the association between anxiety and anticipatory nausea was not statistically significant during the first two chemotherapy cycles but became significant by the sixth cycle. Andrykowski et al.[38] also reported that the relationship between anxiety and ANV should be qualified according to the treatment time frame. To determine if there were different patterns of infusion-related state anxiety and posttreatment nausea prior to AN onset, AN patients were divided into early (i.e., prior to chemotherapy cycle number 7) and late (i.e., following chemotherapy cycle number 7) onset groups. According to this distinction, anxiety appeared to contribute to the development

TABLE 4
Psychological Variables Associated with Anticipatory Nausea and Vomiting

Ref.	n	Anxiety	Depression	Hostility	Coping
Ahles et al.[19]	9	*(state)	—	—	—
Altmaier et al.[39]	9	*(state)	—	x	o
Andrykowski et al.[40]	71	*(state)	—	—	—
Andrykowski et al.[38]	77	+ +(state)	—	—	—
Cohen[25]	31	*(state)	*	—	—
		x(trait)			
Houts et al.[48]	90	*(state)	—	—	—
Ingle et al.[27]	58	*(state)	x	*	*
Nerenz et al.[82]	18	*(state)	—	—	**
Schultz[37]	68	*(state/trait)	—	—	—
van Komen and Redd[28]	100	*(trait)	*	—	—
Wilson[29]	66	+	+	x	—

Note: x indicates that there was no difference between ANV and non-ANV patients. — indicates that the factor was not investigated. * indicates that the measure was significantly elevated in ANV patients. o indicates that the measure was depressed in ANV patients. ** indicates that "more attempts to cope" were made. + indicates that conflicting results were found between measures. + + indicates that anxiety was significantly elevated only in late-onset of ANV patients.

of AN only for patients who were in the late onset group. A clear, direct relationship between anxiety and ANV development has not been found.

Depression was found to be significantly elevated in ANV patients in two out of four studies whereas hostility and coping styles were not found to be consistently different in ANV patients. Altmaier et al.[39] reported that patients with ANV exhibited a coping style which was "inhibitive rather than facilitative in nature". In contrast, Ingle et al.[27] found a greater number of "attempts to cope with chemotherapy and a higher level of hostility in patients with ANV compared to patients without ANV. Hostility and coping styles are, however, difficult hypothetical constructs to operationalize; it is, therefore, possible that these divergent findings reflect measurement variance rather than actual differences in responses.

Summary — Methodological differences in research designs used and assessment techniques employed render firm comparisons among these investigations difficult. In addition, the retrospective nature of studies examining the possible association between single variables and the development of anticipatory side effects limit the conclusions which can be reached from these data.

D. MULTIVARIATE CORRELATES OF ANTICIPATORY SIDE EFFECTS

Several recent studies have built on some of the earlier promising univariate findings and used multivariate procedures to examine potential joint or interactive relationships among variables that might be associated with the development of anticipatory side effects.

Morrow[4] reported results from a two-group discriminate analysis on 225 cancer patients. Overall, an 80% accurate classification was achieved with 42% of patients experiencing ANV and 91% of patients not experiencing ANV correctly classified based on a combination of age, severity and duration of postchemotherapy nausea and vomiting. Cohen[25] reported that the frequency of vomiting during/after chemotherapy sessions and age (younger than 50 years old) accounted for 32% of the variance in the occurrence of anticipatory nausea. Similar patterns were observed in analyses involving anticipatory vomiting. In a follow-up study[25] involving 14 patients with ANV, five variables — nausea, anxiety, noxious sensations, frequency of postchemotherapy vomiting, and age — accounted for 88% of the variance for anticipatory nausea. Four variables — nausea, frequency of vomiting during/after chemotherapy, anxiety and age — accounted for 65% of the variance in anticipatory vomiting. Since complete data were obtained from only 14 patients, these results require cautious interpretation.

Andrykowski et al.[40] studied 26 patients who displayed anticipatory side effects and 45 who did not. While seven variables entered into a hierarchical regression accounted for about half (47%) of the variance in group membership, posttreatment nausea alone accounted for about one quarter (24%). State anxiety and length of time it took to give the chemotherapy drug were the only two other variables giving a significant increment in explained variance.

Dolgan et al.,[41] in a study of 80 pediatric (mean age of 9 years old) cancer patients, identified five variables which accounted for 23% of the variance in group membership. They were: postchemotherapy nausea and vomiting, emetic potential of chemotherapy regimen, administration of the drug cyclophosphamide, time since diagnosis, and parental anxiety.

Ingle et al.[27] used a three-group ("conditioned, may be conditioned, and not conditioned") discriminate analysis involving seven variables from 58 adult cancer patients in order to determine the best set of "predictors" for patients with ANV. These authors reported an overall assignment rate (by regression) of 71% to the three groups based on: age (younger than 50 years old), postchemotherapy nausea and vomiting, anxiety, and "coping effect".

van Komen and Redd,[28] in an invstigation of 59 cancer patients, administered the Millon Behavioral Health Inventory[42] and the Spielberger State-Trait Anxiety Inventory[43] in order to examine potential personality factors hypothesized to be associated with ANV symptomatology. The most important discriminator variables found were social alienation, future despair (depression), and gastrointestinal susceptibility. Trait anxiety was also shown to be higher in patients with ANV compared to patients without ANV. Interestingly, patients who received chemotherapy in a group setting were more likely to experience ANV compared to patients who were treated on an individual basis.

One hundred seventy-six consecutive ambulatory patients with histologically confirmed cancer who were being treated at three geographically separate hospitals at the University of Rochester Cancer Center were studied at the time of their fourth chemotherapy treatment.[32] Patients found to experience anticipatory nausea and vomiting were significantly more likely to have four or more of the following characteristics compared to patients who did not report anticipatory side effects: (1) age (less than 50 years); (2) the experience of nausea and/or vomiting after their last chemotherapy treatment; (3) describe nausea after the last treatment as "moderate, severe, or intolerable"; (4) describe vomiting after the last treatment as "moderate, severe, or intolerable"; (5) report the side effect "warm or hot all over" after their last treatment; (6) susceptibility to motion sickness; (7) experience "sweating after their last treatment"; and (8) experience "generalized weakness after their last chemotherapy treatment".

These results were recently replicated in a prospective study.[44] Five hundred thirty consecutive cancer patients were asked the previously reported eight questions following their first chemotherapy treatment. The outcome measure was whether or not they had developed anticipatory nausea/vomiting by the time of their fourth chemotherapy treatment. Those patients who had four or more of the eight characteristics were predicted to develop anticipatory side effects. Those with three or fewer were predicted not to. While a significant association was found between these characteristics and subsequent development of anticipatory side effects for 345 patients entered into the study and followed through their fourth chemotherapy treatment the prediction was much more accurate in identifying patients who did not develop subsequent ANV than those who did.

IV. PSYCHOLOGICAL MODELS

Theories of how anticipatory nausea/vomiting develops take either a physiologic or psychologic view. The physiologic view is that anticipatory symptoms may be produced by brain metastasis or local cancer involvement of the gastrointestinal tract.[45] This potential explanation is not consistent with at least two findings. The first is that metastatic spread of cancer to the brain or the gastrointestinal tract is significantly less prudent than the greater than 25% prevalence of anticipatory side effects. Second, in a series of randomized clinical trials, we (and collaborating oncologists) carefully screened for any clinical evidence of metastatic spread and found no association between metastatic disease and ANV.[3,4,32,46]

At least three different psychologic viewpoints have been proposed to explain how psychological processes may cause anticipatory side effects. These hypotheses range from a psychodynamic conceptualization to a learning paradigm involving classical conditioning.

A. PSYCHODYNAMIC MODEL

Chang[45] has proposed a psychodynamic origin of anticipatory side effects. According to this view, nausea and vomiting "are not always direct side effects of chemotherapy, but rather may be surfacing manifestations of underlying psychological readjustment problems associated with life-threatening illness". Chang further suggests that these side effects may be caused by "psychological mechanisms, including anger, anxiety, and frustration". This view has received no empirical support and is now largely neglected.[21,47]

B. ANXIETY MODEL

Several investigators have speculated that anxiety may be involved in the development of anticipatory side effects. Houts et al.[48] have proposed four potential ways that anxiety might relate to anticipatory side effects: (a) anticipatory nausea causes pretreatment anxiety; (b) pretreatment anxiety causes anticipatory nausea; (c) anticipatory nausea and pretreatment anxiety are both caused by posttreatment nausea; and (d) pretreatment anxiety facilitates the conditioning process of anticipatory side effects. There are some data that lend partial support to each of the four potential explanations.

However, in order to examine separately each of the potentially competing hypotheses, experiments would have to be designed that would isolate a particular portion of the chemotherapy treatment. This, unfortunately, is not possible in a clinical setting since chemotherapy is given in repeated cycles. Andrykowski et al.[40] recently provided evidence that elevated levels of state anxiety may precede the initial occurrence of anticipatory symptoms. These authors caution, however, that the relationship between anxiety and anticipatory side effects may not be a strictly causal one. Their data also support a view that anxiety may be heightened following a particular chemotherapy treatment and that, in turn, the increased anxiety may increase posttreatment nausea/vomiting which, in turn, may increase susceptibility to conditioning on the next chemotherapy cycle. This circular process may facilitate and promote a conditioning process rather than serve as a direct cause itself. It is likely that some degree of anxiety facilitates the conditioning process by alerting or sensitizing the patient in much the same way that somebody who is mildly anxious may be quite prone to suddenly notice and become concerned over a physical sensation such as irregular heart beats that had probably been present for a period of time.

V. BEHAVIORAL TREATMENT OF SIDE EFFECTS

Neither anticipatory nor posttreatment nausea/vomiting is completely controlled by antiemetic medicines.[4,46,49,50] Three principal interventions (Hypnosis, Progressive Relaxation Training, and Systematic Desensitization) have been investigated for their effectiveness in controlling nausea and vomiting.

A. PROGRESSIVE RELAXATION TRAINING

Progressive Relaxation Training (PRT) is a behavioral technique which involves learning how to relax by actively tensing and relaxing muscle groups in a progressive manner. Typically, an individual is taught deep muscle relaxation by a therapist, a training audiotape is made, and the individual is requested to practice PRT at home in order to acquire the skill. Four case studies and five controlled investigations of PRT have been reported thus far. Results from case studies[51-53] have suggested that PRT can benefit cancer patients by reducing side effects such as postchemotherapy nausea and vomiting, and negative states such as depression and anxiety.

Lyles et al.[54] studied cancer patients experiencing anxiety, depression, nausea, and vomiting; 50 patients were randomly assigned to one of three treatment conditions: (a) relaxation training with guided imagery; (b) therapist control, in which a therapist spent an equal amount of time with the patients as in condition (a); and, (c) no-treatment control. Patients who received PRT were found to be less anxious and nauseated both during and following their chemotherapy treatment sessions compared to the patients in the two other groups. Additionally, patients in the PRT group evidence less physiological arousal (pulse rates) and were less depressed following chemotherapy. The positive treatment effects found in the PRT condition, but not in the therapist attention-control condition, suggest that the improvements were not simply the result of "nonspecific" treatment factors.

These results were supported by Cotanch[52] in a study in which 43 cancer patients were randomly assigned to one of three conditions: (1) PRT, provided by audiotape; (2) tape control, in which patients listened to soothing music and were requested to focus on positive thoughts; and (3) no-treatment control. Patients took part in one baseline session and "varying numbers" of training sessions. Cotanch reported that 67% of the patients in the PRT conditions showed increases in postchemotherapy nausea and vomiting (PCNV), whereas 85% of the patients in the two control groups showed increase in PCNV. This 18% difference between the groups suggests that PRT can be helpful, even with a minimal amount of therapist contact.

In the first reported PRT prevention study, Burish et al.[55] investigated whether PRT could be used to prevent or at least ameliorate chemotherapy side effects through early intervention. Thirty-two cancer patients about to start their first course of emetogenic chemotherapy were randomized to either a PRT group or a no-treatment control group. PRT sessions were held prior to the initiation of chemotherapy and during the first five chemotherapy treatments. Patients in the PRT group reported feeling less nauseated during and following chemotherapy. Additionally, these patients reported fewer occurrences of vomiting and lower physiological arousal (e.g., heart rate and blood pressure) compared to the patients in the control group. PRT also resulted in less dysphoria and a progressive reduction in PCNV symptoms as treatment with chemotherapy continued over time. By the fifth session only 10% of the PRT patients experienced nausea following chemotherapy treatment compared to 54% of the control patients who did. These findings are encouraging.

Overall, the data regarding the use of PRT with cancer chemotherapy patients show that this type of intervention can be effective in reducing side effects which are present during and after cancer chemotherapy sessions. Since nausea symptoms occurring before a treatment session were not assessed in the early work carried out by Burish and associates,[56] any potential impact PRT has on ANV symptoms defined strictly as pretreatment remains uninvestigated. Given the relationship between postchemotherapy side effects and the subsequent development of ANV, using this technique before the initial chemotherapy treatment could potentially block the conditioning process and thereby prevent its occurrence.

B. SYSTEMATIC DESENSITIZATION

Systematic Desensitization (SD) is a well-developed, standardized behavioral technique which has been shown to be useful in altering maladaptive learned responses such as phobias.[57] In SD, patients are first taught a response incompatible with the maladaptive response they presently have to particular stimuli. This alternative response is then paired in imagination with the original stimuli so as to countercondition the maladaptive response.

Two case studies and four controlled investigations of SD have been reported.[5,58-62] Morrow and Morrell,[62] in a study designed to examine the antiemetic efficacy of SD for the control of ANV, randomly assigned 60 patients with ANV to one of three groups: (a) SD; (b) counseling, based on a Rogerian, client-centered approach; and (c) no-treatment control. ANV patients were taught a modified version of Progressive Muscle Relaxation as a competing response to the maladaptive response of anticipatory nausea/vomiting. During the Systematic Desensitization treatment, patients imagine scenes from a hierarchy of events related to chemotherapy treatment (such as driving to the cancer center) while remaining deeply relaxed. In this way, treatment stimuli become associated with relaxation so that when the patient encounters stimuli (such as the clinic nurse), they respond with relaxation rather than nausea and vomiting.

Only patients in the SD group showed a significant reduction in the frequency, severity, and duration of ANV. The efficacy of SD appeared unrelated to antiemetic medications used by the patients. Additionally, patients in the SD group reported no greater expectation for improvement than did the patients in the counseling group. Thus, apparently, nonspecific therapy effects (e.g., attention) were not responsible for the reported positive effects.

In a follow-up study, Morrow[17] compared the effectiveness of SD to (a) relaxation only, (b) counseling, and (c) no-treatment control in order to examine the essential treatment components in the SD procedure. Relative to the other three groups, patients treated with SD reported a significant decrease in the severity and duration of anticipatory nausea from baseline to follow-up sessions. SD and relaxation patients had a significantly greater decrease in the duration and severity of posttreatment nausea compared to patients who were in the other two groups. These results were independent of patients' ratings of their expectations for success or the credibility of the experimenter. Results support a view that *both* the cognitive stimulus hierarchy and relaxation response are necessary components for the successful treatment of ANV.

In another investigation, Dobkin[58] examined the possibility of reducing, retarding, or preventing the development of both post- and anticipatory side effects in new-to-chemotherapy cancer patients. Forty consecutive patients were randomly assigned to either an SD or Waiting-List Control group. SD was administered in two separate 1-h sessions prior to the second chemotherapy cycle. A repeated measures design was employed with one baseline and three follow-up periods; dependent measures included: postchemotherapy nausea and vomiting, anticipatory nausea and vomiting, anxiety (trait at baseline, state at all periods), and tension level postchemotherapy.

Preliminary results showed a downward trend for the SD patients' PCNV side effects in that nausea and vomiting were less frequent, severe, and of shorter duration as chemotherapy progressed. In contrast, there was an upward trend for the control group patients' PCNV side effects in that nausea and vomiting were more frequent, severe, and of longer duration as chemotherapy progressed. In addition, the control patients reported higher levels of tension following chemotherapy compared to SD patients. These preliminary findings suggest that the introduction of SD early in treatment can reduce and retard the development of conditioned side effects resulting from chemotherapy in cancer patients.

In summary, consistent findings regarding the effectiveness of SD have been reported in both case and controlled studies. Although the majority of the SD investigations have been carried out in one research center, two case studies and one controlled investigation[61] in other geographical locations have replicated these promising results.

C. HYPNOSIS

Hypnosis has been defined as a state of intensified attention and receptiveness and an increased responsiveness to an idea or set of ideas.[63] Six case histories of hypnotherapy with cancer patients have reported positive therapeutic results.[64-69] The majority of these investigations have been carried out with a pediatric population probably since children are more readily hypnotized than adults.[68] This may be also because children often experience undesirable side effects from antiemetic drugs and thus some antiemetics are not used with children.[70]

LaBaw et al.[66] studied 27 children and adolescents, aged 4 to 20 years, who were treated with self-hypnosis over a 2-year period (the exact number of treatment sessions per patient was not specified). "Progressive Body Relaxation" was employed as an inductive technique which was followed by "psychic imagery" of fantasied idyllic scenes common in the patient's experience. Dependent measures included patients' self-report and therapist observations. Results indicated that "varying degrees of success" were obtained where "success" was defined as improved sleep, increased caloric intake and retention, increased fluid intake, and greater tolerance for therapeutic procedures. In general, few objective data were collected from these case studies. The "hypnotic" intervention was not standardized and sometimes not described. These methodological limitations preclude definitive conclusions.

Three controlled studies have examined hypnotherapy. Redd et al.[71] treated six patients experiencing ANV with hypnosis in a multiple baseline design. During treatment, each patient was individually instructed in focusing attention, achieving deep muscle relaxation, and imaging pleasant scenes. The training sessions were audiotaped and patients were instructed to practice the treatment daily. Due to unforeseen events, the hypnotic intervention was temporarily interrupted for several of the patients. At this time, the symptoms which had been apparently controlled by hypnosis reappeared, suggesting that the intervention was involved in the initial positive effects. Given the small sample size, these findings require replication before conclusions can be drawn.

Cotanch et al.[70] also combined relaxation training with hypnosis in a study of 12 pediatric inpatients (aged 10 to 18 years) who were referred by oncologists for treatment since they were experiencing troublesome chemotherapy-related nausea and vomiting. The children were randomly assigned to an experimental group (n = 6) or a control group (n = 6) who received standard care. On the day of chemotherapy, the children in the experimental group were trained by a therapist in self-hypnosis. Both groups were followed through two consecutive chemotherapy cycles. Child self-report and nurse observations were obtained on the parameters of nausea and vomiting (intensity, severity, frequency) and on the amount of oral intake 24 h postchemotherapy. Data were collected by staff nurses and research assistants who were unaware which group the child was assigned to. In the experimental group, there was a significant reduction in nausea and vomiting both in terms of intensity and severity, and a significant increase in oral intake. These changes were not evident in the control group. Although this study is suggestive regarding the effectiveness of hypnotherapy, the results could be explained in terms of an attention effect. The children in the experimental group received "extra" attention from a therapist whereas the children in the control group did not. While these findings are suggestive, they require replication with an attention-placebo group to rule out this alternative hypothesis.

Zeltzer et al.[72] compared hypnotherapy to supportive counseling and suggested that nonspecific therapy effects such as demand characteristics and/or attention may contribute to treatment changes found. In their study, 19 children, aged 6 to 17 years, were randomly assigned to a hypnotherapy or a supportive counseling group. Children in both groups reported reductions in nausea and vomiting and rated chemotherapy as "less noxious" following intervention. There were, however, no statistically or clinically significant differences in outcome found between the two approaches.

Overall, it appears that studies using hypnosis for ANV control have shown that this intervention may be beneficial for children. Less evidence is available demonstrating its usefulness for adults. In order to establish the effectiveness of hypnotherapy for cancer chemotherapy patients, studies with larger sample sizes in which patients are randomly assigned to treatment or appropriate control groups are needed.

D. OTHER BEHAVIORAL INTERVENTIONS

Behavioral interventions other than the three discussed above have been directed at the control of chemotherapy side effects. Moore and Altmaier[73] reported a pilot study of nine cancer patients (six females, three males; mean age = 47 years) treated with Stress Inoculation Training (the six-session treatment "package" consisted of Cognitive Behavior Modification combined with PRT and Education). Prior to the intervention, patients were interviewed and completed the Multiple Affect Adjective Checklist (MAACL[74]) which is designed to measure anxiety, depression and hostility. Five of the nine patients exhibited ANV prior to treatment. Since the authors discontinued monitoring the patients at the last training session (i.e., no follow-up data), it is impossible to determine the effectiveness of this approach. Three patients did report, however, that they felt less anxious prior to treatment having learned effectiveness coping skills.

Burish et al.[75] treated a 44-year-old cancer patient with EMG biofeedback combined with relaxation in order to help control anticipatory and posttreatment symptoms. Baseline measures of affect,[74] muscle tension, pulse rate, and blood pressure were taken. Following ten training sessions, the patient was able to reduce her physiological arousal levels (as measured by EMG, pulse rate, and blood pressure) and reported feeling less nauseated. These changes were maintained during three follow-up periods. There were no reported improvements in affect. These results, which are similar to those found for PRT, suggest that EMG Biofeedback may be another means of teaching relaxation to cancer patients.

Three studies, LeBaron and Zeltzer,[76] Kolko and Rickard-Figueroa,[77] and Redd et al.[78] have investigated interventions based on cognitive diversion techniques. The former study involved directing adolescents' attention away from the administration of chemotherapy by having them play games and be actively engaged with a therapist (modified relaxation training was also included in some cases). The latter two studies involved the use of video games to distract pediatric and adolescent patients.

LeBaron and Zeltzer[76] reported a decrease in postchemotherapy nausea, vomiting, and "bother" during the intervention along with fewer disruptions of activities following treatment. These improvements were maintained at follow-up (time period not reported). They concluded that "since a repeated measures design found no symptom reductions prior to intervention, it can be assumed that some aspects of the intervention itself were responsible for the reductions found, rather than attention or expectations related to assessment alone". This conclusion seems premature given a sample size of n = 8, no control groups, and no theoretical rationale of how distraction alone could reduce chemotherapy-related side effects.

Kolko and Rickard-Figueroa[77] used a multiple-baseline (ABAB) design[79] with three pediatric oncology patients (all male, aged 11, 16, and 17 years). Anticipatory "distress", PCNV and state anxiety[43] measures were taken. A Modified-Procedure Behavioral Rating Scale[80] was used to gather observational data 5 min prior to chemotherapy. The introduction of video games concurrent with the administration of chemotherapy was associated with the reduction of self-reported and observer-reported anticipatory symptoms (not ANV) as well as postchemotherapy distress. These improvements were reversed when the return-to-baseline phase was initiated. Symptoms decreased again when the video game procedure was reintroduced in two of the three cases (the third case could not be evaluated due to admission of the patient just before the final condition).

Kolko and Rickard-Figueroa's study[77] addressed the relaxation versus distraction issue regarding the therapeutic mechanisms underlying behavior therapy. Although the results imply that distraction may effectively reduce symptomatology, ANV and PCNV side effects per se were not reduced, only "distress" levels were altered.

Redd et al.[78] conducted two experiments, one of which employed an ABAB design, to evaluate the effect of video game playing in pediatric oncology patients with anticipatory nausea and anxiety. In the first experiment, patients were alternately assigned to either the experimental group or to the control condition. In the second experiment, patients from the first experiment were carried over and exposed to an ABAB design presentation of the video games. Unlike Kolko and Rickard-Figueroa's study,[77] the ABAB presentation took place within the same chemotherapy session, i.e., after a no-video-game baseline assessment (A), patients played video games for 10 min (B), followed immediately by a 10-min no-video-game period (A), and then a second 10-min video game period (B). Nausea and anxiety were assessed using a 10 cm Visual Analog Scale; pulse rate and blood pressure measures were taken to assess physiological indices. Results indicated that anticipatory nausea but not anxiety decreased significantly following video games playing in both studies. Reportedly pulse rates and systolic/diastolic blood pressure rates were variable, with one measure (systolic blood pressure) showing a significant increase from the previous no-game level following the second exposure to video games within the session. The authors interpreted these findings as support for the hypothesis that cognitive distraction, and not relaxation, is the critical component of the intervention.

E. SUMMARY OF TREATMENT STUDIES

Increasing efforts are going in to randomized clinical trials examining the effectiveness of behavioral interventions for both anticipatory and posttreatment nausea and vomiting. Reasonable support has emerged for the view that the behavioral treatment of anticipatory side effects is effective. In broad outline, hypnosis appears to be useful for children but less useful for adults, systematic desensitization has been found effective for management of anticipatory nausea and vomiting in adults, other behavioral techniques have shown less consistent efficacy. One intriguing area for a fruitful future study is the efficacy of behavioral techniques in the management of posttreatment nausea and vomiting. Studies have indicated certain types of behavioral treatment to be effective in the total management of chemotherapy induced side effects. Future controlled trials may focus on the "active ingredient" of these particular interventions.

Chemotherapy induced side effects are a significant challenge to the patients completion of a planned course of treatment for cancer. The adequate management of this treatment related morbidity can significantly influence the patients quality of life. Behavioral interventions for the management of chemotherapy induced nausea and vomiting can have a central role in the adequate management of treatment related morbidity in cancer patients.

ACKNOWLEDGMENTS

This work was supported in parts by Research Career Development Award K04-CA01038 from NCI DHHS, and by R01-NR01905 from National Center for Nursing Research DHH, and PBR 42D, PBR 43 from the American Cancer Society.

REFERENCES

1. **Holland, J.,** Psychological aspects of oncology, *Med. Clin. North Am.,* 61, 1977.
2. **Hoagland, A. C., Morrow, G. R., Bennett, J. M., and Carnrike, C. L. M.,** Oncologists' view of cancer patient noncompliance, *Am. J. Clin. Oncol.,* 6, 239, 1983.
3. **Morrow, G. R.,** Behavioral treatment of anticipatory nausea and vomiting during chemotherapy, *Proc. Am. Assoc. Cancer Res. Am. Soc. Clin. Oncol.,* 22, 396, 1981.

4. **Morrow, G. R.**, Prevalence and correlates of anticipatory nausea and vomiting in chemotherapy patients, *J. Natl. Cancer Inst.*, 68, 585, 1982.

5. **Morrow, G. R.**, Effect of the cognitive hierarchy in the systematic desensitization treatment of anticipatory nausea in cancer patients: A component comparison with relaxation only, counseling, and no treatment, *Cog. Ther. Res.*, 10, 421, 1986a.

6. **Burish, T. G. and Carey, M. P.**, Conditioned responses to cancer chemotherapy: etiology and treatment, in *Impact of Psycho-Endocrine Systems in Cancer Immunity*, Fox, G. H. and Newberry, B. H., Eds., C. J. Hogrefe, Toronto, 1984, 147.

7. **Morrow, G. R.**, Chemotherapy-related nausea and vomiting etiology and management, *CA: J. Clin.*, 39, 89, 1989.

8. **Nicholas, D. R.**, Prevalence of anticipatory nausea and emesis in cancer chemotherapy patients, *J. Behav. Med.*, 5, 461, 1982.

9. **Cella, D. F., Pratt, A., and Holland, J. C.**, Long-term conditioned nausea and anxiety persisting in cured Hodgkin's patients after chemotherapy (abstract), *Proc. Ann. Meet. Am. Soc. Clin. Oncol.*, 3, 73, 1984.

10. **Andrykowski, M. A.**, Definitional issues in the study of anticipatory nausea in cancer chemotherapy, *J. Behav. Med.*, 9, 33, 1986.

11. **Burish, T. G. and Carey, M. P.**, Conditioned aversive responses in cancer chemotherapy patients: theoretical and developmental analysis, *J. Consult. Clin. Psychol.*, 55, 42, 1987.

12. **Duigon, A.**, Anticipatory nausea and vomiting associated with cancer chemotherapy, *Oncol. Nurs. Forum*, 13, 35, 1986.

13. **Morrow, G. R.**, The assessment of nausea and vomiting: past problems, current issues and directions for future research, *Cancer*, 52, 2267, 1948b.

14. **Nicholas, D. R. and Hollandsworth, J. G.**, Assessment of anticipatory nausea and vomiting in cancer patients undergoing chemotherapy: theoretical and methodological considerations, *J. Psychosoc. Oncol.*, 4, 61, 1986.

15. **Wilcox, P. M., Fetting, J. H., Nettesheim, K. M., and Abeloff, M. D.**, Anticipatory vomiting in women receiving cyclophosphamide, methotrexate, and 5-FU (CMF) adjuvant chemotherapy for breast carcinoma, *Cancer Treat. Rep.*, 66, 1601, 1982.

16. **Dobkin, P., Zeichner, A., and Dickson-Parnell, B.**, Concomitants of anticipatory nausea and emesis in cancer chemotherapy, *Psychol. Rep.*, 56, 671, 1985.

17. **Morrow, G. R.**, Behavioral management of chemotherapy-induced nausea and vomiting in the cancer patient, *Clin. Oncol.*, 113, 11, 1986b.

18. **Morrow, G. R., Arseneau, J. C., Asbury, R. F., Bennett, J. M., and Boros, L.**, Anticipatory nausea and vomiting in chemotherapy patients, *N. Engl. J. Med.*, 306, 431, 1982.

19. **Love, R. R., Nerenz, D. R., and Leventhal, H.**, Anticipatory nausea with cancer chemotherapy: Development through two mechanisms, *Proc. Annu. Met. Am. Soc. Clin. Oncol.*, 2, 242, 1982 (abstr.).

20. **Olafsdottir, R., Sjoden, P. O., and Westling, B.**, Prevalence and prediction of chemotherapy-related anxiety, nausea, and vomiting in cancer patients, *Behav. Res. Ther.*, 24, 59, 1986.

21. **Morrow, G. R. and Dobkin, P. L.**, Biobehavioral aspects of cancer treatment side effects, *J. Exp. Clin. Cancer Res.*, in press.

22. **Redd, W. H. and Andrykowski, M. A.**, Behavioral intervention in cancer treatment: Controlling aversion reactions to chemotherapy, *J. Consult. Clin. Psychol.*, 50, 1018, 1982.

23. **Dragoin, W. B.**, Conditioning and extinction of taste aversions with variations in the intensity of the CS and UCS in two strains of rats, *Psychonom. Sci.*, 22, 303, 1971.

24. **Nachman, M. and Ashe, J. H.**, Learned taste aversions in rats and as a function of dosage, concentration, and route of administration of LiCi, *Physiol. Behav.*, 10, 73, 1973.

25. **Cohen, R. E.**, Distress Associated with Anti-Neoplastic Chemotherapy: Prediction, Assessment, and Treatment, unpublished doctoral dissertation, State University of New York, Albany, 1982.

26. **Fetting, J. H., Wilcox, P. M., Iwata, B. A., Criswell, E. L., Bosmajian, L. S., and Shelder, V. R.**, Anticipatory nausea and vomiting in an ambulatory medical oncology population, *Cancer Treat. Rep.*, 67, 1093, 1983.

27. **Ingle, R. J., Burish, T. G., and Wallston, K. A.**, Conditionability of cancer chemotherapy patients, *Oncol. Nurs. Forum*, 11, 97, 1984.

28. **van Komen, R. W. and Redd, W. H.**, Personality factors associated with anticipatory nausea/vomiting in patients receiving cancer chemotherapy, *Health Psychol.*, 4, 189, 1985.

29. **Wilson, J. P., Rahdert, E. R., Black, C. D., Taylor, H. G., and Holloway, H. C.**, Identifying anxiety and/or depression in emesis-prone cancer chemotherapy patients, *Proc. Am. Soc. Clin. Oncol.*, 5, 1986 (abstr.).

30. **Weddington, W. W., Miller, N. J., and Sweet, D. L.**, Anticipatory nausea and vomiting associated with cancer chemotherapy, *N. Engl. J. Med.*, 307, 825, 1982.

31. **Nesse, R. M., Carli, T., Curtis, G. G., and Kleinman, P. D.**, Pre-treatment nausea in cancer chemotherapy: a conditioned response?, *Psychosom. Med.*, 42, 33, 1980.

32. **Morrow, G. R.**, Clinical characteristics associated with the development of anticipatory nausea and vomiting in cancer patients undergoing chemotherapy treatment, *J. Clin. Oncol.*, 10, 1170, 1984c.

33. **Money, K. E. and Cheung, B. S.**, Another function of the inner ear: facilitation of the emetic response to poisons, *Aviat. Space Environ. Med.*, 54, 208, 1983.

34. **Morrow, G. R.**, The effect of a susceptibility to motion sickness on the side effects of cancer chemotherapy, *Cancer*, 55, 2766, 1985.

35. **Morrow, G. R.**, Susceptibility to motion sickness and chemotherapy induced side-effects, *Lancet*, 52, 1098, 1984f.

36. **Morrow, G. R.**, Susceptibility to motion sickness and the development of anticipatory nausea and vomiting in cancer patients, *Cancer Treat. Rep.*, 68, 99, 1984e.

37. **Schultz, L. S.**, Classical (Pavlovian) conditioning of nausea and vomiting in cancer chemotherapy, *Proc. Am. Soc. Clin. Oncol.*, 21, 244, 1980 (abstr.).

38. **Andrykowski, M. A. and Redd, W. H.**, Longitudinal analysis of the development of anticipatory nausea, *J. Consult. Clin. Psychol.*, 55, 36, 1987.

39. **Altmaier, E. M., Ross, W. E., and Moore, K.**, A pilot investigation of the psychologic functioning of patients with anticipatory vomiting, *Cancer*, 49, 201, 1982.

40. **Andrykowski, M. A., Redd, W. H., and Hatfield, A. K.**, Development of anticipatory nausea: a prospective analysis, *J. Consult. Clin. Psychol.*, 53, 447, 1985.

41. **Dolgan, M. J., Katz, E. R., McGinty, K., and Seigel, S. E.**, Anticipatory nausea and vomiting in pediatric cancer patients, *Pediatrics*, 75, 547, 1985.

42. **Millon, T., Green, C. J., and Meagher, R. B.**, The MBHI: a new inventory for the psychodiagnostician in medical settings, *Prof. Psychol.*, 10, 529, 1979.

43. **Spielberger, C. D., Gorsuch, R. L., and Lushene, R.**, *The State-Trait Anxiety Inventory (STAI)*, Consulting Psychologists Press, Palo Alto, CA, 1968.

44. **Morrow, G. R., Waight, J., and Black, P. M.**, Anticipatory nausea development in cancer patients: replication and extension of a learning model, *Br. J. Clin. Psychol.*, in press, 1991.

45. **Chang, J. C.**, Nausea and vomiting in cancer patients: an expression of psychological mechanisms?, *Psychosomatics*, 22, 701, 1981.

46. **Morrow, G. R.**, Prevalence, etiology and treatment of chemotherapy induced anticipatory nausea and vomiting, *Proceedings of the American Cancer Society 4th National Conference on Human Values and Cancer*, 1984d.

47. **Morrow, G. R. and Black, P. M.**, Behavioral interventions reduce available cancer mortality and morbidity, *Cancer Prev.*, 1, 51, 1990.

48. **Houts, P., Morrow, G. R., Lipton, A., Harvey, L. A., and Simmons, M. A.**, The Role of Pretreatment Anxiety in Anticipatory Nausea Among Cancer Patients Receiving Chemotherapy, University of Pennsylvania, unpublished manuscript, 1984.

49. **Laszlo, J.**, *Antiemetics and Cancer Chemotherapy*, Williams & Wilkins, Baltimore, 1983.

50. **Morrow, G. R., Loughner, J., and Bennett, J. M.**, Prevalence of nausea and vomiting (N & V) and other side effects in patients receiving Cytoxan, Methotrexate, Fluorouracil (CMF) therapy with and without Prednisone, *Proc. Am. Soc. Clin. Oncol.*, 3, 105, 1984.

51. **Burish, T. G. and Lyles, J. N.**, Effectiveness of relaxation training in reducing the aversiveness of chemotherapy in the treatment of cancer, *J. Behav. Ther. Exp. Psychiatry*, 10, 357, 1979.

52. **Cotanch, P. H.**, Muscle relaxation versus "attention-placebo" in decreasing the aversiveness of chemotherapy, unpublished manuscript, Duke University, Durham, 1983.

53. **Weddington, W. W., Blindt, K. A., and McCraken, S. G.**, Relaxation training for anticipatory nausea associated with chemotherapy, *Psychosomatics*, 24, 281, 1983.

54. **Lyles, J. N., Burish, T. G., Krozely, M. G., and Oldham, R. K.**, Efficacy of relaxation training and guided imagery in reducing the aversiveness of cancer chemotherapy, *J. Consult. Clin. Psychol.*, 50, 509, 1982.

55. **Burish, T. G., Carey, M. P., Krozely, M. G., and Greco, F. A.**, Conditioned side effects induced by cancer chemotherapy: prevention through behavioral treatment, *J. Consult. Clin. Psychol.*, 55, 1, 1987.

56. **Burish, T. G.**, personal communication, 1985.

57. **Wolpe, J.**, *The Practice of Behavior Therapy*, 3rd ed., Pergamon Press, New York, 1983.

58. **Dobkin, P.**, The Use of Systematic Desensitization, a Behavioral Intervention, in the Reduction of Aversive Chemotherapy Side Effects in Cancer Patients, unpublished doctoral dissertation, University of Georgia, Athens, 1987.

59. **Hailey, B. J. and White, J. G.**, Systematic desensitization for anticipatory nausea associated with chemotherapy, *Psychosomatics*, 24, 287, 1983.

60. **Hoffman, M. L.**, Hypnotic desensitization for the management of anticipatory emesis in chemotherapy, *Am. J. Clin. Hypn.*, 25, 2, 1983.

61. **Meyer, J.**, Systematic Desensitization Versus Relaxation Training and No Treatment (Controls) for the Reduction of Nausea, Vomiting, and Anxiety Resulting from Chemotherapy, unpublished doctoral dissertation, Virginia Commonwealth University, Richmond, 1982.

62. Morrow, G. R. and Morrell, C., Behavioral treatment for the anticipatory nausea and vomiting induced by cancer chemotherapy, *N. Engl. J. Med.*, 307, 1476, 1982.

63. Erickson, M. H., Hypnosis in painful terminal illness, *Am. J. Clin. Hypn.*, 1, 117, 1959.

64. Dempster, C. R., Balson, P., and Whalen, B. T., Supportive hypnotherapy during the radical treatment of malignancies, *Int. J. Clin. Exp. Hypn.*, 24, 1, 1976.

65. Ellenberg, L., Kellerman, J., Dash, J., Higgins, G., and Zeltzer, L., Use of hypnosis for multiple symptoms in an adolescent girl with leukemia, *Am. J. Adol. Health Care*, 1, 132, 1980.

66. LaBaw, W., Holton, C., Tewell, K., and Eccles, D., The use of self-hypnosis by children with cancer, *Am. J. Clin. Hypn.*, 17, 233, 1975.

67. Margolis, C. G., Hypnotic imagery with cancer patients, *Am. J. Clin. Hypn.*, 25, 128, 1983.

68. Olness, K., Imagery (self-hypnosis) as adjunct therapy in childhood cancer: Clinical experience with 25 patients, *Am. J. Pediatr. Hematol./Oncol.*, 3, 313, 1981.

69. Zeltzer, L., Kellerman, J., Ellenberg, L., and Dash, J., Hypnosis for reduction of vomiting associated with chemotherapy and disease in adolescents with cancer, *J. Adol. Health Care*, 4, 77, 1983.

70. Cotanch, P., Hockenberry, M., and Herman, S., Self-hypnosis as antiemetic therapy in children receiving chemotherapy, *Oncol. Nurs. Forum*, 12, 41, 1985.

71. Redd, W. H., Anderson, G. U., and Minagawa, R. Y., Hypnotic control of anticipatory emesis in cancer patients receiving chemotherapy, *J. Consult. Clin. Psychol.*, 50, 14, 1982.

72. Zeltzer, L., LeBaron, S., and Zeltzer, P. M., The effectiveness of behavioral intervention for reduction of nausea and vomiting in children and adolescents receiving chemotherapy, *J. Clin. Oncol.*, 2, 683, 1984.

73. Moore, K. and Altmaier, E. M., Stress inoculation training with cancer patients, *Cancer Nurs.*, October, 389, 1981.

74. Zuckerman, M., Lubin, V., Vogel, L., and Valerius, E., Measurement of experimentally induced affects, *J. Consult. Clin. Psychol.*, 28, 418, 1964.

75. Burish, T. G., Shatner, C. D., and Lyles, L. N., Effectiveness of multiple-site EMG biofeedback and relaxation in reducing the aversiveness of cancer chemotherapy, *Biofeedb. Self-Regul.*, 6, 523, 1981.

76. LeBaron, S. and Zeltzer, L. K., Behavioral intervention for reducing chemotherapy-related nausea and vomiting in adolescents with cancer, *J. Adol. Health Care*, 5, 178, 1984.

77. Kolko, D. J. and Rickard-Figueroa, J. L., Effects of video games in the adverse corollaries of chemotherapy in pediatric oncology patients: A single-case analysis, *J. Consult. Clin. Psychol.*, 53, 223, 1985.

78. Redd, W. H., Jacobsen, P. B., Die-Trill, M., Dermatis, H., McEvoy, M., and Holland, J., Cognitive/attentional distraction in the control of conditioned nausea in pediatric cancer patients receiving chemotherapy, *J. Consult. Clin. Psychol.*, 55, 391, 1987.

79. Kazdin, A. E., *Single-Case Research Designs*, Oxford University Press, New York, 1982.

80. Katz, E. R., Kellerman, J., and Siegel, S. E., Behavioral distress in children with cancer undergoing medical procedures: developmental considerations, *J. Consult. Clin. Psychol.*, 48, 356, 1980.

81. Fdez-Arguelles, P., Guerrero, J., Duque, A., Borrego, A., and Marquez, J., Nauseas y vomitos anticipatorios en pacientes cancerosos sometidos a tratamiento de quimioterapia, paper presented at the meeting in Biobehavioral Oncology, 6th Eupsyca Symposium, Zaragoza, Spain, 1985.

82. Nerenz, D. R., Leventhal, H., Easterling, D. V., and Love, R. R., Anxiety and drug taste as predictors of anticipatory nausea in cancer chemotherapy, *J. Clin. Oncol.*, 4, 224, 1986.

83. Nicholas, D. R., Prevalence of anticipatory nausea and emesis in cancer chemotherapy patients, *J. Behav. Med.*, 5, 461, 1982.

84. Nicholas, D. R., Anticipatory Nausea in Cancer Chemotherapy: Cognitive, Motoric, and Physiological Components, unpublished doctoral dissertation, University of Southern Mississippi, 1983.

85. Palmer, B. V., Walsh, G., McKinna, J. A., and Greening, W. P., Adjuvant chemotherapy for breast cancer: side effects and quality of life, *Br. Med. J.*, 281, 1594, 1980.

86. Scogna, D. M. and Smalley, R. V., Chemotherapy-induced nausea and vomiting, *Am. J. Nurs.*, 79, 1562, 1979.

87. Weddington, W. W., Psychogenic nausea and vomiting associated with termination of chemotherapy, *Psychother. Psychosomat.*, 37, 129, 1982.

88. Weddington, W. W., Miller, N. J., and Sweet, D. L., Anticipatory nausea and vomiting associated with cancer chemotherapy, *J. Psychosomat. Res.*, 28, 73, 1984.

89. Ahles, T. A., Cohen, R. E., Little, D., Balducci, L., Dubbert, P. M., and Kean, T. M., Toward a behavioral assessment of anticipatory symptoms associated with cancer chemotherapy, *J. Behav. Ther. Exp. Psychiatry*, 15, 141, 1984.

90. Hursti, T., Fredrikson, M., Furst, L. J., Johansson, S., Peterson, C., and Stineck, G., Poster presented at the Joint ESPO-BPOG Conference, Royal College of Physicians, London, 1989.

91. Jacobsen, R. and Edinger, J. D., Side effects of relaxation treatment, *Am. J. Psychiatry*, 139, 952, 1982.

Chapter 19

SELECTIVE 5-HT₃ RECEPTOR ANTAGONISTS: A NOVEL CLASS OF ANTIEMETICS

David Warr

TABLE OF CONTENTS

I. INTRODUCTION

The introduction of high-dose metoclopramide brought not only improved control of chemotherapy-induced emesis but also led to the discovery of a new class of antiemetics known as selective 5-HT$_3$ receptor antagonists. This chapter will trace the development of these compounds from the preclinical testing to phase III studies. Although there are relatively few published trials the initial results indicate that these new agents represent a step toward the goal of improving the quality of life for patients with cancer.

II. METOCLOPRAMIDE — THE FIRST 5-HT$_3$ RECEPTOR ANTAGONIST

In the 1980s there was a substantial progress in the management of emesis due to cisplatin with the introduction of high-dose metoclopramide by Gralla.[1] Kris et al. demonstrated that metoclopramide 2 mg/kg for five intravenous doses prevented emesis in 39% (14/39) of patients who received high-dose cisplatin.[2] This activity was confirmed by others and there have been modifications that have made this treatment more convenient to administer and more efficacious.[3]

With the addition of steroids and lorazepam to high-dose metoclopramide, approximately 60% of patients will remain free of emesis in the first 24 h following cisplatin.[4] There is, however, a delayed onset of vomiting in 48% of patients despite maintenance therapy with dexamethasone and metoclopramide indicating that further improvements in efficacy are necessary.[5]

Although there is evidence that the effectiveness of metoclopramide increases with the dose, the side effects of akathisia and extrapyramidal symptoms have been dose limiting especially in younger patients or when this drug is given for several days.[5,6] These toxicities are due to antagonism of dopamine receptors — the receptors that were felt to mediate the antiemetic effect of metoclopramide.[2] The ideal agent would therefore seem to be one that does not penetrate the blood-brain barrier (hence no extrapyramidal effects) yet has strong affinity for the dopamine receptors in the chemoreceptor trigger zone of the area postrema (which is outside of this barrier). Domperidone possesses these properties but demonstrated only modest activity in high doses in an animal model[7] and in man.[8]

An explanation for the efficacy of high-dose metoclopramide in comparison to domperidone might be an interaction with a receptor other than (or in addition to) the dopamine receptor. *In vitro* work had previously established the presence of a serotonin receptor in the nervous system (originally termed 5-HT M but now known as 5-HT$_3$) that could be blocked by relatively high doses of metoclopramide.[9] Miner and Sanger postulated that the antiemetic effect of metoclopramide might be due to its effect on serotonin-induced smooth muscle contractions in the gut.[10] Using the selective 5-HT$_3$ receptor antagonist MDL 72222, they demonstrated virtually complete inhibition of cisplatin-induced emesis in the ferret model. Subsequent work with the other selective antagonists indicated that the emesis in animal models due to doxorubicin, actinomycin D, mechlorethamine, and DTIC could also be abolished.[11] Emesis due to apomorphine[11] (thought to be mediated by dopamine receptors), copper sulfate[11] and motion[12] however were unaffected indicating a selective effect for chemotherapy-induced emesis.

III. PHASE I CLINICAL TRIALS

Table 1 lists the 5-HT$_3$ receptor antagonists for which there are reports of phase I trials. The terminal half-life of these agents in man ranges from 3 to 11 h.[13-16] In phase I trials, the schedules for ondansetron and batanopride (short half-lives) have ranged from a bolus

TABLE 1
5-HT$_3$ Receptor Antagonists for which
Phase I Data is Available

Nonproprietary name	Compound number
Batanopride	BMY25801
Dazapride	?
Granisetron	BRL43694A
Ondansetron	GR38032F or GR-C507/75
None assigned	ICS 205-930

followed by continuous infusions to every 8 h dosing.[13,15,17] ICS 205-930 and granisetron, on the other hand, have usually been given as a single dose in view of their longer terminal half-lives.[14,16] It is not known, however, whether the duration of effect of these agents parallels their pharmacokinetic parameters.

The phase I studies have established that, with two exceptions (electrocardiographic changes and hypotension), the toxicities of these agents are mild and qualitatively similar. A dose-limiting toxicity of prolongation of the QRS, PR, and QT$_c$ intervals has been reported with batanopride[17] but not with other agents. Reports of other cardiovascular adverse events with any 5-HT$_3$ receptor antagonist such as arrhythmias,[14,18] hypertension,[19,20] and hypotension[19,21,22] are rare. Apart from hypotension,[22] at this point, the relation of these events to drug administration is uncertain. There are two reports of bronchospasm (one of which was accompanied by facial edema and a rash)[23,24] and one report of coughing/choking sensation with ondansetron.[19] Fever plus a rash has been observed in one patient with a carcinoid.[21]

One of the most common adverse events reported (up to 45%)[18] is a mild to moderate headache which starts on the day of treatment and usually requires little or no intervention.[19,20,24,25] The reported frequency varies substantially from study to study possibly due to the intensity with which adverse events are sought and the small numbers in most trials. In results from 982 patients treated with granisetron, 13.8% experienced headache as compared to 4.7% of 223 patients in the alternative antiemetic groups from randomized studies.[26] A similar compilation of results with ondansetron indicated that headaches occurred in 19% of 763 patients.[27]

Mild sedation[19,20,28] and elevation of transaminases[18-20] have also been associated with these compounds and are not felt to be dose related. Two reports on batanopride suggest a relatively high incidence of loose stools (9/24[25] and 5/12[29] patients) compared to ondansetron[19] and granisetron.[18] As would be expected from the lack of affinity for dopamine receptors, the 5-HT$_3$ receptor antagonists have not been associated with any extrapyramidal effects. The overall impression is that these agents are well tolerated in comparison with conventional antiemetics.

It is difficult to assess antiemetic efficacy of any drug in phase I studies because of the small numbers of patients involved, the prior treatment of some subjects (rendering them less responsive) and the lack of a comparison group. The presence of complete antiemetic protection in a proportion of patients who have received high-dose cisplatin is encouraging.

IV. PHASE II STUDIES

Phase II studies have been reported for ondansetron[19,31] granisetron[32] and ICS 205-930[20,33] which confirm the efficacy apparent in phase I trials (see Table 2). For batanopride no phase II studies were available, but the results from phase trials have been pooled by Smaldone et al.[17] The issues that have been addressed include schedule-dependency, dose-

TABLE 2
Complete Antiemetic Protection Rates (CR) in Phase II Studies with 50 or More Patients

Drug	No. of subjects evaluable	Chemotherapy	CR[a] (%)	Ref.
Granisetron	288	Cisplatin >49 mg/m² mixed[b]	59	31
	443		79	32
Ondansetron	83	Cisplatin ≥100 mg/m²	75	19
ICS 205-930	100	Cisplatin ≥50 mg/m²	54	20
Batanopride[c]	52	Cisplatin	—[c]	17

[a] Percent of patients with no emetic episodes in the first 24 h.
[b] Anthracyclines, cyclophosphamide, DTIC, cisplatin <50 mg/m², nitrogen mustard.
[c] Pooled results from phase I indicate 0—2 episodes in 67% (% CR not stated).

dependency, maintenance of efficacy with daily dosing and benefit in patients refractory to conventional agents.

A. SCHEDULE-DEPENDENCY

Ondansetron has been reported to show similar efficacy whether given every 2 vs. every 4 h[29] or every 6 h vs. every 8 h.[19] One would anticipate, however, that the differences in efficacy with these modest variations in schedule would be small. The same size of these trials (20 and 83 patients) does not allow one to rule out an effect of schedule on efficacy. For example, in the larger study 95% confidence limits on the difference in complete protection rates extend from −23 to +14% in favor of the more frequent administration.

With single doses of granisetron and ICS 250-930 there are reports that emesis may begin late in the first 24 h.[33,34] This may reflect inadequate blood levels beyond 12 h or breakthrough via another mechanism. Studies are in progress with several of these compounds to determine whether a single dose is as effective as repeated doses or continuous infusions. Based upon pharmacokinetic considerations, one would anticipate that repeat doses are necessary but it has been demonstrated that metoclopramide (terminal half-life of 6 h[35]) may have excellent efficacy even when given as a single dose.[36]

B. DOSE-DEPENDENCY

In phase I trials the escalating doses used to establish the maximal tolerable amount may also provide information about the dose-range or blood levels that are likely to be effective (albeit with wide confidence limits). For example, pooling of the results within a dose-ranging study by Grunberg et al. suggested that doses ≥0.30 mg/kg provided significantly more complete protection than lower doses.[24] A study of ICS 250-930 (5 vs. 10 vs. 20 mg/m²) by Seinen et al. showed no apparent difference in efficacy between dose levels.[33] No information is available thus far which would allow one to comment on the relationship between the dose and effect of batanopride.

In a study of granisetron, Carmichael et al. found higher plasma levels at 5 h in responders than nonresponders.[14] In contrast, Addelman et al. could find no correlation between pharmacokinetic parameters and efficacy.[18] In two large dose-finding studies of this agent, Tabona et al.[32] reported no difference in efficacy or adverse effects over a fourfold range in dose (40 to 60 μg/kg). Thus for granisetron it appears that there is no benefit in exceeding 40 μg/kg. The lowest effective dose has not been well defined for any of these compounds.

C. EFFICACY WITH MULTIPLE DAY CHEMOTHERAPY

There are reports of ondansetron given with multiple day chemotherapy which suggest that, despite maintenance therapy, there is some loss of efficacy on subsequent days.[15,29]

TABLE 3
Phase III Studies

Chemotherapy	No. of subjects	Antiemetics	CR Rate (%)	Ref.
Cisplatin (50—100 mg/m²)	61	hd mcp vs. ondansetron	18 41	42
Cisplatin (80—100 mg/m²)	76	hd mcp vs. ondansetron	16 46	40
Cisplatin (>49 mg/m²)	234	hd mcp + dex vs. granisetron	69 70	43
FAC/FEC	65	md mcp vs. ondansetron	27 66	44
Moderately emetogenic	228	dex + cpz vs. granisetron	49 70	45

Note: Abbreviations: % CR = % of patients free of emesis.
hd mcp = high-dose metoclopramide.
md mcp = moderate-dose metoclopramide.
dex = dexamethasone.
cpz = chlorpromazine.
FAC/FEC = fluorouracil, cyclophosphamide, and doxorubicin (A) or epirubicin (E).

This type of breakthrough also has been reported for patients receiving radiation therapy.[37] These results are compatible with the information that maintenance dexamethasone plus metoclopramide is associated with delayed onset upset after even one dose of cisplatin.[5] The mechanism of this problem is unknown but could be due to an alternative mechanism for delayed onset emesis or tachyphylaxis.

D. EFFICACY IN PATIENTS REFRACTORY TO OTHER AGENTS

There are encouraging reports about the efficacy of these agents in patients who are refractory to conventional antiemetics.[38,39] It is difficult to draw conclusions however because of the lack of information about prior antiemetics and the absence of information about whether or not patients with anticipatory upset were included.

V. PHASE III STUDIES

Thus far few studies have been reported which compare 5-HT$_3$ receptor antagonists with standard antiemetics although many are in progress. Since high-dose metoclopramide blocks receptors for dopamine as well as 5-HT$_3$ it is possible that efficacy would actually be decreased with the more selective agents. The evidence to date suggests that this is not the case. Table 3 summarizes the results of five phase III studies.

De Mulder et al. conducted a double-blind cross-over study of ondansetron vs. metoclopramide (both given by bolus plus infusion), in patients receiving 50 to 100 mg/m² of cisplatin.[40] The results at 24 h were significantly better for the selective antagonist in terms of nausea, emesis and patient preference. In this study, the complete protection rate from emesis with metoclopramide was 18% which is lower than reported by Kris.[2] This may be explained either by the substantially higher proportion of females in this study or random variation. Although the manner of administration of metoclopramide differed from the most commonly used schedules, it was based upon a randomized study that showed superiority over an intermittent schedule.[41] There were no significant differences in adverse events. The frequency of headaches and constipation was greater in the ondansetron group. Metoclopramide was associated with more diarrhea and extrapyramidal effects occurred only with this drug. In a study of similar design, Marty et al.[42] also found that ondansetron was much more effective than high-dose metoclopramide with a complete response rate in both groups that was virtually identical to that reported by De Mulder.

Chevallier has reported the results of a large (234 patients), single-blind study of granisetron given as a single dose vs. dexamethasone plus high-dose metoclopramide for patients receiving >49 mg/m^2 of cisplatin.[43] The proportion of complete responders was 70 and 69%, respectively. The addition of dexamethasone to the metoclopramide (because this represents the best standard therapy) may increase the complete protection rate by 20%.[3] Equivalence with granisetron alone is, therefore, an important result particularly in light of the significant difference in extrapyramidal effects (10.8 vs. 0%) in favor of the granisetron. In this study there was a statistically significant increase in headaches with granisetron (11.4 vs. 3.3%). The conclusion based on these data is that ondansetron and granisetron are as good as or superior to high-dose metoclopramide for high-dose cisplatin therapy.

There have been two studies using these same agents for therapy other than high-dose cisplatin therapy. Bonneterre et al. compared ondansetron with an intermediate dose of metoclopramide (60 mg i.v. plus 20 mg every 8 h) in patients receiving fluorouracil, cyclophosphamide, and either doxorubicin or epirubicin.[44] The trial design was double-blind and there was a cross-over although only the results of the first course were used because of a period effect. The superiority in terms of control of nausea and emesis as well as delayed emesis was statistically significant. This study indicates clear superiority for ondansetron but the standard arm of metoclopramide may be criticized because it is not one that has been previously demonstrated to be effective.

Marty et al. presented results of a randomized, single-blind study comparing a single dose of granisetron to dexamethasone plus chlorpromazine in patients receiving moderately emetogenic therapy.[45] This chemotherapy consisted of a variety of agents (cyclophosphamide, anthracyclines, DTIC, low dose cisplatin, etc.). The 31% difference in the complete emetic response rate in favor of the granisetron was statistically significant. While there were more headaches in the granisetron group (13.9 vs. 6.2%, p value not significant), adverse events were significantly more common overall in the control group. The conclusion from this study is that granisetron is more effective than a standard antiemetic therapy of dexamethasone plus chlorpromazine.

There have been no studies reported thus far that compare the other selective receptor antagonists to standard therapy. No trials have compared these compounds to each other.

Cunningham has reported that dexamethasone plus ondansetron is an effective combination in patients who are not responsive to ondansetron alone and there is reportedly corroboration of additive effects in the ferret model.[46] A randomized, double-blind study by Roila et al. confirms that, for chemotherapy that includes cisplatin, dexamethasone appears to improve the effectiveness of ondansetron.[47] Several studies are underway using other chemotherapy and other 5-HT$_3$ receptor antagonists to test this question.

VI. CONCLUSIONS

The selective serotonin antagonists demonstrate antiemetic activity that appears to be greater than or equal to high-dose metoclopramide and superior to dexamethasone. The experience to date does not allow one to conclude anything about the efficacy of these drugs relative to each other or their optimal schedule. There may be benefit in combining 5-HT$_3$ receptor antagonists with glucocorticoids but controlled trials are required. The side effects appear to be less troublesome than those associated with metoclopramide and, in particular, there are no extrapyramidal effects. For this reason alone these drugs will quickly establish themselves as an important advance in the prevention of nausea and vomiting due to chemotherapy.

REFERENCES

1. Gralla, R. J., Itri, L. M., Pisko, S. E., Squillante, A. E., Kelsen, D. P., Braun, D. W., Jr., Borden, L. A., Braun, T. J., and Young, C. W., Antiemetic efficacy of high-dose metoclopramide: randomized trials with placebo and prochlorperazine in patients with chemotherapy-induced nausea and vomiting, *N. Engl. J. Med.*, 305, 905, 1981.

2. Kris, M. G., Gralla, R. J., Tyson, L. B., Clark, R. A., Kelsen, D. P., Reilly, L. D., Groshen, S., Bosl, G. J., and Kalman, L. A., Improved control of cisplatin-induced emesis with high-dose metoclopramide and with combinations of metoclopramide, dexamethasone, and diphenhydramine: results of consecutive trials in 255 patients, *Cancer*, 55, 527, 1985.

3. Roila, F., Tonato, M., Basurto, C., Bella, M., Passalacqua, R., Morsia, D., DiCostanzo, F., Donati, D., Ballatori, E., Tognoni, G., Franzosi, M. G., and Del Favero, A., Antiemetic activity of high doses of metoclopramide combined with methylprednisolone versus metoclopramide alone in cisplatin-treated cancer patients: a randomized double-blind trial in the Italian Oncology Group for Clinical Research, *J. Clin. Oncol.*, 5, 141, 1987.

4. Kris, M. G., Gralla, R. J., Clark, R. A., Tyson, L. B., and Groshen, S., Antiemetic control and prevention of side-effects of anticancer therapy with lorazepam or diphenhydramine when used in combination with metoclopramide plus dexamethasone: a double-blind, randomized trial, *Cancer*, 60, 2816, 1987.

5. Kris, M. G., Gralla, R. J., Tyson, L. B., Clark, R. A., Cirrincione, C., and Groshen, S., Controlling delayed vomiting: double-blind, randomized trial comparing placebo, dexamethasone alone, and metoclopramide plus dexamethasone in patients receiving cisplatin, *J. Clin. Oncol.*, 7, 108, 1989.

6. Grunberg, S. M., Aler, E., McDremed, J. E., and Akerley, W. L., Oral metoclopramide with or without diphenhydramine: potential for prevention of late nausea and vomiting induced cisplatin, *J. Natl. Cancer Inst.*, 80, 864, 1988.

7. Costall, B., Domeney, A. M., Naylor, R. J., and Tattersal, F. D., Emesis induced by cisplatin in the ferret as a model for the detection of anti-emetic drugs, *Neuropharmacology*, 26, 1321, 1987.

8. Tonato, M., Roila, F., Del Favero, A., Tognoni, G., Franzosi, M. G., and Pampallona, S., A pilot study of high-dose domperidone as an antiemetic in patients treated with cisplatin, *Eur. J. Cancer Clin. Oncol.*, 21, 807, 1985.

9. Bradley, P. B., Engel, G., Fenluk, W., Fozard, J. R., Humphrey, P. P. A., Middlemiss, D. N., Mylecharane, E. J., Richardson, B. P., and Saxena, P. R., Commentary: proposals for the classification and nomenclature of functional receptors for 5-Hydroxytryptamine, *Neuropharmacology*, 25, 563, 1986.

10. Miner, W. D. and Sanger, G. J., Inhibition of cisplatin-induced vomiting of selective 5-hydroxytryptamine M-receptor antagonism, *Br. J. Pharmacol.*, 88, 497, 1986.

11. Smith, W. L., Alphin, R. S., Jackson, C. B., and Sancilio, L. F., The antiemetic profile of zacopride, *J. Pharm. Pharmacol.*, 41, 101, 1989.

12. Lucot, J. B., Blockade of 5-hydroxytryptamine$_3$ receptors prevents cisplatin-induced but not motion- or xylazine-induced emesis in the cat, *Pharmacol. Biochem. Behav.*, 32, 207, 1989.

13. Brady, M. E., Dandekar, K. A., Pfeffer, M., Sartiano, G. P., Alberts, D. S., Plezia, P., and Smaldone, L., Pharmacokinetics of batanopride (BMY-25801). A new antiemetic in cancer patients, *Proc. Am. Soc. Clin. Oncol.*, 8, 330, 1985.

14. Carmichael, J., Cantwell, B. M. J., Edwards, C. M., Zussman, B. D., Thompson, S., Rapeport, W. G., and Harris, A. L., A pharmacokinetic study of granisetron (BRL 43694A), a selective 5-HT$_3$ receptor antagonist: correlation with anti-emetic response, *Cancer Chemother. Pharmacol.*, 24, 45, 1989.

15. Lazarus, H. M., Blumer, J. L., and Bryson, J. C., Antiemetic efficacy and pharmacokinetic (PK) analyses of GR 38032F during multiple day cisplatin (DDP) prior to autologous bone marrow transplantation (ABMT), *Proc. Am. Soc. Clin. Oncol.*, 8, 327, 1989.

16. Tyson, L. B., Gralla, R. J., Kris, M. G., and Clark, R. A., Phase I antiemetic study of the serotonin antagonist ICS 205-930, *Proc. Am. Soc. Clin. Oncol.*, 8, 331, 1985.

17. Smaldone, L., Fairchild, C., Rozencweig, M., Aapro, M., Sartiano, G., Plezia, P., and Alberts, D., Dose-range evaluation of BMY-25801, a non-dopaminergic antiemetic, *Proc. Am. Soc. Clin. Oncol.*, 7, 280, 1988.

18. Addelman, M., Erlichman, C., Fine, S., Warr, D., and Murray, C., Phase I/II trial of BRL43694: a novel 5-HT$_3$ antagonist for the prevention of chemotherapy induced nausea and vomiting, *J. Clin. Oncol.*, 8, 337, 1990.

19. Hesketh, P. J., Murphy, W. K., Lester, E. P., Gandara, D. R., Khojasteh, A., Tapazoglou, E., Sartiano, G. P., White, D. R., Werner, K., and Chubb, J. M., GR38032F (GR-C507/75): a novel compound effective in the prevention of acute cisplatin-induced emesis, *J. Clin. Oncol.*, 7, 700, 1989.

20. Stamatakis, L., Michel, J., Van Bell, S., Cocquyt, V., Keppens, C., Van Hove, R., De Belder, B., and Roosens, W., ICS 205-930: a dose finding study in the prevention of cisplatin induced nausea and vomiting, *Proc. Am. Soc. Clin. Oncol.*, 8, 327, 1989.

21. Coupe, M., Adverse reaction to the 5-HT₃ receptor antagonist ICS 205930, *Lancet*, i, 1494, 1987.
22. Clark, R. A., Kris, M. G., Gralla, R. J., and Tyson, L. B., Serotonin antagonists demonstrate antiemetic (AE) effectiveness without extrapyramidal symptoms: analysis of studies with 3 new agents in 155 patients (pts), *Proc. Am. Soc. Clin. Oncol.*, 9, 322, 1990.
23. Khojasteh, A., Ruble, K., Chambers, J., Coleman, J., and Ahmed, K., The antiemetic response to GR-C507/75 (GR-39032F) (GR) in patients (PTS) receiving multiple-dose cisplatin (DDP) regimens, *Proc. Am. Soc. Clin. Oncol.*, 7, 298, 1988.
24. Grunberg, S. M., Stevenson, L. L., Russell, C. A., and McDermed, J. E., Dose ranging phase I study of the serotonin antagonist GR38032F for prevention of cisplatin-induced nausea and vomiting, *J. Clin. Oncol.*, 7, 1137, 1989.
25. Leibundgut, U. and Lancranjan, I., First results with ICS 205-930 (5-HT₃ receptor antagonist) in prevention of chemotherapy-induced emesis, Lancet, 1 (#8543), 1198, 1987.
26. Plezia, P. M., Davis, L. E., Alberts, D. S., Davis, A., Garewal, H. S., Greenberg, B. R., Smaldone, L., and Fairchild, C., BMY-25801: an effective single agent antiemetic (A) for cisplatin (C)-induced nausea (N) and vomiting (V), *Proc. Am. Soc. Clin. Oncol.*, 7, 294, 1988.
27. Tabona, M. V., Granisetron — a clinical perspective, presented at ECCO 5, The Treatment of Cytostatic Drug-Induced Emesis, London, September 3, 1989, 29.
28. Smith, R. N., Safety of Ondansetron, *Eur. J. Cancer Clin. Oncol.*, 25 (Suppl. 1), s47, 1989.
29. Kris, M. G., Gralla, R. J., Clark, R. A., and Tyson, L. B., Phase II trials of the serotonin antagonist GR38032F for the control of vomiting caused by cisplatin, *J. Natl. Cancer Inst.*, 81, 42, 1989.
30. Sartiano, G. P., Early, W., Early, J., Fairchild, C. J., Crenshaw, R. R., and Schwartz, S. E., BMY-25801-01 (BMY): a non-antidopaminergic agent to prevent cisplatin-induced nausea and vomiting, *Proc. Am. Soc. Clin. Oncol.*, 6, 272, 1987.
31. Cubeddu, L. X., Hoffmann, I. S., Fuenmayor, N. T., and Finn, A. L., Efficacy of Ondansetron (GR 38032F) and the role of serotonin in cisplatin-induced nausea and vomiting, *N. Engl. J. Med.*, 322, 810, 1990.
32. Tabona, M. V., Granisetron in the prevention of cytostatic induced emesis, *Proc. Am. Soc. Clin. Oncol.*, 9, 319, 1990.
33. Seinen, H., Zonnenberg, B. A., Tjia, P., and Neijt, J. P., The effect of three dose levels of ICS 205-930 (a selective 5-HT₃ antagonist) on cisplatin-induced nausea and vomiting, *Eur. J. Cancer Clin. Oncol.*, 25, 1333, 1989.
34. Carmichael, J., Cantwell, M. J., Edwards, C. M., Rapeport, W. G., and Harris, A. L., The serotonin type 3 receptor antagonist BRL 43694 and nausea and vomiting induced by cisplatin, *Br. Med. J.*, 297, 110, 1988.
35. Taylor, W. B., Simpson, J. M., and Bateman, D. N., High-dose metoclopramide by infusion: a double-blind study of plasma concentration-effect relationships in patients receiving cancer chemotherapy, *Eur. J. Clin. Pharmacol.*, 33, 161, 1987.
36. Clark, R. A., Gralla, R. J., Kris, M. G., and Tyson, L. B., Exploring very high doses of metoclopramide (4—6 mg/kg): preservation of efficacy and safety with only a single dose in a combination antiemetic regimen, *Proc. Am. Soc. Clin. Oncol.*, 8, 330, 1989.
37. Priestman, T. J. and Priestman, S. G., Studies with ondansetron in the management of radiation-induced emesis, presented at Ondansetron Symp., London, June 29 to 30, 1989, 34.
38. Cunningham, D., Hawthorn, J., Pople, A., Gazet, J. C., Ford, H. T., and Challoner, T., Prevention of emesis in patients receiving cytotoxic drugs by GR38032F, a selective 5-HT₃ receptor antagonist, *Lancet*, 1 (#8548), 1461, 1987.
39. Green, J. A., Watkin, S. W., Hammond, P., Griggs, J., and Challoner, T., The efficacy of safety of GR38032F in the prophylaxis of ifosfamide-induced nausea and vomiting, *Cancer Chemother. Pharmacol.*, 24, 137, 1989.
40. De Mulder, P., Seynaeve, C., Van Liessum, P., Verweij, J., Vermorken, J., and Lane-Allman, E., A multicentre double blind comparison of ondansetron (GR38032F) and metoclopramide in the prophylaxis of acute emesis induced by cisplatin, presented at ECCO 5, London, September 3, 1989, (#0-0501).
41. Warrington, P. S., Allan, S. G., Cornbleet, M. A., MacPherson, J. S., Smyth, J. F., and Leonard, R. C. F., Optimizing antiemesis in cancer chemotherapy: efficacy of continuous versus intermittent infusion of high-dose metoclopramide in emesis induced by cisplatin, *Br. Med. J.*, 293, 1334, 1986.
42. Marty, M., Pouillart, P., Scholl, S., Droz, J. P., Azab, M., Brion, N., Pujade-Lauraine, E., Paule, B., Paes, D., and Bons, J., Comparison of the 5-Hydroxytryptamine₃ (serotonin) antagonist ondansetron (GR 38032F) with high-dose metoclopramide in the control of cisplatin-induced emesis, *N. Engl. J. Med.*, 322, 816, 1990.
43. Chevallier, B., Granisetron compared with high-dose metoclopramide plus dexamethasone in patients receiving high-dose cisplatin, presented at ECCO 5, The Treatment of Cytostatic Drug-Induced Emesis, London, September 3, 1989, 27.

44. **Bonneterre, J., Chevallier, B., Metz, R., Fargeot, P., Pujade-Lauraine, E., Speilman, M., Tubiana, M., and Bons, J.,** The 5-HT$_3$ antagonist GR38032F is superior to metoclopramide (MCL) in the prophylaxis of FAC/FEC-induced emesis, *Proc. Am. Soc. Clin. Oncol.*, 8, 324, 1989.

45. **Marty, M.,** Graniseton compared with chlorpromazine plus dexamethasone in patients receiving other emetogenic chemotherapy, presented at ECCO 5, The Treatment of Cytostatic Drug-Induced Emesis, London, September 3, 1989, 25.

46. **Cunningham, D., Turner, A., Hawthorn, J., and Rosin, R. D.,** Ondansetron with and without dexamethasone to treat chemotherapy-induced emesis, *Lancet*, 1 (#8650), 1323, 1989.

47. **Roila, F., Tonato, M., Cognetti, F., Cortesi, E., Favalli, G., Marangolo, M., Amadori, D., Cocconi, G., Cellerino, R., Donati, D., Ballatori, E., and Del Favero, A.,** A double-blind multicenter crossover study comparing the antiemetic efficacy and tolerability of ondansetron (ond) vs ond plus dexamethasone (dex) in cisplatin (cddp) treated cancer patients (pts), *Proc. Am. Soc. Clin. Oncol.*, 9, 339, 1990.

Chapter 20

PAIN AND QUALITY OF LIFE: THEORETICAL ASPECTS

Russell K. Portenoy

TABLE OF CONTENTS

I. INTRODUCTION

There is growing recognition that the management of the patient with cancer pain must have goals beyond analgesia alone.[1] These patients often have a degree of psychological distress disproportionate to the severity of pain, as well as multiple symptoms other than pain, each of which may be influenced by physical, psychological, and social factors that change continually and unpredictably over time. This complexity requires a therapeutic approach to the palliation of symptoms that is both flexible and comprehensive.

The shift from an emphasis on pain relief alone to an approach in which the treatment of pain is considered within a larger clinical context depends on an accurate assessment of the patient.[2-7] Many of the issues raised by this assessment are fundamentally similar to those long considered to be central to the evaluation of "quality of life".[8] These include the relationship of pain to the physical, psychological, social functioning of the patient; the role of pain treatment among multiple other therapies; and the meaning of "satisfactory" symptom control in the large proportion of patients who never achieve "complete" relief. The interplay between physical and psychological factors that is fundamental in this process determines the global well-being of the patient, as well as the experience of the pain itself.

Unfortunately, the recognition that a comprehensive approach to cancer pain management links it directly to larger issues in quality of life has not been mirrored by a theoretical or empirical realignment of either the pain or quality of life literature. Indeed, it is likely that cancer pain specialists and those whose focus is quality of life discuss many of the same issues, but use different nomenclature. For example, the terms that appear prominently in the pain literature to suggest a focus on a broader evaluation of patient well-being, such as "suffering"[9,10] and "total pain",[11,12] or the concepts defined by "continuing care",[1] "supportive care",[13,14] "palliative care",[15] and "hospice care",[16] are not discussed in writings about quality of life; similarly, quality of life itself, which would seem a core construct in any discussion about the well-being of the cancer patient,[17-22] is seldom mentioned in the pain literature.

II. PAIN AND QUALITY OF LIFE: PROBLEMS OF ASSESSMENT

The potential confusion that may arise from the use of different terms to describe the same phenomena is compounded by the lack of research that specifically explores the interrelationships among the various dimensions of pain and quality of life. This continues despite general agreement that the perception of pain is an important element in the overall well-being of the patient with cancer.[1,17,21,23-27] To a large extent, the process has been hindered by the difficulties encountered in defining and measuring the clinical phenomena of pain and quality of life.

A. DEFINITION AND ASSESSMENT OF QUALITY OF LIFE

From a theoretical standpoint, most discussions of quality of life implicitly endorse a multidimensional view of health that encompasses both the lack of disease and the experience of well-being. The experience of well-being, in turn, is clearly influenced by many factors, some of which are directly related to medical illness and others independent of it. This view appears in the definition of health adopted by the World Health Organization: "not only the absence of infirmity and disease but also a state of physical, mental and social well-being".[28]

The physical, psychological, and social dimensions included in this definition of health are widely accepted components of the construct, "quality of life".[17-19,21,24,26,29-31] Each of these dimensions is itself complex, however, and measurement of each requires careful consideration of the specific information desired. As the first step, it is useful to describe each dimension with respect to the types of disturbances that occur with disease and its treatment. Thus, the physical dimension is typically depicted in terms of the experience of symptoms (including pain), the integrity of body image, the ability to be freely mobile, and the capacity to perform activities of daily living or work. The psychological dimension usually incorporates any of several affective disturbances (e.g., depression and anxiety) and the ability to cope. The social dimension often includes reference to the integrity of the family, financial status, and both medical and nonmedical support networks.

The complexity of these factors, any combination of which may predominate in determining the global well-being of the patient, is augmented by the existence of other dimensions that are even more difficult to define operationally and measure in a reliable and valid way. The influence of a spiritual domain is accepted by many investigators,[17,30] and others, such as a cultural perspective, may also be important.[17]

Notwithstanding the multiple factors that contribute to quality of life, it is also true that the patient with chronic illness is typically able to integrate these perceptions into a global description of well-being. Indeed, the degree of "satisfaction" or "well-being," which has been usefully defined as the perceived difference between personal desires and current status,[17] is generally considered to be a critical feature in quality of life assessment.

This description of the construct, "quality of life", suggests the features that would have to be included in an optimal assessment. Since quality of life is inherently subjective, an assessment should employ self-report measures;[21,30,32] some objective measures, however, such as performance status, may contribute to the overall evaluation. There should be both a general measure of well-being or satisfaction and independent measures of the various dimensions that may contribute to this perception.[21,22,30] Indeed, it is likely that additional information could be obtained if a scale of global satisfaction were applied to each domain independently (e.g., psychological, social, physical, etc.), as well as to the overall perception of quality of life. Instruments to assess these factors must be sensitive to changes over time and should be able to record positive elements and improvement in quality of life, as well as the factors that can comprise well-being. Finally, it is generally agreed that an optimal assessment tool for measuring quality of life should be reliable and valid, capable of providing subscale scores (each reflecting a different domain of experience), and acceptable to the patient.[22,30]

Despite substantial advances in methodology, efforts to integrate a quality-of-life assessment into clinical trials of antineoplastic therapies has only just begun. Most clinical trials have not measured any component of quality of life, and most of those that have addressed the issue have relied solely on measures of physical functioning (e.g., Karnofsky Performance Status Scale).[19,29,30] Although a determination of performance status may be all that is possible in trials of patients with far advanced disease, whose deteriorating physical and cognitive status can preclude the use of even simple self-assessment scales,[33] both the limitations of performance status scales[34] and the need for a more comprehensive quality-of-life assessment are becoming increasingly clear.[21,26,35-38] It is therefore encouraging to note that quality-of-life assessment tools have been successfully implemented in a few recent studies.[39-41]

1. Pain in Quality-of-Life Assessment

Pain assessment has usually,[42-46] but not always,[47] been incorporated into scales designed to evaluate symptom distress and general health status. These instruments do not specifically measure quality of life, but there is clearly overlap between the constructs they attempt to assess and the dimensions commonly considered to be fundamental to quality of life. These measures typically include several items that determine pain intensity; one also evaluates the experience of uncontrolled pain.[45] None has been employed in clinical trials.

Instruments designed specifically to assess quality of life have also usually incorporated some measure of pain. The QL-Index,[48] an early and validated tool that is often used to cross-validate new instruments, is an important exception. Most others include a pain-related question or two. For example, a relatively popular instrument, the Functional Living Index-Cancer,[27] uses visual analog scales completed by the patient to rate the amount of pain related to the cancer and the degree to which pain interferes with daily activities. Of note, a recent controlled trial of chemotherapy in patients with advanced non-small cell lung cancer attempted to implement this scale as an outcome measure, but found that the physical and cognitive impairments in this population limited compliance.[33,40]

This experience with the Functional Living Index-Cancer underscores the difficulties inherent in the assessment of pain within the context of a more general quality of life determination. Since patients with advanced disease are the group most likely to experience pain, any procedure designed to assess the relationship between pain and quality of life must be able to be implemented in this population. The need to be brief and simple, in turn, demands that very few questions relate to any single factor, such as pain. This may create more problems, since the effort to shorten and refine pain-related questions, and thereby capture the most important information precisely, may unintentionally introduce qualifiers that can confuse the severely ill patient and compromise data collection still further.

Other quality-of-life scales assess diverse aspects of the pain experienced by the cancer patient. Some determine only the presence of pain and its intensity. Others also evaluate the distress associated with the pain.[25,39] The degree of pain relief experienced by the patient is measured in an instrument developed by the European Organization for Research and Treatment of Cancer Study Group on Quality of Life.[24]

B. DEFINITION AND ASSESSMENT OF PAIN

Pain, like quality of life, is a subjective and multidimensional perception.[4,6,49-53] One clinically relevant conceptualization suggests that pain has three major dimensions, comprising a sensory-discriminative component (including severity, location, and quality), an affective-motivational component (including pain-related distress and associated mood disturbances), and a cognitive-evaluative component (attitudes and beliefs about the pain).[49] The severity of pain, which can be assessed using valid instruments and methodologies[54-56] and is the characteristic grasped most readily by patients and clinicians, represents only one facet of this complex experience. Indeed, the report of pain severity is itself determined by numerous interacting factors, including some that are inherent in the stimulus (such as its intensity or type) and some that originate with the patient (such as the degree of anxiety).

Another paradigm that reflects the complexity of clinical pain and is particularly relevant to the cancer population conceptualizes pain as a perception related to nociception and suffering.[5] Nociception refers to the activity induced in afferent neural pathways by stimuli that are potentially tissue damaging. It is almost invariable that the pain of cancer patients is associated with a lesion capable of producing nociception. Nociception, however, is not equivalent to pain, and indeed, is neither necessary nor sufficient for pain perception. Pain may be absent despite evident nociception (immediately after trauma for example), or may be severe with little or no nociception. This observation reflects the potential contribution of multiple non-nociceptive processes in the pathogenesis of pain. These non-nociceptive factors may be related to identifiable changes in the function of the nervous system, or reflect the impact of psychological factors. Thus, although most cancer patients have ongoing nociception as the predominating factor in sustaining pain (this has been termed nociceptive pain[57]), many other factors — physical, psychological, and social — can influence this process and alter the severity or other characteristics of the pain.

This distinction between nociception and pain is usually discussed with reference to a third level of experience, which has been termed "suffering" in the pain literature.[5,8-10] Suffering can be defined as a more global aversive experience that relates to numerous perceptions, one of which may be pain. The suffering of a patient with cancer pain may range from slight to profound, and often appears to be only loosely related to the presence or severity of pain. Suffering may relate to the experience of symptoms other than pain, the loss of physical functioning, isolation from family, financial concerns, fear of death, or any number of other issues. The potential for numerous contributing factors is evidenced in the observation that amelioration of any single problem, such as pain, may not change the level of suffering.

From this description, it is evident that the construct of suffering overlaps that of quality of life. Indeed, suffering may be viewed operationally as impairment of quality of life, whereas the relief of suffering can be considered to be improvement in quality of life. The degree of suffering cannot be equated with quality of life, however. The absence of suffering does not indicate a sense of well-being or satisfaction, a positive side of experience that is included within the quality-of-life construct. There have been no efforts to empirically evaluate suffering, and though the construct is intuitively meaningful to clinicians, it is probably preferable to focus on quality of life, rather than suffering, in future investigations of these issues.

Thus, notwithstanding great improvements in the epistemology and assessment methodologies for both pain and quality of life, it is evident that the information directly accessible about the relationship between these phenomena, as determined from the assessment of pain in quality-of-life instruments or the evaluation of quality of life in measures of pain, is very limited. Furthermore, currently available instruments highlight the problems that must be overcome to elucidate these issues. Any useful assessment must provide patient-generated data, be brief and simple enough for a severely ill population, and yield comprehensive information adequate to characterize and relate the multiple dimensions of quality of life and pain. Although it is likely that the pain assessment included in most quality-of-life instruments could be improved, studies capable of substantively illuminating the relationship between these phenomena will probably require the use of multiple tools or the development of a quality-of-life measure that sacrifices some types of information to gain more about pain.

III. PAIN AND QUALITY OF LIFE: CLINICAL OBSERVATIONS AND CURRENT RESEARCH

The relationship between pain and quality of life in patients with cancer must ultimately be evaluated through surveys that systematically assess the various dimensions described by these two constructs. Given the complexity of this assessment, the procedures for future studies must be carefully scrutinized to ensure the collection of valid and generalizable data. This is facilitated by the elaboration of hypotheses, which clarify the important issues and can be tested through specific analyses. Hypotheses, in turn, can be derived from two broad types of information, (1) clinical observations of patients with cancer pain and (2) inferences relevant to quality of life drawn from research in the pain population.

A. CLINICAL OBSERVATIONS

It is often taken as axiomatic that pain has a prominent influence on quality of life and that the direction of this influence is intuitively obvious, i.e., more pain always worsens, and relief of pain always improves, quality of life. Many clinical observations suggest that these assumptions neither describe the situation of most pain patients nor predict the outcome of those who develop pain or are relieved of it.

Some observations are particularly relevant:

1. As suggested previously, the severity of pain in the cancer patient is related to the degree of nociception, but nociception is insufficient to explain the severity of pain

or the degree of distress it produces. It is common to encounter patients with nociceptive lesions (e.g., a pathological fracture of a bone) who report minimal or no pain, or equally remarkable, patients with stable nociceptive lesions whose pain wanes without treatment or fluctuates widely with the degree of psychological distress.

2.   The severity of pain is directly related to the degree of psychological distress associated with the pain, but severity alone is not sufficient to explain the degree or type of this distress. Support for the independence of pain severity and distress can be adduced from the experimental literature, in which it has been demonstrated that pain severity and unpleasantness following an analgesic intervention can be measured separately.[58] Implicit in these observations is the notion that patients may express psychological distress that they relate to the experience of pain, and that this can be distinguished from psychological distress driven by other factors, or at least attached to other factors by the patient. This is an extension of the multidimensional model of pain discussed previously,[49] which postulated an affective-motivational component to the experience. Cancer patients have many reasons to experience psychological distress, and if possible, pain assessment should determine whether pain is the overriding element, one of several experiences sustaining distress, or a minor factor compared to others.

3.   In addition to pain severity, chronicity is a critical factor that influences the distress associated with the pain. Importantly, chronicity refers to the *perceived* duration of the pain, and includes the length of time pain has already been experienced, the course of the pain during that time (getting better or worse), the anticipation that the pain will lessen or cease, the expected interval before improvement will begin, and the anticipated time required for substantial improvement. The relative importance of these various elements of perceived chronicity is unknown, and represents another important area for investigation. To the extent that these temporal influences can be distinguished from the many other facets of the pain, it can be conjectured that the distress associated with pain is relatively great soon after onset (during the acute phase), declines for a time thereafter, but increases again with the realization that pain will be a chronic problem.

4.   The meaning of the pain to the patient may also strongly influence the psychological distress associated with the pain, and perhaps, pain severity as well. The meaning to the patient includes the beliefs and attitudes about the pain, among the most important of which is the perceived relationship to the progression of the cancer. Both uncertainty of diagnosis and the knowledge that pain relates to the progression of disease can be profoundly distressing. Indeed, the anxiety noted soon after pain onset often appears to relate less to any difficulty coping with the pain itself than to the meaning of the pain in terms of the underlying disease. In this situation, pain-related distress, and sometimes pain severity, may greatly improve if the patient can be informed that pain is not due to progressive disease. More remarkable, the distress of many patients diminishes as soon as the cause of the pain becomes an issue to the physician, well before the diagnosis is established. In these cases, knowledge that the uncertainty is being addressed may be the most salutary aspect. As another indication of the importance of meaning, some patients strongly resist therapy that will completely eradicate the pain, stating that they rely on pain to monitor the disease and would be more distressed by the knowledge that pain was completely ''suppressed'' than by the experience of pain itself.

5.   The perceived availability and efficacy of measures to relieve the pain is another major influence on pain-related distress, and perhaps pain severity. This factor is closely related to the perceived chronicity of the pain. A corollary observation is that the modality of treatment may be an important determinant in this process. For example, some patients are comforted by the availability of opioid analgesics to relieve the pain,

whereas others are significantly distressed by the use of this approach, either as a result of properties they perceive in the drugs themselves (e.g., addiction) or from the knowledge that they treat the pain but not the underlying cause, which is presumably progressing.

6. The severity, chronicity, and meaning of the pain, the perceived availability of relief, and the degree of psychological distress specifically associated with the pain are all related to the more global experience of suffering, or alternatively, to impaired quality of life. Although these factors are interrelated, it is herein suggested that each may have an independent effect on quality of life. The manner by which these phenomena affect quality of life is usually predictable (e.g., more severe pain is associated with greater impairment in quality of life), but there are many patients who demonstrate unusual patterns, and these may be important in understanding the complexity of the relationships. For example, some patients, usually those whose pain is not severe, will evince a greater degree of suffering when pain is relieved through treatment.

7. All these phenomena, including suffering or quality of life, vary dynamically and can change rapidly or more slowly, on a day-to-day or week-to-week basis. They may vary together or independently.

8. In some patients, specific intervening variables can be identified that appear to relate the characteristics of the pain to either the distress associated with the pain or the overall impairment in quality of life. For example, pain may produce immobility, and this loss may become the predominating factor in undermining the patient's quality of life. From the clinical standpoint, these intervening variables are important to discern, since they may be amenable to treatment that can provide a means to improve quality of life even if pain relief is difficult to achieve.

9. The behavior of significant others in the patient's environment can influence the characteristics of the pain, including severity and pain-related distress, and can have a profound impact on the degree of suffering. This influence may or not be beneficial.

B. CURRENT RESEARCH WITH IMPLICATIONS FOR PAIN AND QUALITY OF LIFE

The foregoing observations suggest numerous hypotheses and the type of information that will have to be collected to adequately characterize the complex relationship between pain and quality of life. These hypotheses, some of which are discussed in the following section, can be refined through the application of data obtained from studies performed in the cancer pain population. Although only one study directly addresses the relationship between pain and quality of life, and none is adequate to either validate or refute these clinical observations, all provide information that clarify the salient issues and highlight the need for specific types of information.

A recent survey[59] attempted to identify the important determinants of quality of life in patients with cancer pain. Content analysis of the verbal responses of 41 patients to four open-ended questions (three about the meaning of quality of life and one about the importance of pain) yielded three general categories of attributes, each of which contributed to the patient's perceived quality of life: physical well-being, psychological well-being, and interpersonal well-being. Each of these categories comprised numerous perceptions. For example, physical well-being was related to the overall ability to function and to specific factors associated with the disease and its treatment. The latter included the experience of symptoms, of which pain was by far the most prominent in this sample. When asked a general question about quality of life, 25 patients reported that the experience of pain caused a poor quality of life and 8 patients stated that the lack of pain produced an improved quality of life. When subsequently queried specifically about the pain, 37 of the 41 patients intensely avowed that pain undermined quality of life; 4 patients explained that pain-related impairment

TABLE 1
Symptoms Spontaneously
Volunteered by 90 Patients
with Advanced Cancer
Approximately 4 Weeks
Prior to Death[a]

Symptom	No. (%)
Fatigue	52 (58)
Pain	49 (54)
Weakness	39 (43)
Sleepiness	22 (24)
Mental clouding	22 (24)
Anxiety	19 (21)
Leg weakness	16 (18)
Shortness of breath	15 (17)
Nausea	11 (12)
Decreased hearing	8 (9)
Depression	7 (8)
Loss of appetite	7 (8)
Insomnia	6 (7)
Arm weakness	6 (7)
Cough	5 (6)
Restlessness	5 (6)
Difficulty speaking	5 (6)

[a] Twenty other symptoms were reported by less than 5% of patients and are not included.

Adapted from Coyle, N. et al., *J. Pain Symptom Manage.*, 5, 83, 1990.

of quality of life was mediated by increased fear of the disease or treatment (e.g., becoming an addict). Interestingly, four patients also noted that pain had positive effects on quality of life (e.g., by contributing to improved family interactions).

The use of patient report in this survey to inductively identify the important attributes of quality of life lends strong support to the multidimensional view of this construct advanced by theorists. Unfortunately, specific characteristics of pain, such as severity or chronicity, were not assessed, and this complicates interpretation of the data. Nonetheless, the results suggest that the quality of life of patients with cancer pain relates strongly, but by no means exclusively, to the experience of pain. Functioning in other broad domains of experience — physical, psychological, and social — are extremely important in these patients, as they are believed to be in those without pain. Moreover, the reaction to pain is complex. Although the aversive perceptions related to pain were usually described in general terms, or in terms related to function, some patients dwelled on the meaning of the pain to the underlying disease, and some even perceived there to be positive elements in the pain.

Other data similarly indicate the importance of pain. Pain is extremely prevalent in the cancer population,[60] and two well-conducted prospective surveys identified a relationship between pain and depression.[61,62] One of these studies noted that pain was more prevalent only among patients who were both depressed and had substantial physical disabilities.[62]

Other surveys, however, also affirm the common observation that pain, despite its prominence, is only one of numerous symptoms that potentially influence quality of life. Most patients with advanced cancer experience multiple symptoms concurrently (Table 1), and though pain is usually among the most common,[63,64] it may or may not be perceived as the major impediment to function. For example, a recent survey of 90 cancer patients one month prior to death observed that these individuals had very limited activity (98% with a Karnofsky Performance Scale score of 50 or below and 77% in bed or chair continuously), but that this was attributed to pain only by those whose pain was relatively severe;[63] only 2 of 24 patients (8%) with mild pain stated that activity was pain limited, whereas 19 of 31 patients (61%) with moderate pain and 17 of 18 patients (94%) with moderate to severe pain endorsed this belief. This suggests that pain, albeit very common, is not uniformly associated with factors, e.g., limited activity, that may correlate with poor quality of life.

The finding that pain severity is an important determinant of the impact of pain on quality of life was also adduced in a large prospective survey that correlated pain severity scores with scores on a series of numeric scales that assessed the degree of interference caused by the pain in various spheres of physical, psychological, and social functioning.[6] Patients who scored above the halfway point on the pain severity measure were observed to have a disproportionate degree of interference by the pain. That is, patients whose pain severity was perceived to be half as bad as it could possibly be or worse noted that pain substantially interfered with many experiences (e.g., physical activity, mood, relations with other) related to quality of life, whereas patients who perceived their pain to be less than this reported little interference.

The relationship between psychological distress and pain characteristics has also been explored in several studies. Psychological distress, like physical limitations, presumably contributes to impaired quality of life. With rare exception, however, these reports do not distinguish between psychological distress that is specifically associated with the pain and more global distress. As discussed previously, most psychologically distressed patients with cancer pain can estimate the degree to which pain contributes to this experience, and it is often observed that some patients demonstrate prompt improvement in psychological status following relief of pain, whereas others continue to manifest severe distress despite improved comfort. Clearly, important information could be gained if these distinctions between pain-related distress and more global distress were evaluated systematically, and the impact of each on overall quality of life was determined.

Notwithstanding this important limitation, studies of psychological distress in cancer pain patients can provide important insights into the relationship between pain and quality of life. The increased prevalence of depression in patients with pain has already been noted.[61,62] A prospective survey that used visual analog scales and categorical scales to quantitate pain demonstrated that pain severity correlated with the fatigue and confusion subscales of the Profile of Mood States;[55] importantly, there was no significant relationship between pain severity and the depression subscale or the total score, which is often taken to reflect global psychologic distress. Thus, although there is clearly a relationship between the report of pain and psychological symptomatology, and the relationship is determined in part by pain severity, these data do not support the conclusion that pain severity is the overriding factor in the psychological distress experienced by the patient.

Other data clarify this relationship and suggest that the perception of pain relief may be another important determinant of psychological distress. The strongest relationship recorded in the aforementioned survey[55] was between scores on a visual analog scale for pain relief and the total score on the Profile of Mood States. Recently, a retrospective study demonstrated a significant inverse relationship between suicidal ideation (determined by affirmative responses to questions related to suicide on two depression inventories) and the scores on a visual analog scale for pain relief in 185 patients with cancer pain;[65] there was no association between suicidal ideation and scores on a visual analog scale for pain severity.

Even more compelling are data from another retrospective study that reanalyzed the scores on visual analog scales of pain severity, pain relief, and mood from two previous studies of patients with cancer pain, one a survey and the other an analgesic trial.[66] Zero-order and partial correlations revealed that the moderate inverse correlation between pain severity and mood disappeared when the pain relief was partialed out, whereas the partial correlation between pain relief and mood (with pain severity removed) remained significant. Of note, previous studies indicate that the mood visual analog scale correlates highly with the total score on the Profile of Mood States, and hence, can be viewed as a global measure of psychological distress.[55]

Although it is necessary to infer a relationship between quality of life and the dependent measures of psychological distress used in these studies, the data suggest that perceived pain relief should be considered an important potential determinant of quality of life. Interestingly, a pain relief scale has also been found to be a more sensitive measure than pain severity scales in clinical trials of analgesic drugs.[67] It is essential to note, however, that the precise attribute measured by a pain relief scale in the routine clinical setting is not entirely clear, as it is in an analgesic trial, wherein the score reflects the degree of relief produced by the study intervention at a specified moment in time. The use of the scale as a more global measure may be reflecting the patient's perception of anticipated relief or the availability of the methods to provide relief. Future investigations of pain and quality of life will need to both incorporate a pain relief instrument and attempt to assess the specific elements it measures.

The meaning of the pain to the patient was previously postulated to be an important factor on the basis of clinical observation. This possibility was also indicated by several patients interviewed during the aforementioned survey of quality of life attributes;[59] these patients noted that fear of disease progression mediated pain-related distress. The only other empirical demonstration of this influence is found in a survey of breast cancer patients, whose pain severity was significantly associated with the degree to which the patient believed that the pain reflected progression of disease.[68]

IV. THEORETICAL IMPLICATIONS

These clinical observations and survey data have begun to elucidate the complex relationship between pain and quality of life. It is important to emphasize, however, that the observed correlations do not imply causation, and it would be incorrect to assume that any finding, such as the relationship between pain relief and mood, suggests an explanation for the association. All the available information about pain and quality of life should, therefore, be considered useful material for the elaboration of hypotheses that remain to be tested in future studies. Some of the most important hypotheses, and their implications for research, can be summarized as follows:

1. The relationship between pain severity and quality of life is inverse and not linear. A pain severity perceived to be approximately halfway along a self-described scale anchored by no pain at one end and worst possible pain at the other may be fundamental to understanding this relationship. It may be speculated that a pain severity less than this halfway point has either no relationship with quality of life or a relationship defined by a flat curve, such that changes in pain severity have little to no impact; a strong relationship exists at pain severities above this point. The implication of this hypothesis is clear: pain severity must be scaled in surveys evaluating the relationship between pain and quality of life. The assessment of pain as a quantal phenomenon ("present-absent") is not adequate in these studies.

2. Since perceived pain relief and perceived pain chronicity are likely to be important determinants of quality of life, studies should incorporate instruments to measure these characteristics. Given available information, it is reasonable to hypothesize that perceived pain relief is a more important factor than pain intensity, and furthermore, that

the influence of pain chronicity on quality of life operates through its impact on perceived pain relief, rather than pain severity.

3. It has also been speculated that the psychological distress of the cancer pain patient is determined by many factors, only one of which is pain, and that careful assessment can identify psychological distress that the patient associates specifically with the pain. Two hypotheses derive from these observations: (1) changes in pain over time may or may not parallel psychological disturbances, and (2) quality of life may or may not improve as pain declines. The most valid assessment of these hypotheses will require longitudinal studies, which incorporate repeated evaluation of pain, psychological status and quality of life. Again, it would be important to follow several specific pain characteristics (e.g., severity, perceived relief, and chronicity) and evaluate a variety of psychological factors (e.g., mood disturbance and coping ability) in this assessment.

4. It may be conjectured that pain-related psychological distress and impairment in quality of life correlate with the meaning of the pain to the patient, and specifically with the degree to which pain is ascribed to cancer progression. Future studies should consider a systematic assessment of patient's beliefs about the relationship between pain and the underlying disease and a concomitant determination of disease-related anxiety.

5. The counterintuitive observation that pain may have no effect on quality of life, and indeed, may occasionally serve a positive function,[59] suggests several additional hypotheses relating pain to psychological distress. Longitudinal studies with multifactorial assessment may be able to address these considerations. For example, some patients, such as those predisposed to opioid side effects or those with an inappropriate fear of addiction, may experience pain therapy as so stressful that psychological distress produced by the treatment overwhelms the improvement in quality of life that might have occurred with enhanced comfort. Alternatively, some patients appear to be enmeshed in a family dynamic characterized by psychological support contingent on the report of pain; for this group, relief of pain may induce increased isolation from family, and consequently, impaired quality of life. Finally, some patients appear to "bind" anxiety about the underlying disease, or limit rumination about other losses, by focusing on the pain and efforts to manage it; relief of pain may be followed by increasing psychological distress, and thereupon, worsening quality of life.

V. CONCLUSION

The ability of future research to provide a cogent understanding of the many factors that contribute to the relationship between pain and quality of life will depend on the sophistication of the methodologies employed. Elucidation of the complex interaction between these two dynamic and multidimensional constructs will require concurrent evaluation of numerous pain characteristics, pain-related interference with psychological integrity and other function, overall well-being, functioning within several domains of experience that contribute to perceived well-being, and other factors, such as cognitions about pain and disease. Multivariate statistical techniques will identify many interrelationships among these factors, and should be able to clarify the contribution of various combinations of factors to overall quality of life.

REFERENCES

1. Ventafridda, V., Continuing care: a major issue in cancer pain management, *Pain*, 36, 137, 1989.
2. Ventafridda, V., Tamburini, M., Selmi, S., and DeConno, F., Pain and quality of life assessment in advanced cancer patients, in *Assessment of Quality of Life and Cancer Treatment*, Ventafridda, V., Van Dam, F. S. A. M., Yancik, R., and Tamburini, M., Eds., Excerpta Medica, Amsterdam, 1986, 183.
3. Ventafridda, V., Tamburini, M., and DeConno, F., Comprehensive treatment in cancer pain, in *Advances in Pain Research and Therapy*, Vol. 9, Fields, H. L., Dubner, R., and Cervero, F., Eds., Raven Press, New York, 1985, 617.
4. Foley, K. M., Assessment of pain in patients with cancer, in *Cancer Pain*, Swerdlow, M. and Ventafridda, V., Eds., MTP Press, Lancaster, 1987, 37.
5. Portenoy, R. K., Practical aspects of pain control in the patient with cancer, *Ca*, 38, 327, 1988.
6. Daut, R. L. and Cleeland, C. S., The prevalence and severity of pain in cancer, *Cancer*, 50, 1913, 1982.
7. Donovan, M. I., Clinical assessment of cancer pain, in *Cancer Pain Management*, McGuire, D. B. and Yarbro, C. H., Eds., Grune & Stratton, New York, 1987, 105.
8. Portenoy, R. K., Pain and quality of life: clinical issues and implications for research, *Oncology*, 4, 172, 1990.
9. Portenoy, R. K. and Foley, K. M., Management of cancer pain, in *Handbook of Psychooncology*, Holland, J. C. and Rowland, J. H., Eds., Oxford University Press, New York, 1989, 369.
10. MacDonald, N., Report and recommendations: pain management, *J. Palliat. Care*, 5, 40, 1989.
11. Saunders, C., The philosophy of terminal care, in *The Management of Terminal Malignant Disease*, 2nd ed., Saunders, C., Ed., Edward Arnold, London, 1984, 232.
12. Twycross, R. G. and Lack, S. A., *Symptom Control in Far Advanced Cancer*, Pitman, London, 1983, 32.
13. Coyle, N., A model of continuity of care for cancer patients with chronic pain, *Med. Clin. North Am.*, 71, 259, 1987.
14. Townsend, C. M., Report and recommendations: continuing care/care at home, *J. Palliat. Care*, 5, 48, 1989.
15. Latimer, E. J., The impact of palliative care: present and future, *J. Palliat. Care*, 1, 35, 1985.
16. Mount, B. M., Editorial: hospice care, *J. R. Soc. Med.*, 73, 471, 1980.
17. Calman, K. C., Definitions and dimensions of quality of life, in *The Quality of Life of Cancer Patients*, Aaronson, N. K. and Beckmann, J. H., Eds., Raven Press, New York, 1987, 1.
18. deHaes, J. C. J. M. and van Knipperberg, F. C. E., *Quality of Life of Cancer Patients: A Review of the Literature*, Aaronson, N. K. and Beckman, J. H., Eds., Raven Press, New York, 1987, 167.
19. deHaes, J. C. J. M. and van Knipperberg, F. C. E., The quality of life of cancer patients: a review of the literature, *Soc. Sci. Med.*, 20, 809, 1985.
20. van Dam, F. S. A. M., Assessment of quality of life in cancer patients, in Organizing Committee of the Workshop of Quality of Life in Cancer Patients, Takeda, F., Ed., in Chief, Quality of life in cancer patients: a current topic in cancer treatment and care, Office of the Organizing Committee of the Workshop on Quality of Life in Cancer Patients, Saitama, Japan, 1984, 55.
21. Moinpour, C. M., Feigl, P., Metch, B., et al., Quality of life end points in cancer clinical trials: review and recommendations, *J. Natl. Cancer Inst.*, 81, 485, 1989.
22. van Knipperberg, F. C. E. and deHaes, J. C. J. M., Measuring the quality of life of cancer patients: psychometric properties of instruments, *J. Clin. Epidemiol.*, 41, 1043, 1988.
23. Tannock, I., Gospodarowicz, M., Meakin, W., et al., Treatment of metastatic prostatic cancer with low-dose prednisone: evaluation of pain and quality of life as pragmatic indices of responses, *J. Clin. Oncol.*, 7, 590, 1989.
24. Aaronson, N. K., Bakker, W., Stewart, A. L., et al., Multidimensional approach to the measurement of quality of life in lung cancer clinical trials, in *The Quality of Life of Cancer Patients*, Aaronson, N. K. and Beckmann, J. H., Eds., Raven Press, New York, 1987, 63.
25. Ferrell, B. R., Wisdon, C., and Wenzl, C., Quality of life as an outcome variable in management of cancer pain, *Cancer*, 63, 2321, 1989.
26. Schipper, H. and Levit, M., Measuring quality of life: risks and benefits, *Cancer Treat. Rep.*, 69, 1115, 1985.
27. Schipper, H., Clinch, J., McMurray, A., et al., Measuring the quality of life of cancer patients: the functional living index-cancer: development and validation, *J. Clin. Oncol.*, 2, 472, 1984.
28. World Health Organization: The first ten years of the World Health Organization, World Health Organization, Geneva, 1958.
29. Fayers, P. M. and Jones, D. R., Measuring and analyzing quality of life in cancer clinical trials: a review, *Stat. Med.*, 2, 429, 1983.
30. Donovan, K., Sanson-Fiser, R. W., and Redman, S., Measuring quality of life in cancer patients, *J. Clin. Oncol.*, 7, 959, 1989.

31. **Hornquist, J. O.**, The concept of quality of life, *Scand. J. Soc. Med.*, 10, 57, 1982.
32. **Najman, J. M. and Levine, S.**, Evaluating the impact of medical care and technologies on the quality of life: a review and critique, *Soc. Sci. Med.*, 15, 107, 1981.
33. **Ganz, P. A., Figlin, R. A., Haskell, C. M., et al.**, Supportive care versus supportive care and combination chemotherapy in metastatic non-small cell lung cancer, *Cancer*, 63, 1271, 1989.
34. **Orr, S. T. and Aisner, J.**, Performance status assessment among oncology patients: a review, *Cancer Treat. Rep.*, 70, 1423, 1986.
35. **Brinkley, D.**, Quality of life in cancer trials, *Br. Med. J.*, 291, 685, 1985.
36. **Skeel, R. T.**, Quality of life assessment in cancer clinical trials—it's time to catch up, *J. Natl. Cancer Inst.*, 81, 472, 1989.
37. **Yancik, R. and Yates, J. W.**, Quality of life assessment of cancer patients: conceptual and methodologic challenges and constraints, *Cancer Bull.*, 38, 217, 1986.
38. **Aaronson, N. K., Bullinger, M., and Ahmedzai, S.**, A modular approach to quality of life assessment in cancer clinical trials, *Rec. Results Cancer Res.*, 111, 231, 1988.
39. **Levine, M. N., Guyatt, G. H., Gent, M., et al.**, Quality of life in stage II breast cancer: an instrument for clinical trials, *J. Clin. Oncol.*, 6, 1798, 1988.
40. **Ganz, P. A., Haskell, C. M., Figlin, R. A., et al.**, Estimating the quality of life in a clinical trial of patients with metastatic lung cancer using the Karnofsky performance status and the functional living index: cancer, *Cancer*, 61, 849, 1988.
41. **Coates, A., Gebski, V., Bishop, J. F., et al.**, Improving the quality of life during chemotherapy for advanced breast cancer. A comparison of intermittent and continuous treatment strategies, *N. Engl. J. Med.*, 317, 490, 1987.
42. **McCorkle, R.**, The measurement of symptom distress, *Semin. Oncol. Nurs.*, 3, 248, 1987.
43. **Stewart, A. L., Hays, R. D., and Ware, J. E.**, The MOS short-form general health survey: reliability and validity in a patient population, *Med. Care*, 26, 724, 1988.
44. **Hunt, S. M., McKenna, S. P., McEwen, J., Williams, J., and Papp, E.**, The Nottingham health profile: subjective health status and medical consultations, *Soc. Sci. Med.*, 15A, 222, 1981.
45. **Schag, C. C., Heinrich, R. L., and Ganz, P. A.**, Cancer inventory of problem situations: an instrument for assessing cancer patients' rehabilitation needs, *J. Psychosoc. Oncol.*, 1, 11, 1983.
46. **Kaplan, R. M., Bush, J. W., and Berry, C. C.**, Health status: types of validity for an index of well-being, *Health Serv. Res.*, 11, 478, 1976.
47. **Gilson, B. S., Gilson, J. S., Bergner, M., et al.**, The sickness impact profile: development of an outcome measure of health care, *Am. J. Public Health*, 65, 1304, 1975.
48. **Spitzer, W. O., Dobson, A. J., Hall, J., et al.**, Measuring the quality of life of cancer patients: a concise QL-index for use by physicians, *J. Chronic Dis.*, 34, 585, 1981.
49. **Melzack, R.**, Neurophysiological foundations of pain, in *The Psychology of Pain*, 2nd ed., Sternbach, R. A., Ed., Raven Press, New York, 1988, 1.
50. **Ahles, T. A., Blanchard, E. B., and Ruckdeschel, J. C.**, The multidimensional nature of cancer-related pain, *Pain*, 17, 277, 1983.
51. **Melzack, R.**, The McGill pain questionnaire: major properties and scoring methods, *Pain*, 1, 277, 1975.
52. **Turk, D. C.**, Assessment of pain: the elusiveness of latent constructs, in *Advances in Pain Research and Therapy*, Vol. 12, Chapman, C. R. and Loesser, J. D., Eds., Raven Press, New York, 1989, 267.
53. **Cleeland, C. S.**, Measurement of pain by subjective report, in *Advances in Pain Research and Therapy*, Vol. 12, Chapman, C. R. and Loesser, J. D., Eds., Raven Press, New York, 1989, 391.
54. **Syrjala, K. L.**, The measurement of pain, in *Cancer Pain Management*, McGuire, D. B. and Yarbro, C. H., Eds., Grune & Stratton, New York, 1987, 133.
55. **Fishman, B., Pasternak, S., Wallenstein, S. L., et al.**, The Memorial pain assessment card: a valid instrument for the assessment of cancer pain, *Cancer*, 60, 1151, 1987.
56. **Wallenstein, S. L., Heidrich, G., Kaiko, R., and Houde, R. W.**, Clinical evaluation of mild analgesics: the measurement of pain, *Br. J. Clin. Pharmacol.*, 10, 319S, 1980.
57. **Arner, S. and Meyerson, B. A.**, Lack of analgesic effect of opioids on neuropathic and idiopathic forms of pain, *Pain*, 33, 11, 1988.
58. **Gracely, R. H., Dubner, R., and McGrath, P. A.**, Narcotic analgesia: fentanyl reduces the intensity but not the unpleasantness of painful tooth pulp sensations, *Science*, 203, 261, 1979.
59. **Padilla, G. V., Ferrell, B., Grant, M. M., and Rhiner, M.**, Defining the content domain of quality of life for cancer patients with pain, *Cancer Nurs.*, in press.
60. **Portenoy, R. K.**, Cancer pain: epidemiology and syndromes, *Cancer*, 63, 2298, 1989.
61. **Bukberg, J., Penman, D., and Holland, J.**, Depression in hospitalized cancer patients, *Psychosom. Med.*, 46, 199, 1984.
62. **Derogatis, L. R., Morrow, G. R., Fetting, J., et al.**, The prevalence of psychiatric disorders among cancer patients, *JAMA*, 249, 751, 1983.

63. **Coyle, N., Adelhardt, J., Foley, K. M., and Portenoy, R. K.,** Character of terminal illness in the advanced cancer patient: pain and other symptoms during the last four weeks of life, *J. Pain Symptom Manage.*, 5, 83, 1990.

64. **Walsh, T. D.,** Control of pain and other symptoms in advanced cancer, *Oncology*, 1, 5, 1987.

65. **Saltzburg, D., Breitbart, W., Fishman, B., Stiefel, F., Holland, J., and Foley, K.,** The relationship of pain and depression to suicidal ideation in cancer patients, *Proc. Am. Soc. Clin. Oncol.*, 8, 312, 1989.

66. **Fishman, B., Houde, R. W., Wallenstein, S., and Foley, K. M.,** Appraisal of pain relief mediates the relationship between pain intensity and emotional distress in cancer pain, *Pain*, Suppl. 4, S415, 1987.

67. **Littman, G. S., Walker, B. R., and Schneider, B. E.,** Reassessment of verbal and visual analog rating in analgesic studies, *Clin. Pharmacol. Ther.*, 38, 16, 1985.

68. **Spiegel, D. and Bloom, J. R.,** Pain in metastatic cancer, *Cancer*, 52, 341, 1983.

Chapter 21

PAIN ASSESSMENT IN CANCER

Charles S. Cleeland

TABLE OF CONTENTS

I. INTRODUCTION

Poorly controlled pain has such deleterious effects on the cancer patient and the patient's family that its proper management ought to have the highest priority in the routine care of the patient with cancer. Not only do mood and quality of life deteriorate in the presence of pain, but pain has adverse effects on such measures of disease status as appetite and activity. Pain of severe intensity may be a primary reason why both patients and their families decide to abandon treatment.

Unfortunately, despite the many treatment options that exist for cancer pain management,[1] under treatment of cancer pain is a significant public health problem throughout the world.[2] Even in the most medically sophisticated countries, as many as 50% of patients may not get optimal cancer pain management.[3] The reasons that patients are undertreated are multiple, and involve patients, health care providers, and health care delivery systems. In order to develop strategies for reducing these barriers to adequate cancer pain treatment, we need appropriate measurement instruments for evaluating pain, its impact on the patient, and its response to various treatment efforts. We also need to consider how a selection of these instruments can be made to address specific clinical and research questions. Without pain measurement tools, we cannot expect to understand how many cancer patients have pain and how pain impairs patient function. Without such tools, the clinical assessment of pain is greatly hampered. Finally, pain measurement methods are critical to the conduct of clinical trials which might answer questions about what pain therapies are the most effective. This chapter will examine some of the methodological issues in the measurement of pain and its impact, and illustrate how specific measurement techniques might be used in prevalence and risk studies, in clinical and quality assurance applications, and in the conduct of clinical trials in cancer pain.

Pain can be defined in terms of several different theoretical perspectives, each of which will dictate a specific set of measurement techniques. For example, some investigations rely heavily on physiological changes which take place when pain is present. Others may focus on the behavior of subjects in pain. For the types of application that we will consider (prevalence studies, clinical assessment, clinical trials), the subject's report of pain and of functional impairment caused by the pain will be the primary variables that we will be interested in.

Pain, in the sense of something we ask people about, is a construct, much in the same realm and with the same measurement problems as other constructs of distress or pleasure, such as anxiety, sadness, anger, and euphoria.[4] Subjective report is also the major tool for measurement of these other constructs. As with related constructs, we will never be able to measure pain to everyone's satisfaction. From our own experience, however, we do know that we can judge when pain is present. We can make judgments about when pain is more or less severe, and whether or not pain is interfering with how we feel and what we want or have to do.

Traditionally, the subjective nature of pain measurement has caused some to argue that pain (as well as many other variables related to well being or quality of life) can never be measured in a meaningful way. The basis for this skepticism is usually based on the high degree of variability associated with the typical situation of asking patients about pain in the clinic. The usual clinical interchange between health care provider and patient about pain is often so casual or unstructured that variability is assured.[5] For instance, it may be left up to patients to mention pain in the first place. Even if patients are asked about pain, they may be left entirely on their own to come up with a format for communicating the characteristics and intensity of their pain. This type of unstructured communication maximizes the chances that personality, cultural, stylistic, and situational variables will contribute their weights to the communication. Such an interchange is not a measurement situation in any sense. Variability in response will be dramatically reduced if order is placed on the communication by standardizing the set of questions asked and by introducing measurement scales designed to measure subjective response.

II. SUBJECTIVE MEASUREMENT SCALES

Whatever the eventual application, pain measurement and measurement of functional impairment will use measurement scales which allow for at least ordinal ratings of the severity of pain or impairment. Three general types of pain measurement scales have proven to be useful in a variety of clinical and research settings; the categorical scale, the visual analog scale, and the numeric scale. Since, from a practical standpoint, these scales provide roughly equivalent data,[6] a choice of which scale to use will usually depend on such factors as investigator preference, appropriateness of the scale for the study design, and ease of administration.

The categorical scale — Categorical scales have a long history in pain research.[7] The subject is asked to pick a verbal category, such as "none," "mild," "moderate," "horrible," and "excruciating" which best describes severity. Pain relief can be categorized in a similar way, such as "none," "slight," "moderate," "lots," and "complete." While these categorical scales have proven useful in numerous laboratory and clinical studies, such scales assume that subjects have roughly the same meaning in mind when picking the word most describing their pain. This assumption may be tenuous when a given study will sample patients of diverse educational, cultural, or linguistic backgrounds.

The visual analog scale — Visual analog scales have long been used in research comparing the effectiveness of analgesic drugs.[8] The patient makes a judgement of how much of the scale, usually a horizontal straight line of 10 cm in length, is equivalent to (or analogous with) the severity of the pain. One end of the line represents no pain and the other some concept such as "pain as bad as you can imagine." These scales have proven their usefulness in analgesic assay studies comparing different types of doses of analgesic medications. Visual analog scales require that the patient understands the analog concept. This may require substantial instruction of subjects and monitoring by study personnel. Visual analog scales have recently been adapted for more routine clinical use in the Memorial Pain Assessment Card.[9]

The numeric scale — Patients can be asked to rate their pain on numeric scales. Because of the use of numbers, some have classified numeric scales as a type of categorical scale. Numeric scales most often have a range from 0 to 5, 0 to 10, or 0 to 100. As with the visual analog scales, numeric scales are bounded by "no pain" and, at the extreme, by "pain as bad as you can imagine" or "pain as bad as it possibly can be." Numeric scales are presented horizontally or vertically, and are thus displayed much like visual analog scales. Numeric scales are often more intuitively understood by patients than visual analog scales, and their use of numbers instead of words may remove some sources of cultural and linguistic variation.[4]

A. PROPERTIES OF PAIN SCALES

All of the pain intensity scales described above perform reasonably well in both the clinical and research application and are relatively easy to administer and score. Most investigators tend to treat these ratings as interval or ratio data, although it is rarely possible to demonstrate that subjects in fact treat the units of these scales in a way that would justify such assumptions. On the contrary, it is easy to argue that a unit change at the higher end of visual analog or numeric scales may not be logically equivalent to a unit change at the lower ends. While there have been several pain measurement techniques devised to deal with such problems as response bias and inequality of intervals, most of these techniques are either statistically or administratively too cumbersome to be used in the clinic or in clinical research. If by default alone, these three simple scales will be the ones used in most clinical research. It is of some assurance that findings from multiple studies using these scales produce coherent results that discriminate along the measurement dimensions of most interest.

III. SELECTION OR CONSTRUCTION OF A MEASUREMENT SCALE

Rarely will a single item (such as "rate your worst pain in the last day") give enough information to satisfy a research or clinical question. When one selects a pain measurement tool, one has to reach a compromise between asking all the questions that could be asked about the experience of pain and what is theoretically and practically possible to expect of a pain assessment. Since pain is such a complex experience, involving personality, learning, and situational elements, it is tempting to try to capture the flavor of these several dimensions of pain in clinical studies. On the other hand, studies using factor analysis typically find two or three dimensions which describe most of the variance among multiple items which people respond to when describing their pain. For instance, Melzack and Casey suggest three dimensions; sensory-discriminative, motivational-affective, and cognitive-evaluative.[10] Much more common is the finding that two dimensions account for most of the variance. These two dimensions have been variously called by Beecher "pain" and "reaction to pain,"[11] by Clark and Yang "sensory-discriminative" and "attitudinal"[12] and, in our own work (following Beecher) "sensory" and "reactive."[13] Some have equated the reactive dimension with the distress caused by pain. Despite some variance in terminology, the agreement among these studies suggest that we should be somewhat modest in what we attempt to capture in studies of pain which rely on subjective report. If we can provide quantitative information on a "sensory" dimension and a "reactive" dimension, that is about the best that we can do.

It might be argued that the sensory dimension might be thought of as closer to "true pain," and that ratings on this dimension ought to stand alone as a criterion for clinical and research decisions. On the other hand, a reduction in the reactive component (or distress or affective component), even in the absence of a reduction in the sensory component, should be viewed as a positive outcome. For example, a significant reduction in the sensory intensity of pain might be difficult to achieve in some circumstances, yet the impact of pain (the reactive dimension) might be amenable to an intervention. A judgment as to which dimension should get the predominant weighting in outcome research should be left to the set of questions to be asked by the study.

IV. ATTRIBUTES OF A PAIN MEASUREMENT INSTRUMENT

When selecting or designing a pain measurement instrument, there are certain principles which can guide decisions. These considerations come from both measurement experience and common sense.[4] These include:

1. The intent of items should be unambiguous. Subjects need to understand what information is wanted. Sometimes conceptual muddiness is confused with psychological subtlety or sophistication. Measurement is hopeless if the subject is lost concerning what you want reported or how to use the scales that you provide. If simple scales will work, they should be used. More complex scales need to be justified, both in terms of their theoretical contribution as well as by data which substantiate that subjects understand how to use them. If subjects know what you want, their ability to respond

seems to be robust across a wide variety of scale types, including numeric, categorical, or visual analog.[6]

2. Limit the dimensions of subjective experience that will be assessed in any given measurement situation. In most pain assessments, one of these dimensions will be the intensity of the sensory dimension of pain, giving you at most one or two more dimensions to tap. Expect these dimensions to be correlated, almost always in the range of .30 to .50. This correlation appears to be part of subjective reporting of experience, and trying to force the dimensions to be orthogonal will distort the nature of the process. The natural correlation among dimensions of subjective reporting obtained in a given assessment suggests an obvious potential trap for interpretation: the confusion between association and causality. If the set of questions to be answered suggests that there are multiple relevant dimensions which need to be sampled, sequential studies may have to be designed.

3. If other constructs, such as anxiety or depression, are liable to cloud the interpretation of outcome data, the design must provide ways to minimize conceptual confusion. Ask specific questions pertinent to these other constructs so that their contribution might be estimated. In some instances, these constructs might be the primary focus of interest in persons who have pain. The theory underlying an experimental design should specify this.

4. As is true with any measurement using subjective report, it is important to estimate what percentage of the variance in responding may be due to variables totally extraneous to the questions under consideration. This includes consideration of such issues as the social desirability of possible responses and the subjects' perception of possible consequences of their response. Often, a well-prepared preamble to the assessment can be very effective in minimizing these potential biases. Another obvious source of extraneous variability in studies involving sick patients in pain is the subject's ability to endure the subjective reporting process. The patient in pain may not be able to tolerate a long procedure which is otherwise theoretically interesting and psychometrically sound.

V. PAIN QUESTIONNAIRES OR INVENTORIES

Based on the set of questions to be answered, and keeping the considerations just discussed in mind, a questionnaire or inventory can be constructed by assembling a set of items. Several questionnaires for patients with pain have been developed over the last three decades. The design of most of these questionnaires has been mindful of the multiple domains of pain expression. Probably the most thoroughly researched of these scales is the McGill-Melzack Pain Questionnaire.[14,15] This questionnaire takes a long time to complete, which makes it difficult for many cancer patients. Other pain questionnaires, designed for patients with nonmalignant pain, are also too demanding for the cancer patient with moderate to severe pain.

A description of the composition of the Brief Pain Inventory (BPI),[16] a questionnaire specifically designed to assess pain in cancer, should illustrate some of the issues already discussed.[6] This questionnaire, initially called the Wisconsin Brief Pain Questionnaire, attempts to cover many of the content areas sampled by the McGill-Melzack and other instruments, but takes only about 15 min to complete. Depending on the patient, it can be self-administered or used in a clinical interview. The form of administration has little effect on the outcome.[17] A review of its items will illustrate some of the important assessment dimensions that need to be sampled in a clinical and research questionnaire. The Inventory was designed to provide information on the intensity of pain (the sensory dimension) as well as the degree to which pain interferes with function (the reactive dimension). The BPI also

TABLE 1
Functions Reported as Impaired by Pain
Severity Level

Function	Rating of worst pain
Enjoyment of life	3
Work	4
Mood	5
Sleep	5
General activity	5
Walking	7
Relations with others	8

Note: Impaired = mean score of 4 or greater on 0—10 scales.

asks questions about pain relief, pain quality, and the patient's perception of the cause of pain.

A. PAIN SEVERITY

It is more important to know the intensity of a person's pain than to know only whether or not pain is present. Many adults, including cancer patients, function quite effectively with background levels of pain which, for the most part, are not attended to. As pain increases, however, it passes a threshold beyond which it can no longer be ignored. At this point, it becomes disruptive to many aspects of the person's life. When it is very severe, pain generally becomes a primary focus of attention and prohibits most non-pain-related activity.

The BPI uses 0 to 10 numeric scales for item rating. Since pain due to cancer can be quite variable over a day, the BPI asks patients to rate their pain at the time of responding to the questionnaire *(pain now)*, and also at its *worst, least,* and *average* over the previous week. The ratings can also be made for the last 24 h. The design of the study will dictate the most appropriate period to rate. The *pain worst* rating can be chosen to be the primary response variable, with the other items serving as a check on variability, or, alternatively, these ratings can be combined to give a composite index of pain severity.[18,19]

B. PAIN INTERFERENCE

While it is necessary to limit the dimensions of assessment, it is critical to estimate the degree to which pain limits patient function. Interference of function can be thought of as a reactive dimension. An effective intervention for cancer pain control should demonstrate its effectiveness on more than a reduction in pain intensity alone. Using numeric 0 to 10 scales, with 0 being "no interference" and 10 being "interferes completely," the BPI asks for ratings of how much pain interferes with mood, walking and other physical activity, work, social activity, relations with others, and sleep. The mean of these scores can be used as a pain interference score. This mean is highly correlated with an interference factor derived from a common factor analysis solution. As ratings on *pain worst* increase, additional pain interference items are rated as impaired.

Table 1 portrays the level of pain severity at which these dimensions begin to be impaired as pain becomes more severe. As detailed in the table, several items are responded to as impaired once pain reaches the mid-point on rating of *worst pain.* Several studies using both numeric and visual analog have demonstrated that the mid-point of pain rating scales seems to represent a critical value beyond which patients report disproportionate impairment of functional status. Because of these findings, it is possible to define "significant pain" as pain which is rated at or higher than the midpoint on pain intensity scales.

TABLE 2

Factor Loading Comparison — Wisconsin, Vietnamese, Mexican, and Philippine Cancer Patients

	Wis. 138		Viet. 36		Mex. 93		Phil. 244	
Sample Size	I	II	I	II	I	II	I	II
Severity Items								
Pain worst	.34	.55	.52	.86	.55	.67	.44	.78
Pain least		.89		.81		.83		.82
Pain average		.97		.95		.86		.78
Pain now		.62		.41		.72		.79
Interference Items								
General activity	.80		.79		.86		.77	
Mood	.77		.75		.83		.72	
Walking	.73		.87		.70		.76	
Work	.91		.91		.89		.78	
Relations with others	.87		.82		.82		.67	
Sleep	.57		.64		.60		.67	

Note: BPI Severity (Factor II) and Interference (Factor I) Items.

Mexican data courtesy of Dr. Juan Romero Romo. Philippine data courtesy of Dr. Cennon R. Cruz.

C. RELIABILITY AND VALIDITY

Any questionnaire must demonstrate that it performs in a stable manner and that it measures what it was intended to measure. The BPI has demonstrated respectable test-retest item correlations (reliability), at least over short intervals. Evidence for the validity of the BPI comes from several studies using the instrument with cancer patients and patients with other diseases who had pain. Expected differences in pain severity were found between groups of patients with pain who differed in the presence or absence of metastases. Ratings of pain interference with various activities were highly correlated with ratings of pain severity. The proportion of patients receiving opioid analgesics increased with increased severity rating. Finally, the intercorrelations among the items differed in a logical way from one disease to another, suggesting that the BPI is sensitive to differences in pain characteristics associated with different diseases.[17]

Using translations of the BPI, the responses of cancer patients from several countries, including the Dominican Republic, Mexico, the Philippines, and Vietnam have been compared with each other and with responses of patients from the U.S. Common factor analysis demonstrates two factors, with the intensity and pain interference items loading separately on one of the factors in each of the samples. Furthermore, the factor structure is similar in each of the samples. Table 2 portrays the severity and interference factors obtained from these samples.

These data suggest that cancer patients in pain from widely different cultural and linguistic backgrounds respond to rating the severity of their cancer-related pain and the interference caused by their pain in a similar fashion. In the non-U.S. samples, where adequate analgesia was not available at the time patients were studied, the magnitude of pain severity ratings and pain interference ratings was quite similar. For all the samples, the intensity of pain is rated somewhat independently from ratings of the interference that the pain causes in important dimensions of the patients lives, suggesting that the two sets of items are not redundant. These cross-cultural and cross-linguistic data, coupled with reliability and validity data, indicate that the portrayal of pain using the BPI's simple scales is quite robust.

D. OTHER BPI ITEMS

Like most pain questionnaires, the BPI asks the patient to provide a graphic representation of the location of pain. The patient is given a front and back view of a human figure and asked to shade in the area of pain. This item can provide a wealth of information about possible physical mechanisms contributing to the pain. For example, patients may draw the pain in the distribution of a particular nerve, suggesting that the mechanism of pain is tumor impingement on that nerve. A more diffuse representation of pain might suggest radiation-induced fibrosis or myelopathy.

The BPI asks patients to rate the percentage relief they feel that their current pain treatments provide. This might be thought of as an item which taps satisfaction with treatment. The BPI also asks patients to report the duration of pain relief that they get following taking their pain medications. Patients are asked to attribute the cause of their pain, either to the disease, the treatment of the disease, or to conditions unrelated to the disease.

Finally, the BPI asks patients to select words which best describe the quality of their pain. The list of words that patients choose from were selected from McGill-Melzack descriptors used by most cancer patients in a survey study of more than 500 patients.[3] The particular words that a patient chooses may be helpful in approximating the type of pain the patient has. For example, patients with pain from stimulation of pain receptors frequently use "aching" or "gnawing", while those with damage to neural structures might chose "numb" or "shooting."

E. ADDITIONAL INFORMATION

Pain assessment, whether for clinical or research purposes, should include more information than a patient questionnaire can provide. Much of this information is not obtainable from the standard medical record, and a special assessment effort has to be made. Response to pain therapies will be dependent on a number of factors, including the physical basis or cause of the pain, the temporal pattern of the pain, the history of prior attempts to manage pain, and the prognosis for both the disease and the conditions which create the pain.

F. PHYSICAL BASIS OF CANCER PAIN

Cancer pain is caused by different physical mechanisms, and given treatments will be more or less effective for pain of different types. Cancer patients may have pain due to invasion of tumor, pain due to treatment, or pain unrelated to the disease due to a co-morbidity such as arthritis or chronic headache. More than two thirds of patients who are specifically evaluated for pain will have pain related to tumor. As many as 25% may have pain related to the treatment of the disease. A small number (less than 10%) will have pain not related to their disease or its treatment.[20] When pain is related to the disease or its treatment, it can usually be classified as one of a number of recognized pain syndromes.[21] An important distinction needs to be made between primary nociceptive pain (pain caused by stimulation of pain receptors) with neuropathic or deafferentation pain (painful sensations that are caused by injury to peripheral or central nervous system structures). Since nociceptive pain responds to different pharmacological interventions than does deafferentation pain, this distinction is critical for both clinical management and for the design of clinical trials. Either the trial should examine pain of one type or the other, or pain type (cause) should be a stratification variable. It is critical to exclude patients with pain due entirely to co-morbidities from cancer pain clinical trials.

Not all cancer pain remains at a constant level over a 24-h period, and it is important to capture the temporal pattern of pain. Some patients will have significant exacerbation of their pain with movement, especially if the pathologic process responsible for the pain is influenced by movement (pain in the back or in or near a joint). This movement-related pain (sometimes called incident pain) may require increases in analgesia when movement is anticipated. Other types of pain (usually deafferentation pain) may have periods when pain spontaneously becomes more intense. In designing clinical trials it may be necessary to stratify on the temporal pattern of pain.

The patient's response to prior pain treatment and prognosis are additional variables that need to be considered in both patient management and in clinical research. Patients whose pain has been refractory to prior pain treatment attempts present especially difficult management problems and may require alternate routes (epidural, intrathecal, subcutaneous) of analgesic administration. Such patients will obviously require greater clinical attention and should be treated separately in designs for clinical trials. Prognosis will often be related to pain treatment choices. For example, neuroablative techniques (destroying the pain pathway) may be a treatment choice, but is not indicated for patients with a longer prognosis. These invasive techniques present a risk for functional impairment. The effectiveness of these treatments is also of limited duration (weeks or months).

V. APPLICATIONS OF PAIN MEASUREMENT

Pain measurement methods are the basis of several applications, including studies of the epidemiology of cancer pain, the routine clinical assessment of pain, efforts to assure the quality of pain management, and the conduct of clinical trials examining the effectiveness of cancer pain treatments. A review of each of these areas will illustrate the application of pain measurement and assessment techniques.

A. PREVALENCE AND SEVERITY OF CANCER PAIN

The use of pain measurement questionnaires in several clinical surveys has provided a much clearer view of the nature and extent of the cancer pain problem. These issues were only known in broad outline through the 1970s. Studies published in the 1980s have documented that significant pain is a problem for large numbers of patients with metastatic cancer.[22-26] These descriptive studies have established the relative risk for significant pain that patients face, often dictated by the primary site of cancer, the site of metastases, and disease progression. They have also forced us to rethink the time course of significant pain associated with cancer. In the past, pain was typically associated with end-stage cancers. We now realize that significant pain can be present for long periods of time, especially with the continuing development of treatments that prolong life.

As discussed above, we are also beginning to understand what "significant" pain is. Most persons face mild pain periodically (some on a daily basis) with little intereference with their daily life. As pain becomes more severe, it contaminates more domains of the patient's daily functioning. Using the operational definition of significant pain as that which is rated at the midpoint or higher on conventional pain severity scales, we can now estimate the percentages of patients who will have pain at this level, dependent on disease site and disease progression.

It has long been accepted that the majority of cancer patients with advanced cancer will need careful pain management. Estimates are that between 60 and 80% of such patients will have significant pain.[21] Less attention has been paid to pain as a problem for patients before end-stage disease has been reached. As increasing numbers of patients live longer, proportionately greater numbers of patients face longer periods of having to cope with pain. A significant percentage of those who achieve a cure will face indefinite periods of treatment-related pain.

Severe pain is rarely a problem before metastatic disease is present. Most immediate postoperative pain can be managed without difficulty. Only 5 to 10% of patients report persistent disease-related pain at this stage.[22] When the disease has metastasized, however, the percentages increase dramatically. Fully 30 to 40% of hospitalized patients with metastatic disease report significant pain as we have defined it. Preliminary studies indicate that similar percentages are found among outpatients. Both the presence and severity of pain will be dictated by several factors, including the primary site of the disease and metastatic location. Many cancers which were painless at onset will have a high incidence of pain as the disease progresses. Breast disease is an excellent example: while rarely painful in the early stages, half of those affected will report pain after metastatic disease is present. One survey study, using analgesic requirement as a criterion, found 85% of patients with primary bone tumors, 52% of patients with breast carcinoma, and 45% of patients with lung cancer required analgesics. Patients less frequently requiring analgesics included those with lymphomas (20%) and leukemias (5%).[27]

The prevalence and severity of pain will obviously vary as a function of adequacy of treatment. Using patient estimates of how much relief they achieve with their pain treatments, studies in the U.S. and the U.K., and Japan indicate that less than half of those patients sampled reported that their pain was effectively managed.[3] It is also important to keep in mind that the patients surveyed in the studies reviewed above were *all* receiving analgesic treatment for their pain. Prevalence studies have not attempted to estimate whether pain was being adequately treated. It is possible to index adequacy of pain management, at least in a crude fashion. In one study,[28] an index of pain management was derived from a combination of patient pain report and the World Health Organization's[2] recommendations for cancer pain management. The WHO's "step ladder" of analgesic prescription specifies aspirin-class analgesics for mild pain, codeine-class analgesics for moderate pain, and morphine-class analgesics for severe pain. The index ranged from 0 to 3, with 3 (a patient with severe pain receiving no analgesics) representing extreme mismanagement. This index does not take into account whether or not the appropriate dose of the primary analgesic (or adjuvant drug) is being ordered. However, this simple index is able to differentiate patients being seen in different treatment settings. Using even this conservative index, 27% of patients in the total sample (n = 423) were mismanaged. Both codeine and morphine-level analgesics were under-utilized. Mismanagement, as estimated by the index, was significantly correlated with mood disturbance (depression, tension, anger as measured by the Profile of Mood States) and with sleep disturbance in patients who had moderate to severe pain.

B. CLINICAL APPLICATIONS

Standard pain measurement techniques are increasingly becoming used in the clinical assessment of cancer pain. Their use minimizes some of the barriers that exist in the typical communication between patient and health care provider (HCP) concerning pain. HCPs may not ask patients about pain at all. Or, once an analgesic has been started, they may assume that the pain has been taken care of. Individuals with cancer may have resistances to reporting pain not found in other clinical conditions. For instance, they may not wish to acknowledge the spread of disease that new pain can signal, they may not want to report that mild analgesics are no longer effective, they may be frightened about addiction and side effects, and they may be concerned that complaining of pain will divert the doctor from the task of curing the tumor. Finally, patients want to be liked by those taking care of them, and know that persistent complaining is viewed as troublesome.[5]

Using pain assessment instruments minimizes many patient reporting biases and assists HCPs in obtaining complete information. Using pain scales which assign a metric to pain intensity and interference makes pain more of an "objective" symptom, more like other signs and symptoms such as blood pressure and heart rate. By making pain "objective", standard questions make patients feel freer to report its presence, severity and also to report when treatment is not working. Patients are often less concerned about responding openly to a questionnaire than to questions put to them by staff who care for them. Using pain questionnaires or pain measurement scales also can serve to minimize *staff biases* in recognizing when pain is present or in estimating its severity.[13] Using pain measurement tools reduces staff time in the assessment process. Finally, assigning a metric to pain allows for monitoring the effectiveness of pain treatment.

Because pain is so debilitating, poorly treated pain should be considered a quality assurance issue. Patients should be guaranteed the best possible pain management. Pain assessment tools provide a method for monitoring pain in the clinic setting. Quality assurance depends on indicators of performance which can easily be monitored. If quality assurance is to encompass pain relief, a major first step will be the introduction of pain measures into routine practice, coupled with charting of the results on a routine basis. Once this is done, it is quite reasonable to establish an "incident" of poorly controlled pain that calls for review. An incident might be defined as the presence of significant pain, defined as we have, as pain which is rated at the midpoint or higher on an accepted pain rating scale.

Williamson[29] has suggested that quality assurance monitoring could be programmed to trigger corrective educational measures. He has argued that education for health practice change must be based on an evaluation encompassing both outcomes and process. Only when outcome data indicate deficiencies is process evaluation warranted and educational intervention mandated. His strategy begins with a standard of care which can be reasonably operationalized, such as a given percentage of patients with significant pain. Each institution would set a maximum acceptable level for this percentage. If outcome index data were above this level, process evaluation and education would be invoked. The outcome evaluation process would then be repeated to determine the extent of improvement.

C. CLINICAL TRIALS APPLICATIONS

A major barrier to cancer pain management has been a lack of traditional controlled clinical trials in cancer pain management. Most of our information about the effectiveness of analgesics has come from the single dose acute analgesic assay model.[30] In this model, a test drug and a standard drug are studied in randomized, double blind cross-over design. Subjects are assessed by trained research personnel (usually research nurses) immediately before and at specified times after the administration of the test or standard drug. On the second day of the study, the subject receives the other drug. These elegant single institution studies have provided the basis for judging the comparative effectiveness of various analgesics. One argument advanced for this study model is that pain assessment is tightly controlled by the use of trained observers highly familiar in instructing patients in making pain ratings. Inherent in this model is the suspicion that multi-institutional studies done without these trained observers would produce measurement information so highly variable as to be of little use.

There are many important clinical questions that cannot be answered by the single dose assay. For instance, if is often important to judge the efficacy of analgesics over repeated administrations. Some pharmacologic interventions may take several days to reach maximum effectiveness, and the latency of their effectiveness may vary from patient to patient. Non-pharmacological interventions for pain control, including physical therapy, behavioral therapy, and temporary and permanent disruption of pain pathways do not lend themselves to evaluation by this model. Finally, it is increasingly apparent that optimal cancer pain management may involve the simultaneous applications of different pain control methods.[31] These questions could be addressed in multi-institutional clinical trials *if* it can be demonstrated that pain could be measured using simple assessment tools following easily understood protocols specifying principles of pain measurement.

Support for the feasibility of clinical trials using this type of measurement comes from several sources. First, most of the cancer pain prevalence and severity studies cited above have followed this model. Simple pain rating scales, either visual analog[26] or numeric,[22,25] were given to patients by observers who were minimally trained in pain assessment. These studies have demonstrated that pain ratings obtained in this way vary in a logical fashion with such characteristics as disease progression, extent of metastases, and appropriateness of pain treatment. Second, clinical trials of pain relief measures in other diseases using simple pain scales in multi institutional trials have demonstrated reliable discrimination between more and less effective treatments.[32,33]

Multi-institutional trials in cancer pain management should obviously adhere to the highest standards of multi-institutional clinical trials in general.[34] Designs should include randomized assignment to treatment or control groups, and should be double-blind designs. In addition to criteria we have discussed concerning subjective response measures, subjective response measures should be obtained by a data manager or other person not a part of the treatment team. Criteria for measures to be derived from record review or special assessment should be unambiguous and high inter-rater reliability should be demonstrated. The question that the trial is designed to answer should be stated in such a way that the data will provide clear confirmation or disconfirmation of the question.

Clinical trials in cancer pain management generate the need for some special considerations. Since cancer pain is progressive, often rapidly so, planning for the duration of the trial must consider the possibility that worsening disease progression will obscure real differences in the treatments being contrasted. Analgesics, especially the more potent ones like morphine, will produce side effects readily apparent to the patient, especially patients who have a history of taking analgesics. When such drugs are studied, it may be appropriate to include a so-called "active placebo", a drug which is similar in its side-effect profile to the study drug, but has minimal or no analgesic action. Such active placebos will be difficult to construct for the evaluation of nondrug therapies, such as the blocking of pain pathways or behavioral treatments.

VII. RESUME

While there remain doubts about the perfection of pain measurement tools and pain assessment, a growing body of literature documents that simple pain scales can be combined in measurement tools that can answer meaningful questions about the nature of cancer pain and the effectiveness of various treatment techniques. Perhaps too much energy has been expended in disputes about measurement technology and not enough in creative applications of the techniques that we already have.

ACKNOWLEDGMENT

Preparation of this chapter was supported by grant CA 26582 from the U.S. Public Health Service.

REFERENCES

1. Foley, K. M., Treatment of cancer pain, *N. Engl. J. Med.*, 313, 84, 1985.
2. World Health Organization, Geneva, *Cancer Pain Relief*, 1986.
3. Cleeland, C. S., The impact of pain on the patient with cancer, *Cancer*, 58, 2635, 1984.
4. Cleeland, C. S., Measurement of pain by subjective report, in *Issues in Pain Measurement*, Chapman, C. R. and Loeser, J. D., Eds., Raven Press, New York, 1989.
5. Cleeland, C. S., Effects of attitudes on cancer pain control, in *Drug Treatment of Cancer Pain in a Drug-Oriented Society: Adequate or Inadequate?*, Hill, C. S., Jr. and Fields, W. S., Eds., Raven Press, New York, 1989.

6. **Kremmer, E., Atkinson, J. H., and Ignelzi, R. J.,** Measurement of pain: patient preference does not confound pain measurement, *Pain*, 10, 241, 1981.

7. **Lasagna, L.,** Analgesic methodolgy: a brief history and commentary, *J. Clin. Pharmacol.*, 20, 373, 1980.

8. **Houde, R. W., Wallenstein, S. L., and Beaver, W. T.,** Clinical measurement of pain, in *Analgesics*, deStevens, G., Ed., Academic Press, New York, 1965, 75.

9. **Fishman, B., Pasternak, S., Wallenstein, S., Houde, R. W., Holland, J., and Foley, K. M.,** The memorial pain assessment card: a valid instrument for the evaluation of cancer pain, *Cancer*, 60, 1151, 1987.

10. **Melzack, R. and Casey, K. L.,** Sensory, motivational and central control determinants of pain: a new conceptual model, in *The Skin Senses*, Kenshalo, D., Ed., Charles C. Thomas, Springfield, IL, 1968.

11. **Beecher, H. K.,** *Measurements of Subjective Responses*, Oxford University Press, New York, 1959.

12. **Clark, W. C. and Yang, J. C.,** Applications of sensory decision theory to problems in laboratory and clinical pain, in *Pain Measurement and Assessment*, Melzack, R., Ed., Raven Press, New York, 1983.

13. **Cleeland, C. S.,** Assessment of pain in cancer: measurement issues, in *Advances in Pain Research and Therapy*, Vol. 16, Foley, K. M. et al., Eds., Raven Press, New York, 1990.

14. **Melzack, R. S.,** The McGill pain questionnaire: major properties and scoring methods, *Pain*, 1, 277, 1975.

15. **Melzack, R. and Torgerson, W. S.,** On the language of pain, *Anesthesiology*, 34, 50, 1971.

16. **Cleeland, C. S.,** Measurement and prevalence of pain in cancer, *Semin. Nurs. Oncol.*, 1, 87, 1986.

17. **Daut, R. L., Cleeland, C. S., and Flannery, R. C.,** Development of the Wisconsin Brief Pain Questionnaire to assess pain in cancer and other diseases, *Pain*, 17, 197, 1983.

18. **Cleeland, C. S., Shacham, S., Dahl, J. L., and Orrison, W.,** CSF beta-endorphin and the severity of clinical pain, *Neurology*, 34, 378, 1984.

19. **Shacham, S., Dar, R., and Cleeland, C. S.,** Relationship of mood state to the severity of clinical pain, *Pain*, 18, 1984.

20. **Payne, R.,** Pathophysiology of cancer pain, in *Advances in Pain Research and Therapy*, Vol. 16, Foley, K. M. et al., Eds., Raven Press, New York, 1990.

21. **Portenoy, R. K.,** Cancer pain: epidemiology and syndromes, *Cancer*, 63, 2298, 1989.

22. **Daut, R. L. and Cleeland, C. S.,** The prevalence and severity of pain in cancer, *Cancer*, 50, 9, 1913, 1982.

23. **Bonica, J. J.,** Treatment of cancer pain: current status and future needs, in *Proc. 4th World Congress of Pain*, Fields, H. L., Dubner, R., and Cerveo, F., Eds., Vol. 9, Raven Press, New York, *Adv. Pain Res. Ther.*, 56, 2337, 1985.

24. **Peteet, J., Tay, V., Cohen, G., and MacIntyre, J.,** Pain characteristics and treatment in an outpatient cancer population, *Cancer*, 57(6), 1259, 1986.

25. **Donovan, M. I. and Dillon, P.,** Incidence and characteristics of pain in a sample of hospitalized cancer patients, *Cancer Nurs.*, 10(2), 85, 1987.

26. **Greenwald, H. P., Bonica, J. J., and Bergner, M.,** The prevalence of pain in four cancers, *Cancer*, 60, 2563, 1987.

27. **Foley, K. M.,** Pain syndromes in patients with cancer, in *Advances in Pain Research and Therapy*, Vol. 2, Bonica, J. J. and Ventafridda, V., Eds., Raven Press, New York, 1979, 59.

28. **Zelman, D. C. and Cleeland, C. S.,** A Preliminary Index of Cancer Pain Management/Mismanagement: A Cross-Institutional Investigation, presented at the 1987 Int. Association for the Study of Pain, Hamburg, Germany.

29. **Williamson, J. W.,** Evaluating quality of patient care: a strategy relating outcome and process assessment, *JAMA*, 218, 564, 1971.

30. **Wallenstein, S.,** Measurement of pain and analgesia in cancer patients, *Cancer*, 53, 10 (Suppl.), 2260, 1984.

31. **Cleeland, C. S., Rotondi, A., Brechner, T., Levin, A., MacDonald, N., Portenoy, R., Schutta, H., and McEniry, M.,** A model for the treatment of cancer pain, *J. Pain Sympt. Manage.*, 1, 209, 1986.

32. **Bombardier, C., Ware, J., Russell, I. J., Larson, M., Chalmers, A., and Read, J. L.,** Auranofin therapy and quality of life in patient with rheumatoid arthritis, *Am. J. Med.*, 81, 4, 565, 1986.

33. **Parr, G., Darekar, B., Fletcher, A., and Bulpitt, C.,** Joint pain and quality of life; results of a randomized trial, *Br. J. Clin. Pharmacol.*, 27, 235, 1989.

34. **Friedman, L. M., Furberg, C. D., and DeMets, D. L.,** *Fundamentals of Clinical Trials*, PSG Publishing, Littleton, MA, 1985.

Chapter 22

CLINICAL TRIALS IN PAIN CONTROL

Eduardo Bruera and R. Neil MacDonald

TABLE OF CONTENTS

I. INTRODUCTION

Pain occurs in 60 to 80% of cancer patients before death.[1,2] It is one of the most feared consequences of cancer for patients and their families. For this reason, when present, pain should be the main target of the efforts of the medical team.

In 1973, Marks and Sachar[3] reviewed the patterns of pain treatment in a medical ward. Their findings were very disappointing: the doses of narcotic analgesics that patients were receiving were too low, the intervals between doses too long, there was an abuse of ''PRN'' administration, and as a result, more than two thirds of the patients were in poor pain control while admitted to the hospital. After this initial report, several other authors made reference to the poor management of pain in different populations, with particular emphasis in cancer pain.[4-7] As a result of these publications, increased awareness of the poor management of cancer pain developed. Several authors wrote excellent reviews on the proper treatment of cancer pain, and increased interest in the design and execution of clinical trials in cancer pain emerged.[1,8-10]

The purpose of this chapter is to discuss the main obstacles limiting the design and execution of clinical trials in cancer pain. We will focus on three main areas of concern: the proper staging of cancer pain, the design of trials on narcotic analgesics, and the design of trials on adjuvant drugs.

II. THE STAGING OF CANCER PAIN

Staging systems have proven to be an invaluable resource for research and treatment of cancer.[11] They provide a common language for a rapid and reproducible description of patient characteristics and for the comparison of new therapies. Until recently, no such system existed for assessing cancer pain. Yet the simple description ''pain due to cancer'' is probably as simplistic and difficult to assess and interpret as ''carcinoma of the breast''. For the latter, we know that estrogen and progesterone receptors, positive or negative axillary nodes, menopausal status, and pattern of dissemination are all of prognostic importance.

In pain, too, there are numerous factors that influence the prognosis for management:

- Its origin (neuropathic, visceral, etc.)
- Whether it is incidental or continuous in nature
- The possible development of tolerance
- Whether the patient has been previously treated with high doses of narcotics
- Concern about addiction
- Psychological distress
- The presence or absence of poor prognostic factors (e.g., metabolic compromise) will have a major effect on the results of treatment

Our group has recently developed the Edmonton Staging System for Cancer Pain[12] (Table 1). This system classifies patients as Stage 1 (good prognosis), Stage 2 (intermediate), or Stage 3 (poor prognosis), according to the presence or absence of a series of seven different prognostic factors. Initial application suggests that this system has significant specificity, sensitivity, and positive and negative predictive value.[12] After 3 weeks of treatment by highly experienced medical personnel adequate pain control was achieved in only 22% of patients with Stage 3 pain as compared to more than 80% of patients with Stage 1 pain.

The system needs to be tested independently by other groups and perhaps modifications of the initial design will be needed. However, we believe that the development of a common language could have the same impact on the treatment of cancer pain as staging systems had on the therapy of various malignancies. A common language may also help explain the

TABLE 1
Edmonton Staging System for Cancer Pain

A. Mechanism of pain
  1. Visceral
  2. Bone or soft tissue
  3. Neuropathic
  4. Mixed
  5. Unknown

B. Pain characteristics
  1. Nonincidental
  2. Incidental

C. Previous narcotic exposure
  1. < 60 mg oral morphine/day
  2. 60—300 mg
  3. >300 mg

D. Cognitive function
  1. Normal
  2. Abnormal

E. Psychological distress
  1. Absent
  2. Present

F. Tolerance
  1. <5% of initial dose/day
  2. >5% of initial dose/day

G. Past History of Drug Addiction or Severe Alcoholism
  1. Absent
  2. Present

Stage 1 (good prognosis)
  A1-2 B1 C1 D1 E1 F1 G1

Stage 2 (intermediate prognosis)
  A5 C2 D2 (if not Stage 3)

Stage 3 (poor prognosis)
  A3-4 (independently of the results of B C D E F & G)
  B2 (independently of the results of A C D E F & G)
  C3 (independently of the results of A B D E F & G)
  E2 (independently of the results of A B C D F & G)
  F2 (independently of the results of A B C D E & G)
  G2 (independently of the results of A B C D E & F)

difference in study results of various analgesic techniques, such as oral and parenteral narcotics, anesthesiologic procedures, neurosurgical procedures, and acupuncture. With a better knowledge of the potentially responsive population, we will be able to better define the indications for different procedures.

III. NARCOTIC ANALGESICS

Opiate drugs are among the oldest remedies of mankind. References to the use of extracts of the poppy are contained in ancient Greek and Sumerian writings.[13] Opium was probably introduced into Europe by the Crusaders. Its use was popularized by Paracelsus who promoted Laudanum — a mixture of opium, alcohol, and spices for a wide variety of disorders.[13] The popularity of opiates with physicians continued into the 19th century.[14]

Following the synthesis of heroin in 1889, society, which had recognized but tolerated the addictive potential of opiates, came down hard on them and a series of laws were introduced in most countries which tended to discourage physician use, community understanding, and consequently research on the opioid drugs.

While morphine and its congeners continued to be used to alleviate the pain of cancer patients, the fashion in which these drugs were used was based on earlier incorrect patterns of practice. Because of the influence of the hospice movement and the research of pain study groups in a few academic centers, the use of opiate drugs has recently been established on a more rational basis. Clinical research primarily involves studies on established opiates as, in contrast to cancer chemotherapy, no new clinically useful opiates have emerged in the last 20 years.

The toxicity and efficacy of correctly used opiates has been established. However, comparison trials between different drugs are relatively uncommon, as are trials comparing different routes of administration. For example, most statements on the relative efficacy of diamorphine and morphine in cancer patients are based on two studies[15,16] which have been criticized on methodologic grounds,[17] while a study comparing the two most commonly employed potent narcotics in Canada (hydromorphone and morphine) has never been conducted. The relative place of long-term epidural opioids in the management of cancer pain remains uncertain as comparison trials between epidural and systemic opiates in matched groups of patients have not been carried out.

The absence of classification systems facilitating the interpretation of pain studies has already been commented upon. Other factors which limit the conduct of opiate clinical trials include:[18]

1. The lack of information linking biologic characteristics of tumors with their propensity to induce pain
2. The absence of an interinstitutional structure for the conduct of trials, resulting in inadequate enrollment of sufficient patients in many trials
3. Inherent problems in controlling variables in patients with unstable states of disease, notably the confounding presence of other drugs which influence opioid efficacy and side effects in a patient with a changing metabolic base
4. The lack of long term follow-up (in this respect, pain studies suffer in comparison to phase III cancer chemotherapy trials whose end-points concentrate on long-term objectives such as disease remission or longevity)
5. Ethical problems involved in the recruitment of advanced cancer patients into clinical trials
6. The absence of stratification that may influence small group study interpretation

Examples of areas where clinical impression substitutes for scientifically established principles include:

1. The degree of cross-tolerance between various narcotics
2. The rationale of including more than one narcotic in a patient's drug profile
3. The clinical significance of opiate metabolites
4. The relative advantages of different routes of administration
5. The profile of optimal and harmful adjuvant drug interaction in the clinical setting

A. IS ONE NARCOTIC ANALGESIC CLEARLY SUPERIOR TO ANOTHER IN MANAGING CANCER PAIN?

Clinically available opiates have differential effects on selective subsets of opioid receptors in the central nervous system. The side effects of opiate drugs may be selectively mediated by different receptors.[19] It is theoretically possible to develop an analgesic with a specific affinity for the proposed mu-one receptor which is thought to mediate analgesia but not sedation or respiratory depression. The kappa receptor is also thought to be a mediator of pain transmission at the spinal level. A number of kappa agonists have been developed, a few of which are undergoing clinical trial. Concern exists that kappa agonists may be associated with increased psychotomimetic effects.[20]

While the development of receptor selective opiates with specific analgesic properties in the absence of the other side effects is the "holy grail" of opiate research, at the present time clinically useful new opiates have not been developed. Consequently, current clinical research has concentrated on the optimal use of the opiates which have been available to mankind for many years.

Unsubstantiated claims of superiority of one opiate over another have been made by politicians and the lay press and, occasionally, by clinicians. Few Phase III type trials exist and therefore clinical impression rules the day. The following conclusions arise from influential studies, but in view of the size of the trials, their conclusions require buttressing by larger interinstitutional trials:

1. Heroin (diamorphine) is not a superior analgesic to morphine, although its solubility and related lack of tissue irritation are useful properties in patients requiring high subcutaneous doses of opiates and/or who have reactions to subcutaneous administration of other opiates.
2. Methadone is equivalent in effective analgesic action to morphine although it produces a slightly longer period of analgesia at the cost of more sedation. Methadone's low cost (at least in Canada) makes it an interesting alternative agent for more widespread use. Methadone has a variable half-life, certainly longer than that of morphine. Clinicians have been cautioned that the use of Methadone is fraught with increased risk of respiratory compromise.[21]
3. Mixed agonist-antagonist opiates are not indicated for the management of cancer. This advice is based on studies demonstrating the psychotomimetic effects of the most commonly available drug in this class, Pentazocine, the lack of readily available oral forms of other members of the class, and the possible presence of an analgesic ceiling (advocates of bupremorphine would debate this stricture).

B. WHAT IS THE RATIONALE OF SWITCHING FROM ONE OPIATE TO ANOTHER?

As cross tolerance between opiates, even those thought to act on the same class of opioid receptors, is not absolute,[1] a shift from one opiate to another is recommended when the side effect-analgesic equation is skewed towards the side effect component. The clinical impressions of experienced clinicians clearly support this view although opinions on the formula for dose interchange varies from one group to another.[1,22,23]

It may be that the existence of several opioid receptors mediating pain can be exploited to limit the onset of tolerance and to reduce opioid side effects. Russell and Chang[24] have demonstrated, in a rat model, that the alternative use of a predominant delta agonist (DADLE (D-Ala[2], D-Leu[5]) enkephalin) and a mu agonist (morphine) can limit and even reverse opioid tolerance. Levorphanol, which shares an affinity for the delta receptor with DADLE was studied by Moulin and Pasternak.[19,25] They observed, again in a rat model, that animals tolerant to morphine exhibited an excellent response to Levorphanol, although the reverse switch of Levorphanol tolerant animals to morphine was not successful in reversing analgesic tolerance, presumably due to the mixed delta and mu agonist action of Levorphanol in contrast to the more specific mu agonist action of morphine at the doses used.

The transfer of animal data derived from experiments using pain models which do not mimic human cancer pain is clearly inexact. Nevertheless, the evidence is strong that humans share with their mammalian brethren multiple opioid receptor subsets. Therefore, it may be possible to sequence opioids in order to limit tolerance development. The use of opiates in combination, or their prospective sequential alteration in an effort to limit side effects and tolerance has never been studied and represents an area for logical clinical trial implementation.

C. WHAT IS THE ROLE OF OPIATES IN NEUROPATHIC PAIN?

The efficacy of opiates in the treatment of neuropathic cancer pain syndromes is debated. Although the classification systems for neuropathic pain vary considerably from author to author, all of them are characterized by the presence of neurologic damage, either to the peripheral nervous system, the spinal cord, or within the brain itself.

Current clinical wisdom holds that the various neuropathic pain syndromes are poorly responsive to opiates. This concept is clearly articulated by Arner and Myerson,[26] based on a carefully designed study of patients with a variety of nerve damage syndromes (none of the patients had cancer). They demonstrated, in a placebo controlled study, that, in contrast to a group of patients with nociceptive pain, the patients with neuropathic pain failed to show any response to opiates at "unusually effective doses". They concluded that opiates are likely to be of little use in the management of these pain syndromes. However, they did not treat the patients to the point of intolerable side effects, and it is possible that some of these patients may have achieved satisfactory analgesia with higher doses of opiates.

In contrast, it is the view of Portenoy and colleagues[27] that the pathophysiology of the various pain states which are included under the rubic of "neuropathic pain" is poorly understood and that this group of conditions may include subsets that are opioid sensitive. Portenoy and colleagues favor the concept of a continuum between no response and good response — the position of a patient on this continuum to be established after an opiate trial. They stress that the individual response to opioids varies, and for reasons stated in the previous section "data relevant to opioid responsiveness obtained with one drug should not be generalized to all opioids". They also believe that opiates can be used in selected patients with nonmalignant pain.[28]

The long-term behavioral effects of opiates may influence clinical response in any situation. In addition, studies on opiates in neuropathic pain must not only consider pain factors, but also patient factors including factors of individual variation (v.i.), propensity to develop opiate side effects (renal or other metabolic impairment), and prior opiate exposure.[33]

In summary, adequately controlled studies on the role of opiates in cancer-induced neuropathic pain do not exist. The successful design and implementation of a clinical trial in this area is dependent upon the adoption of a transferable classification system for neuropathic pain, the formation of an interinstitutional consortium allowing for the enrollment of a sufficient number of patients and adoption of a trial design which meets Portenoy's requirement for ensuring that patients receive doses of opiates carried to levels where side effects preclude further efforts to obtain pain relief. Until these studies are carried out, as there are a number of small clinical trials which conclude that a proportion of patients with neuropathic pain will respond to opiates, it is reasonable to titrate several opiates before concluding that they are ineffective.

D. IS THERE A ROLE FOR PATIENT-CONTROLLED ANALGESIA?

Conventional teaching on cancer pain calls for regular use of analgesics at a set time period with provision for breakthrough therapy as required. However, often cancer pain relates to activity or fluctuates in severity for unknown reasons. It is possible that regular use of opiates is not right in every situation; intermittent use adjusted to fluctuating periods of pain may enable selected patients to take lower doses of opiates with consequent less risk of side effects.

The option to use oral opiates in a flexible fashion is available to palliative care patients at the present time and many patients and their families tailor their physician's opiate

TABLE 2
Drugs Suggested to have Adjuvant Effects

Nonsteroidal anti-inflammatories	Antibiotics
Laxatives	Baclofen
Antiemetics	Amphetamines
Phenothiazines	Corticosteroids
Benzodiazepines	Diphosphonates
Tricyclic antidepressants	Calcitonin
Diphenylhydantoin	Clonidine
Carbamazepine	Anti-arrhythmics
Sodium valproate	Sympatholytics
	Cholinergic drugs

recommendations to adjust to their perceived daily needs. The authors are only aware of one small study on oral patient-controlled analgesia in chronic cancer pain.[29]

The availability of subcutaneous techniques for opiate administration has opened the door for consideration of parenteral patient-controlled analgesia (PCA). PCA analgesia using nonportable hospital pumps is increasingly used for acute postoperative pain and enables patients to receive timely and safe postoperative pain control.

Only a few studies have been conducted on the suitability of parenteral PCA for chronic cancer pain.[30] Hill and colleagues, in a 2-week study on bone marrow transplant patients with stomatitis, concluded that patient-controlled opiate analgesia produced equivalent analgesia, achieved with lower doses of morphine.[31] Bruera et al. studied 25 patients with chronic cancer pain in a cross-over trial comparing PCA administered by a Pharmacia Pump with continuous infusion of opiates.[32] They concluded there was no significant difference in pain intensity between the two groups and noted that half the patients preferred a PCA mode to that of physician-controlled continuous infusion therapy. Although we did not study psychologic characteristics of their patients, the literature on the management of acute pain suggests that patients with a need for a high locus of personal control prefer a PCA option.[33] A major tenet of palliative medicine is to return as much autonomy as possible to the patient. The use of PCA techniques fit very well with this philosophy, and deserves further study.

IV. ADJUVANT DRUGS

Opiate analgesics are the most important drugs for the treatment of chronic pain.[1,2] Although these drugs can control severe pain in most cases, they can cause or aggravate pre-existing symptoms such as nausea or somnolence.[1,2,34] This problem is particularly severe in the case of patients with advanced cancer. The combination of severe pain, anorexia, chronic nausea, asthenia, and somnolence in the same patient is a frequent finding in the daily treatment of advanced cancer.[34]

An adjuvant drug should be able to (1) increase the analgesic effect of narcotics (adjuvant analgesia); (2) decrease the toxicity of narcotics; or (3) improve the associated symptoms of terminal cancer. In some cases, when epidemiological data suggest that some patients are at high risk of developing toxicity after starting a narcotic treatment (e.g., constipation after chronic narcotic therapy), the adjuvant treatment should be started before there is any clinical evidence of toxicity.

Many drugs have been suggested to have adjuvant analgesic effects (Table 2). Unfortunately, most of the evidence for the effects of these drugs is anecdotal. Controlled clinical trials are needed to define the indications and risk:benefit ratios of these agents, some of which have significant toxicity and could potentially aggravate the toxicity of narcotics. Research is complicated by the multiple end-points that need to be measured during such a trial. Although some of these end-points are likely to remain constant (e.g., constipation or pain), others are likely to change as a function of time (sedation, nausea). The duration of the clinical trial and the design will also be affected by the characteristics of the adjuvant drugs being tested.

A. GUIDELINES FOR CLINICAL TRIALS ON ADJUVANT DRUGS

For the proper design and execution of clinical trials on adjuvant drugs, the investigator will have to consider the characteristics of the drugs under investigation, the patient population, and the nature of the effects that will be measured. In the following paragraphs we will address some of these issues.

1. The Drug

As we previously discussed, an adjuvant drug may be useful either because it potentiates the analgesic effect of a narcotic, i.e., nonsteroidal anti-inflammatory drugs (NSAIDs), because it decreases narcotic-induced toxicity (i.e., laxatives), or both (i.e., amphetamines).

One constant characteristic of these trials will be that the patients will already be receiving narcotic drugs. The adjuvant drug under study might have effects on the bioavailability of the narcotic. A recent report suggested that orally administered imipramine can increase the bioavailability of morphine, possibly by reducing its rate of elimination.[35] Studies of antiemetics that can increase gastric emptying can also change the rate of absorption of orally administered narcotics.[36] In these two cases, the interaction between the narcotic and the adjuvant drug might significantly affect the final results. In the second case (antiemetics that increase gastric emptying) the potential bias can be easily eliminated by studying the antiemetic effects only in patients receiving parenteral narcotics. In the first case (drugs that could increase the bioavailability of narcotics) one possible way of correcting the bias would be to study individuals on patient-controlled analgesia. Once the patients have reached stable pain on a placebo the blood level of the narcotic may be determined. Again, after patients achieve stable pain on the studied drug, blood levels of narcotics are repeated. If the "narcotic-sparing effect" with similar blood level of pain control occurs in the absence of any change in blood level of the drugs, it can be assumed that the adjuvant narcotic only works by increasing the bioavailability of the narcotic. On the other hand, if the "narcotic-sparing effect" with similar symptom control occurs in the presence of the lower steady state blood level of the narcotic, it can be assumed that there is a genuine analgesic potentiating effect.

One of the most sensitive areas of interaction between narcotic and adjuvant drugs is the possibility of increased sedation or confusion when the drugs are combined. Comparisons between oral morphine solutions and the Brompton's Cocktail[37] showed that the addition of other drugs in the cocktail did not result in increased pain control An increased level of obtundation or confusion in patients will result in decreased perception or communication of pain intensity. Therefore, the simple measurement of "narcotic-sparing effect" is a dangerous conclusion, particularly when the symptom assessment and the administration of the drugs are done by a third person. If the adjuvant drug has as possible side effects sedation or confusion (i.e., benzodiazepines, phenothiazines, and antihistaminics), it is important to assess in a prospective manner the cognitive status and the level of sedation of the patient population during each of the two phases of the study. If the "narcotic-sparing effect" or the "blinded" choice by the patient and the investigator are accompanied by significant cognitive deterioration or increased sedation, it cannot be ruled out that the effects are just a consequence of increased central toxicity by the adjuvant drug. If the adjuvant drug is likely to potentiate narcotic induced sedation, patients should be asked if they feel they are receiving the adjuvant drug or placebo and why, in order to assess the effectiveness of the blinding. One double-blind placebo-controlled cross-over study of cyproheptadine by our group was cancelled after 13 consecutive patients easily recognized the drug phase because of somnolence. This failure might have been avoided by doing a short-term pilot study in a small number of patients. Some studies mask the sedating effect by controlling the results not only with a placebo, but also with other drugs with sedative effects.[38,39] This is likely to improve the blinding and also to be able to differentiate "narcotic-sparing effect" from simple sedation or confusion, but it is also likely to make the trial longer and more complicated.

a. Long-Acting Drugs

For drugs with a long latency to maximal effect, such as tricyclic antidepressants, patients will need to receive the drug or placebo for several days before an assessment can take place. If a cross-over design is tried under these conditions, the status of the patients' symptoms may change significantly before the completion of the trial (i.e., development of tolerance to opiate-induced analgesia, sedation or nausea, or development of confusion or bowel obstruction in cancer patients). In trials in advanced cancer, the number of nonevaluable patients at the end of the study may be large enough to invalidate the results. For these reasons, authors such as Walsh[40] chose a parallel design for the comparison of the effects of the adjuvant drug. The main problem associated with this choice is that the power of the trial decays very significantly. A deterioration in the cognitive status or sedation in the patient population receiving the study drug may not be easily perceived, and the final choice of the patient and investigator as an overall assessment of satisfaction is lost. Considering a drug with a potentially long latency to maximal effect, it is important to consider that this long latency may not necessarily be true for all the effects of the drug. For example, although the antidepressant effect of tricyclics takes place over approximately 2 or 3 weeks after starting the treatment, analgesic effects on post-herpetic neuralgia may take place as early as 48 and 72 h after they are started.[41] Although the maximal effect of an NSAID in the treatment of rheumatic conditions usually takes several weeks, their effect on cancer pain usually can be measured after just a couple of days.[42] Before enrolling ourselves in a long-lasting and expensive controlled trial of a new adjuvant, we find it extremely useful to perform a pilot uncontrolled trial in a reduced number of patients trying to determine the onset of action and duration of the different effects of the new adjuvant. During this pilot uncontrolled trial, it is also possible to test different doses of the drug under study. Although the placebo effect cannot be ruled out, these pilot trials provide information about the characteristics of the drug and about the accuracy of the whole trial that is being designed. Comparing the results of the use of the adjuvant drug with our historical controls we are able to plan our controlled trial in a much more accurate way.

b. Short-Acting Drugs

In the case of short-acting drugs the design is much more simple. A double-blind cross-over trial is almost mandatory for proper assessment of these drugs. The power of this design is much higher than that of parallel design, and it also allows for a blinded choice by patients and investigators. This blinded choice provides an overall estimation of the patient and investigators satisfaction with the new agent.

However, some drugs cannot be tested on a double-blind cross-over trial although they may have a short effect. We have previously described our experience with drugs with sedating effects. The patient and investigator are much more able to discriminate on the effects and side effects of drugs on a cross-over trial. Therefore, drugs with a significant number of side effects may need to be given in a very low dose or to be tested in a parallel trial, where the ability to compare on the same patient with placebo does not exist.

Other drugs that may not be used in a short-term cross-over trial are those that have a rapid onset of action but a long-lasting effect. For example, a study of antibiotics on the pain on ulcerated tumors could not be designed on a cross-over basis because of the significant effect that 3 or 4 days of antibiotic therapy would have on the natural history of local infection and therefore, on the subsequent placebo phase.

2. The Patient Population

Clinical trials should be performed in a population that resembles as much as possible, the population that will clinically benefit from the use of the drug on a daily basis.

Unfortunately, in an effort to better characterize the biological effects of certain agents and to simplify the clinical trial, investigators frequently study a population of patients in more stable conditions than those patients who would ultimately benefit from the new treatment. One example of this problem is the development of long-acting morphine preparations. Most of the studies on these new agents were done in a population of very stable patients requring an overall low dose of narcotics.[43-45] The results from these trials cannot be applied to a population of patients with severe pain, requring much higher doses of narcotics, who have significant impairment of gastrointestinal motility and in whom the bioavailability of the long-acting preparation may be significantly different from that of patients in an earlier stage of the disease.

Sometimes, because of the characteristics of the drug, the study cannot be performed in the population that is most likely to benefit from it. If this is the case, the investigators should report this fact in the "patients and methods" section and should also discuss the possible impact of the patient population on the final results of the study.

The patient population should be properly characterized using all known prognostic parameters. In the case of a cross-over trial, it will help other investigators and clinicians to properly understand the population in which the trial was performed. In the case of a parallel trial, a proper characterization of the population becomes much more important. The population of patients should be stratified according to the most important prognostic factors before randomization takes place. The distribution of neuropathic vs. non-neuropathic pain, incidental vs. continuous pain, and patients on very high doses of narcotics, with rapid development of tolerance, or with severe psychological distress should be balanced between patients receiving placebo and patients receiving the adjuvant drug. We have previously discussed the importance of proper staging in cancer pain research. The effects of any adjuvant drug may be significantly less evident in patients who are experiencing a rapid development of tolerance. Patients with a history of severe alcoholism or drug addiction or with cognitive impairment should be detected prior to admission to the trial and considered ineligible. Unfortunately, the statement "pain due to cancer" is considered an acceptable characterization of the pain syndrome by most medical journals. After we have defined the criteria for eligibility, it is important to consider how many of these potentially eligible patients we can enter in our trial within a reasonable period of time. The assistance of a biostatistician is invaluable at this stage of the planning of a trial. By determining what we would consider a clinical relevant difference, a biostatistician would be able to define for us the number of cases that we need in order to significantly reject a Type 2 error (the possibility that a real adjuvant effect exists even if our study does not find it). The strength with which our study will be able to reject this Type 2 error is defined as the "power" of the study. The number of cases that we will need to have a powerful study will be larger if we choose a parallel design than if we choose a cross-over design. Sometimes in order to answer some fundamental questions concerning the effects of different drugs, large numbers of patients are required. Even the largest individual centers may not be able to perform such trials. In cancer medicine this problem has been overcome very successfully by the creation of cooperative groups. These groups are able to design a significant number of clinical trials, and all the member institutions cooperate by accruing patients to these large trials. Unfortunately, no such group exists for clinical research in pain. If the problem under study occurs very rarely and patients remain stable for long periods of time, the "n of 1" design can be used. This has been discussed in depth in a previous chapter (see Chapter 5).

3. The End-Points of the Study

An adjuvant drug by definition is an additional drug that is given to a patient who is already receiving a narcotic analgesic. Therefore, this drug will (1) change the effects of the narcotic on the patient (i.e., analgesia, nausea, sedation, constipation, etc.), and (2) have therapeutic and side effects of its own (in the case of the tricyclic antidepressant it will have antidepressant effects as well as autonomic effects, dry mouth, hypotension, arrhythmias). For these reasons, the effects of an adjuvant drug on a patient who is already receiving a narcotic can be extremely complex.

These different effects will have a different latency of action (in the case of a tricyclic, dry mouth and sedation can take place immediately, analgesia can take place after 3 or 4 days of administration, and an antidepressant effect can take place after 2 weeks of administration). The effects will also have a different duration and a different intensity. From this, it is easy to conclude that no single study would be able to properly characterize the adjuvant effects of a given drug. Short-term, intensive cross-over trials will provide ample information on the acute effects of an adjuvant drug while missing some of the important long-term effects. Less intensive, long-term studies will focus on long-term effectiveness and side effects, while missing early effects. Research on amphetamines provides a useful example of these problems. Forrest et al. proved in an elegant double-blind study that a single dose of dextroamphetamine was able to potentiate morphine-induced analgesia and to decrease sedation.[46] However, it is not possible to conclude from this study that repeated doses of amphetamines are useful adjuvants for cancer pain. Our group found in two short-term cross-over trials that amphetamines could decrease narcotic-induced sedation in cancer patients and potentiate analgesia,[47,48] but significant toxicity and a rapid development of tolerance were detected. The results of our studies suggest that amphetamines can be useful adjuvants in a selected proportion of patients with pain due to advanced cancer. However, from our studies it cannot be assumed that amphetamines will be useful for long-term use in patients with chronic benign pain.

The finding of a significant improvement in one or more isolated variables does not necessarily mean that an adjuvant drug will be clinically useful: at the end of our double-blind, cross-over trial of mazindol, patients had significantly better pain control and lower analgesic consumption on mazindol as compared to placebo.[47] However, their final choice was equally distributed between "drug", "placebo", and "no-choice". In the case of mazindol, the lower level of patient satisfaction with the drug was probably due to the fact that it caused a significant deterioration in anxiety, appetite, and food intake.[47] This fact could be determined because we were measuring several other variables in addition to pain. However, even the simultaneous measurement of several variables will not give an adequate idea of global satisfaction: it is always possible that deterioration occurs in a variable that we are not measuring. It is also possible that the patient's choice reflects in some studies the improvement or deterioration of several variables that independently do not reach statistical significance. A recent trial on clonidine in the treatment of anticipatory nausea in patients receiving chemotherapy probably reflects this fact: although clonidine was able to decrease anticipatory nausea, patients preferred not to receive it in subsequent courses of chemotherapy.[49]

Although it is useful to combine objective (daily dose of narcotics, number of rescue doses, number of vomiting episodes, etc.) and subjective variables (pain intensity, nausea, somnolence, confusion, etc.) in these trials, it must be clear that the clinical usefulness of an adjuvant drug will depend on its ability to modify the subjective parameter: a "narcotic-sparing effect" is only important for the patient's comfort if it is associated with decreased toxicity (decreased narcotic-induced toxicity without significant toxicity by the adjuvant), or improved pain control. Because of the importance of the subjective parameters in these studies, a placebo or alternative drug phase is crucial: in both our trials on methylprednisolone[50] and methylphenidate,[48] pain intensity decreased significantly during the placebo phase as compared to the baseline assessment.

4. Future Research

Numerous studies of adjuvant drugs are needed. Some of the most important are as follows:

1. Non-narcotic analgesics: a better definition of the effects of these drugs in different types of pain is needed (i.e., visceral, neuropathic, incidental, etc). Because of their different side effects and mechanism of action, a comparison between acetaminophen and different NSAIDs in cancer pain would be useful. Among NSAIDs, the best type and dose has not been defined as yet.

2. Tricyclics: research on these drugs is complicated by their long latency to maximal effects and their high incidence of side effects. Although several controlled trials were started on these drugs as adjuvants for cancer pain, only one was published in abstract form.[41] A potential study on these drugs will be even more complicated in view of their recently suggested effect on bioavailability of morphine.[51] However, because they are frequently used as an adjuvant by some groups[52] and rarely used by others,[53] these drugs should be studied in a controlled trial. Such a study could very likely require a multicenter effort.

3. Corticosteroids: the nature and duration of effects of these drugs needs to be better characterized. The best drug and dose of corticosteroid should be established. The potential for additive toxicity suggests that they should not be combined with NSAIDs, a comparison on both drugs as narcotic adjuvants would be desirable.

4. Amphetamines: the indication for their use, as well as the proper type and dose should be better defined.

5. Antiemetics: comparative trials in order to assess the effectiveness and toxicity should be performed between metoclopramide, haloperidol, prochlorperazine, and corticosteroids. The newer antiemetics such as modified benzamides[54] or anti-serotonergic drugs[55] should be tried as narcotic adjuvants. This is an area in which prospective studies are almost nonexistent.

6. Laxatives: prospective comparative trials should be designed in narcotic-induced constipation to assess effectiveness, toxicity, and patient satisfaction and compliance. The last two end-points are very important given the need for long-term use of laxatives in patients receiving narcotics. These patients frequently experience anorexia and chronic nausea that make the treatment more difficult.

7. Other drugs: the rest of the drugs included in Table 2 have been suggested to have adjuvant analgesic effects. Osteoclast-inhibiting agents such as diphosphonates[56] or calcitonin[57] are potentially useful drugs for bone pain. Because of the potential role of local infection, antibiotic trials should be performed in patients with ulcerated tumors who present with sudden and severe increase in pain due to ulcerated tumors.[58] Because information on the potential adjuvant effects of these drugs is extremely limited, uncontrolled trials of different dosages of these drugs should be tried before long-term, expensive controlled trials. These uncontrolled trials would help to define type and duration of effects, and the end-points of the controlled trial.

V. SUMMARY AND CONCLUSIONS

During recent years, major progress has taken place in the treatment of cancer pain. This progress has been the result of both improved medical education and aggressive clinical research. In this chapter we have focused on what we believe are the three most important areas where the development of consensus among researchers is vital. The next step for those of us interested in cancer pain management will be to work closely with other disciplines. We need to interact with basic cancer scientists to better define the mechanisms by which cancer pain occurs and its association with different characteristics of tumors. We must interact with epidemiologists and biostatisticians to define a new common language that will allow us to compare the results of our work. We also need to cooperate with neurologists, pharmacologists, and gastroenterologists to better characterize the effects of narcotics, the other symptom complexes that are present in the cancer patient, and the effects of different adjuvant drugs. The integration of pain within the overall picture of quality of life will increase our knowledge on the impact of pain on the whole person.

Hopefully, new and exciting therapeutic alternatives for cancer pain will evolve from this interaction.

REFERENCES

1. **Foley, K.,** The treatment of cancer pain, *N. Engl. J. Med.*, 313, 84, 1985.
2. Cancer Pain: A monograph on the management of cancer pain, Health and Welfare Canada, Minister of Supply and Services Canda, H42-2/5-1984E.
3. **Marks, R. and Sachar, F.,** Undertreatment of medical inpatients with narcotic analgesics, *Ann. Intern. Med.*, 78, 173, 1973.
4. **Angel, L. M.,** The quality of mercy, *N. Engl. J. Med.*, 306, 98, 1982.
5. **Morgan, J. and Plett, D.,** Opiophobia in the United States: the undertreatment of severe pain, in *Society and Medication: Conflicting Signals for Prescriptions of Patients*, Morgan, J. and Kagan, D., Eds., Lexington Press, Lexington, Massachusetts, 1983, 313.
6. Pain and the dissatisfied dead (editorial), *Br. Med. J.*, 1, 459, 1978.
7. **Swerdlow, M. and Stjernsward, J.,** Cancer pain relief — an urgent problem, *World Health Forum*, 3, 325, 1982.
8. **Stimmel, B.,** Pain, analgesia and addiction: an approach to the pharmacologic management of pain, *Clin. J. Pain*, 1, 14, 1985.
9. **Payne, R. and Foley, K.,** Advances in the management of cancer pain, *Cancer Treat. Rep.*, 68, 173, 1984.
10. **Beaver, W.,** Management of cancer pain with parenteral medication, *JAMA*, 744, 2653, 1980.
11. **Patersen, A. H. G.,** Clinical staging in its prognostic significance, in Stage B, in *Pointers to Cancer Prognosis*, Martinus Nijoff, Dordrecht, 1988, 37.
12. **Bruera, E., Macmillan, K., Hanson, J., et al.,** The Edmonton staging system for cancer pain, *Pain*, 37, 203, 1989.
13. **Levinthal, C. F.,** Milk of Paradise — Milk of Hell — The history of ideas about opium, *Perspect. Biol. Med.*, 28, 4, 561, 1985.
14. **Brecher, E.,** *Licit and Illicit Drugs*, Little, Brown, Boston, 1972.
15. **Kaiko, R. F., Wallenstein, S. L., Rogers, A. G., Gravinski, T. Y., and Houde, R. W.,** Analgesic and mood effects of heroin and morphine in cancer patients with post-operative pain, *N. Engl. J. Med.*, 304, 1501, 1981.
16. **Twycross, R. G.,** Choice of strong analgesic in terminal cancer: diamorphine or morphine?, *Pain*, 3, 933, 1977.
17. **Levine, M. N., Sackett, D. L., and Bush, H.,** Heroin vs. Morphine for cancer pain, *Arch. Intern. Med.*, 146, 353, 1986.
18. **MacDonald, R. N. and Bruera, E.,** Clinical trials in cancer pain research, in *Recent Advances in Pain Research*, Foley, K. and Ventafridda, V., Eds., Raven Press, New York, 1990.
19. **Pasternak, G. W.,** Multiple MU opiate receptors: biochemical and pharmacological evidence for multiplicity, *Biochem. Pharmacol.*, 35(3), 361, 1986.
20. **Pfeiffer, A., Brantl, V., Herz, A., and Emrich, M.,** Psychotomimesis medicated by kappa opiate receptors, *Science*, 233, 774, 1983.
21. **Ettinger, D. S., Vitali, P. J., and Trump, D. L.,** Important clinical pharmacologic considerations in the use of methadone in cancer patients, *Cancer Treat. Rep.*, 63, 457, 1979.

22. Levy, M. H., Pain management in advanced cancer, *Semin. Oncol.*, 12(4), 3394, 1985.
23. McGivney, W. T. and Crooks, G. M., The care of patients with severe chronic pain in terminal illness, *JAMA*, 251 (9), 1182, 1984.
24. Russell, R. D. and Chang, K. J., Alternated delta and mu receptor activation: a strategem for limiting opioid tolerance, *Pain*, 36, 381, 1989.
25. Moulin, D. E., Ling, G. S. F., and Pasternak, G. W., Unidirectional analgesic crosstolerance between morphine and levorphanol in the rat, *Pain*, 33, 233, 1988.
26. Arnér, S. and Myerson, B. A., Lack of analgesic effect of opioids in neuropathic and idiopathic forms of pain, *Pain*, 33, 11, 1988.
27. Portenoy, R. K., personal communication.
28. Portenoy, R. K. and Foley, K. M., Chronic use of opioid analgesics in non-malignant: a report of 38 cases, *Pain*, 25, 171, 1986.
29. McGuire, D. B., Barbour, L., Boxler, J., et al., Fixed interval dosing vs. as-needed analgesics in cancer outpatients, *J. Pain Sympt. Mgmt.*, 2(4), 199, 1987.
30. Barkas, G. and Duafala, M. E., Advances in cancer pain management: a review of patient-controlled analgesia, *J. Pain Sympt. Control*, 3(3), 150, 1988.
31. Hill, H. F., Chapman, R. C., Cornell, J. A., Sullivan, K. M., Sager, L. C., and Benedetti, C., Self administration of morphine in bone marrow transplant patients reduces drug requirement, *Pain*, in press.
32. Bruera, E., Brenneis, C., Michaud, M., Macmillan, K., Hanson, J., and MacDonald, R. N., Patient-controlled hydromorphone versus continuous subcutaneous infusion for the treatment of cancer pain, *J. Natl. Cancer Inst.*, 80, 1152, 1988.
33. Johnson, L. R., Magnani, B., Chan, V., and Ferrante, F. M., Modifiers for patient controlled analgesia efficacy. I. Locus of control, *Pain*, 39, 17, 1989.
34. Foley, K. M., Portenoy, R., MacDonald, R. N., and Bruera, E., Cancer pain, *Am. Soc. Clin. Oncol. Educational Booklet*, 1988, 79.
35. Feinman, C., Pain relief by antidepressants: possible modes of action, *Pain*, 23, 1, 1985.
36. Manara, A., Shelly, M., Quinn, K., et al., The effect of metoclopramide on the absorption of oral controlled release morphine, *Br. J. Clin. Pharmacol.*, 25, 518, 1988.
37. Twycross, R., Effect of Codeine in the Brompton Cocktail, in *Advances in Pain Research*, Bonica, J. and Ventafridda, V., Eds., Raven Press, New York, 1979, 627.
38. Woodcock, A., Gross, E., and Gellery, A., A comparison of diazepam and promethazine in the treatment of breathlessness in patients with chronic obstructive lung disease, *Br. Med. J.*, 1, 96, 1982.
39. Woodcock, A., Gross, E., Gellery, A., et al., Effects of dihydrocodeine, alcohol and caffeine on breathlessness and exercise tolerance in patients with chronic obstructive lung disease, *N. Engl. J. Med.*, 305, 1611, 1981.
40. Walsh, T. D., Controlled study of imipramine and morphine in chronic pain due to cancer, *Proc. ASCO*, 5, 237, 1986.
41. Watson, C., Evans, R., Reed, K., et al., Amitryptiline versus placebo in post-herpetic neuralgia, *Neurology*, 32, 671, 1982.
42. Ferrer-Brechner, T. and Ganz, P., Combination therapy with ibuprofen and methadone for chronic cancer pain, *Am. J. Med.*, 77, 78, 1984.
43. Hanks, G., Twycross, R., and Bliss, J., Controlled release morphine tablets: a double-blind trial in patients with advanced cancer, *Anaesthesia*, 42, 840, 1987.
44. Walsh, T. D., Clinical evaluation of slow release morphine tablets, *Proc. Am. Soc. Clin. Oncol.*, 4, 266, 1985.
45. MacDonald, R. N., Bruera, E., Brenneis, C., et al., Long acting morphine in the treatment of cancer pain: a double-blind cross-over trial, *Proc. Am. Soc. Clin. Oncol.*, 6, 1054, 1987.
46. Forrest, W., Brown, B., Brown, C., et al., Dextroamphetamine with morphine for the treatment of postoperative pain, *N. Engl. J. Med.*, 296, 712, 1977.
47. Bruera, E., Carraro, S., Roca, E., et al., Double-blind evaluation of mazindol in enhancing the comfort of terminally ill cancer patients, *Cancer Treat. Rep.*, 70, 295, 1986.
48. Bruera, E., Chadwick, S., Brenneis, C., et al., Methylphenidate associated with narcotics for the treatment of cancer pain, *Cancer Treat. Rep.*, 71, 67, 1987.
49. Fetting, J., Stefanek, M., Sheidlen, J., et al., Noradrenergic activity in anticipatory nausea, *Proc. Am. Soc. Clin. Oncol.*, 7, 284, 1988.
50. Bruera, E., Roca, E., Cedaro, L., et al., Action of oral Methylprednisolone in terminal cancer patients: a prospective randomized double-blind study, *Cancer Treat. Rep.*, 69, 751, 1985.
51. Ventafridda, V., Ripamonti, C., DeConno, F., et al., Antidepressants increase bioavailability of morphine in cancer patients, *Lancet*, i, 1204, 1987.
52. Brodie, G., Indomethacin and bone pain, *Lancet*, 2, 1180, 1988.
53. Ventafridda, V., Spaldi, E., Caraceni, A., and De Conno, F., Intraspinal morphine for cancer pain, *Acta Anaesthesiol. Scand.*, 31 (Suppl. 85), 47, 1987.

54. **Smaldone, L., Fairchild, C., Rozencweig, M., et al.,** Dose-range evaluation of BMY-25801, a non-dopamenergic antiemetic, *Proc. Am. Soc. Clin. Oncol.*, 7, 280, 1988.
55. **Kris, M., Gralla, R., Tyson, L., et al.,** Phase I study of the serotonin antagonist GR-C507 when used as an antiemetic, *Proc. Am. Soc. Clin. Oncol.*, 7, 283, 1988.
56. **Chung, A., Chantrinia, A., et al.,** Use of diphosphonate in metastatic bone disease, *N. Engl. J. Med.*, 308, 1499, 1983.
57. **Vaughn, C. and Vaitkevicius, K.,** The effects of calcitonin in hypernidemia in patients with malignancy, *Cancer*, 34, 1268, 1974.
58. **Bruera, E. and MacDonald, R. N.,** Intractable pain in patients with advanced head and neck tumors: a possible role for local infection, *Cancer Treat. Rep.*, 70, 691, 1986.

Chapter 23

QUALITY-OF-LIFE RESEARCH IN THE EUROPEAN PALLIATIVE CARE SETTING

Sam Ahmedzai

TABLE OF CONTENTS

I. INTRODUCTION: WHAT IS 'PALLIATIVE CARE'?

The expression 'palliative care' is not new in medical terminology, but it has recently acquired a more specific meaning, particularly in the context of cancer treatment.[1] There is still debate about the exact boundaries of this emerging discipline.[2] The term is derived from the Latin 'pallium', for 'cloak'. The implication is that the disease process, which is accepted as being incurable (and usually has a very poor or 'terminal' prognosis), is being 'cloaked' or covered. More importantly it implies that the problems caused by the disease (which may be physical symptoms, or emotional, social, or spiritual distress) are also 'cloaked' — that is, they are alleviated or rendered or rendered harmless to the patient, without trying to eradicate their causes.

A crucial ingredient of the modern approach to palliative care is the recognition of the patient as just one part of the family, of which other members may be also suffering.[3] ('Family' is freely interpreted as including not only blood or marriage relations, but close friends, neighbors, and other nonprofessional carers.) Their distress may be caused by observing the effects of disease on the patient; the strain of an increasing nursing burden; the consequences of social and financial embarrassment; or the emotional stresses of impending loss, with the accompanying feelings of guilt and shame which often arise in families.

Of course, not all patients with terminal cancer come from close-knit families. Especially for those without relatives or close friends and who are socially isolated, there are aspects of the illness which cannot be understood and managed in purely medical terms. Palliative care embodies 'holistic' care, i.e., the patient is approached as a whole person and consequently much of the 'therapy' is oriented along the lines of nursing, or psychosocial support, rather than the prescription of drugs or other oncological regimens.[1]

Most clinicians working in palliative care would emphasize that the specialty is not restricted to cancer patients, and although malignancy is the subject of this book, nearly all of the issues raised in this chapter apply equally well to other diagnostic groups.

II. DEVELOPMENT OF PALLIATIVE CARE IN EUROPE

Although the term 'palliative care' is new in this specific sense, there is a long tradition in European medicine of its underlying tenets. The origins of the 'modern' hospice movement may be traced to early Christian times,[1] and at the time of the Crusades in the Holy Land there arose both military and religious orders which built fine 'hospitals' throughout southern Europe. Some of these medieval foundations are still surviving, although the edifices may have been rebuilt. The words 'hospital' and 'hospice' are derived from the Latin 'hospes', which means 'guest' or 'host'.

The first truly modern hospice, which was specifically established for the 'dying' (as opposed to the poor and needy sick) was Our Lady's Hospice, opened in 1876 in Dublin, Eire. St. Joseph's Hospice followed in the East End of London, founded by the same order of Catholic nuns. St. Christopher's Hospice was opened by Cicely Saunders in 1967, again in London. In the U.K. now there are over 120 free-standing hospice establishments, most of which are to varying degrees independent from the National Health Service. A recent survey of British in-patient units by Johnson et al.[4] has shown that it would be a mistake to regard these as a homogeneous group — the most significant variations arose in the context of the medical staffing level of hospice units.

Alongside this expansion of in-patient hospice units in Britain, there have been three significant related developments. In the community, 'home care' has rapidly become a major priority for the allocation of resources and skilled manpower,[5] sometimes taking precedence over in-patient facilities. This compares with the evolving situation in North America, where community-based 'hospice programs' are also increasing.[6] In mainland Europe too, the organization of health care in many countries has been conducive to the development of community-based palliative care.[7]

Attached to many British hospice buildings are the 'day hospices', which allow for the care of patients who do not need admission, but who may benefit from a more socially orientated program.[8] Many day-patients however have major physical problems, which may be amenable to skilled input from physiotherapists and occupational therapists, as well as doctors and nurses.

The third new area of palliative care provision is the 'hospital support team'. The model is particularly well developed in some of the major London teaching hospitals.[9] This type of care can more readily reach patients with recently diagnosed incurable cancers, and is particularly applicable where the proportion of deaths occurring in hospitals is high, or where there is no in-patient hospice establishment nearby. In other European countries without the well-established infrastructure of charitable and voluntary resources which prevails in Britain, the hospital support team may become an attractice model for providing palliative care. In late 1989 Paris opened its first Centre de Soins Palliatif — appropriately enough, in the Hotel Dieu, which is one of the most beautiful surviving examples of the early Christian 'hospital'.

III. RESEARCH IN PALLIATIVE CARE

It was inevitable that in its early years, palliative care would strive to establish itself as a 'respectable' discipline. This has been done up till now mainly by the educational efforts from hospice staff who have impressed medical and nursing colleagues in 'mainstream' oncology, of the benefits of the intensive palliative approach. In the 1980s, however, it became clear that in order to justify its very existence in the increasingly expensive and competitive health care 'marketplace', palliative care — like oncology as a whole — had to prove its worth more rigorously, by means of published research.[10,11]

The fields of research in this subject fall broadly into two categories: operational (concerned with the models of care, the provision of services, the requirements of staff, etc.), and clinical.[12] Within clinical research, there has been in the past a tendency to dwell on empirical observations (particularly by means of single-center surveys or retrospective series), rather than on prospective and controlled trial designs. Very large empirical series, however, especially those which are multicenter such as the National Hospice Study in the U.S.A.,[13] may yield valuable information about the prevalence of symptoms and other problems in terminal cancer.

Clinical research in European palliative care has focused, not unexpectedly, mainly on the problems of pain management.[14] But while great strides in the understanding of pain mechanisms and analgesic regimes may have come from European research, the wider issues of 'quality of life' in the advanced cancer patient have not been formally addressed with anything like as much enthusiasm. Thus, in spite of the 'holistic' nature of palliative care, there has been a tendency to present the results of management of a single or range of physical symptoms,[15,16] which leads the reader to make the assumption that this automatically resulted in improved 'quality of life'.

There is clearly no shortage of clinical parameters which could be measured in studies of palliative care. First, there are the direct noxious tissue effects of the disease process and the multitude of treatment toxicities which can give rise to symptoms and degrees of physical impairment and disability. Oncologists have for years recorded these problems using *ad hoc* symptom scores and standardized instruments such as the WHO toxicity scales.[17] Palliative care services must clearly also attempt to measure physical suffering, but it would be sad if they stopped at that, as so often oncologists do.

Second, there are more diffuse and subtle 'paraneoplastic' syndromes (many of which are hormonally mediated), which may cause upsets of physical, mental, or psychological functioning as well as shorten life.[18] The commonest and often most devastating syndrome is 'cancer cachexia', which affects patients with both solid tumors and hematological malignancies. Its cause is still poorly understood, although the roles of abnormal tissue metabolism, cytokines, and psychological factors have been emphasized.[19,20] Recently the administration of a progestogen such as megestrol acetate has been found to reverse many of the features of cachexia, but not without significant dose-related toxicity.[21] As another example, hypercalcemia, which ultimately may be fatal, is the cause of significant loss of well-being due to nausea, vomiting, confusion, and debility. It can now be readily controlled for weeks with intravenous regimes.[22] This obviously raises ethical issues about the use of i.v. treatments in patients who may be dying — another aspect that needs to be explored and evaluated.

Third, it is now well accepted that patients with malignant disease at any stage are susceptible to major psychological or psychiatric disorders.[23,24] They may precede the malignant disease and are often then exacerbated by it, or they arise secondarily to the diagnosis of cancer and its treatment. In palliative care of terminally ill patients, these disorders have a great impact not only on the patients' lives, but also on their carers and other family members.

The influx of 'technological' procedures for palliation in oncology, such as endoscopic laser treatment for tracheobronchial or rectal lesions,[25,26] or the introduction of stents for tracheobronchial obstruction,[27] will soon be felt in palliative care. Just as McNeil et al.[28] showed that patients with laryngeal cancer could be critical of their surgeons' approach, it is valid to challenge the place of these new technologies when they start to be applied in more advanced cancer patients. Quality-of-life evaluation (certainly also with some assessment of financial costs) would be the ideal way of undertaking this.

IV. DIRECTIONS OF QUALITY-OF-LIFE RESEARCH

Even in the latter half of the 1980s, there were relatively few publications focusing on the broad aspects of quality of life in advanced cancer patients receiving palliative care, compared with those in the early stages of disease and receiving 'radical' or 'curative' regimes of surgery, radiotherapy, or chemotherapy.[29,30]

It is interesting to note that some of the studies which appear to focus on 'quality of life' aspects in hospice patients tend to be really more concerned with evaluating the process and quality of care in specialist settings.[15,31] Once again, this may be valid and useful if there is a multicenter comparison of outcomes,[31] but single-center studies are inevitably open to bias and will have mainly localized relevance. Unlike the large-scale National Hospice Study in the U.S.,[32] so far there has not been an objective attempt to compare outcomes between palliative care settings and 'mainstream' hospitals or oncology centers in Europe.[33]

The National Hospice Study used, among other tools, standard 'oncology' approaches to measuring facets of quality of life in hospice patients, notably the Spitzer[34] and Karnofsky[35] scales. The former was designed for use with 'advanced' cancer patients (but has been used extensively in early cancer); the latter acknowledges the possibility of the patient's death, but only in terms of progressive loss of functioning. While comparability with oncology settings is important, it is clear that more specific measures also need to be employed for research in the modern palliative care setting.

One recent candidate for this application is an instrument published by MacAdam et al.[36] This new questionnaire had 43 items, scored with a five-point verbal self-rating scale. The authors performed a factor analysis based on a pilot study with 259 patients, which led to the identification of five main factors: 'mood', 'gastrointestinal symptoms', 'fears and family worries', 'knowledge and involvement', and 'support'. The patients in this study had 'advanced cancer', and were taken from acute hospitals in Perth, Western Australia. From these results a shorter 20-item questionnaire was formulated.

It is interesting to compare MacAdam's five factors with the nine identified in the piloting of three new site-specific measures for assessing quality of life in 'advanced cancer', conducted by Cella et al.[37] among 45 cancer patients. They found the nine separate content domains rated in order of priority by patients were: 'physical function', 'family relationships', 'emotional function', 'spirituality', 'treatment satisfaction', 'future orientation', 'intimacy/sexuality', 'social relationships', and 'work'.

Fowlie et al.[38] have described the validation and application of MacAdam's shortened scale. They compared it with the Spitzer scale and a 10 cm linear analog scale completed by patient, doctor, and nurse. For analysis purposes they divided the 20-item MacAdam questionnaire into four sections, covering 'symptoms', 'spirits', 'knowledge', and 'support'. This study had the added feature of a comparison between a continuing care unit and a general hospital medical ward in Aberdeen, Scotland. The MacAdam scale was found by Fowlie et al. to be a "useful diagnostic and therapeutic tool, particularly in the areas relating to a patient's mood or spirits".

The assertion that the questionnaire was 'therapeutic' is intriguing, and the authors qualify it so: "There was a sense in which the administration of the questionnaire was therapeutic, allowing patients to consider and explore areas of difficulty which might otherwise not be readily accessible. Several patients from each unit admitted that this was the first time they had talked to anybody about certain aspects of their illness." Fowlie et al. are to be congratulated on their honesty over this point: many would find it strange that patients in a continuing care ('hospice') unit had not previously had the opportunity to talk openly of their concerns. However, those who have worked in this setting will acknowledge that even the open atmosphere that prevails in a hospice does not always immediately allow everybody the ability to communicate freely. The thoughtful and selective use of a questionnaire may thus be seen not as intrusive, but rather as a positive gesture facilitating communication between patients and staff.

The Spitzer scale was also used by Higginson et al.[39] in their development of the 'Support Team Assessment Schedule' (STAS). This schedule has particular relevance to community care of patients with cancer, and also of AIDS patients. The STAS has the benefit of using clear definitions for its 16 items, which are graded on a 0—4 scale. The range of subjects in the schedule is also impressive — they include symptom control, anxiety, insight, communication and planning, practical and financial needs, communication between professionals, and the support and advice needed for other professionals. The scale was based on a North London team's goals for providing care. The items are completed weekly by the team staff.

The STAS has been piloted and is being validated in a number of British community teams, against instruments such as the Karnofsky and a modified Spitzer scale. It would be interesting to see if this method, which relies heavily on its verbal description of responses, can adapt to the needs of other European countries in translation. Further tests for this approach would be its use in in-patient hospice settings; and in controlled clinical trials.

The STAS, like the original version of the Spitzer scale, is based on the observations and scores of staff members. This approach may be more practical in some settings, and could have the benefit of less 'missing data' as patients become sicker and less able or motivated to complete self-rated questionnaires.[12] Moreover, in one multicenter study comparing home care nursing teams in the north of England, it was found that the Spitzer scale functioned as a useful predictor of future nursing needs.[40] However, it is now acknowledged that patients themselves (and relatives to some extent) must contribute significantly to their own quality-of-life measurement.[30,41]

Prospective controlled studies using patient-rated instruments have not emerged in the European palliative care literature. This may be because of the 'newness' of such instruments (at least to the staff in palliative care settings), or because they have been mostly designed from the point of view of the cancer clinical trial. The former excuse will become less valid as the usage of self-rated forms becomes accepted in European clinical research. The latter is not so easily rectified, and calls for the design of new specific scales for palliative care usage, or validated modifications of existing 'oncology' instruments.

Other formal methods of assessing patients' health care needs can tell us indirectly about their quality of life. Thus, a Swedish study by Beck-Friis et al.[42] of patients with advanced cancer living at home and focusing on their 'activities of daily living' which used the traditional 'ADL' instrument of Katz,[43] has given good insight into the problems of dying with failing independence. Another approach which avoids the 'medical' model is the nursing assessment of patient and family dependency (acuity);[44] this is particularly relevant in view of the significant nursing role in palliative and terminal care. Such forms of assessment can very reasonably be seen as contributing to 'quality of life' research: ideally all studies in this field should be multidisciplinary.

A different way again of looking at quality of life, which is in tune with modern 'marketplace' attitudes to health care provision,[45] is the measurement of 'consumer satisfaction'. (It could be argued that the rise of the hospice movement itself is a good example of a consumer-led health care provision, at least in Britain where there has been considerable reliance on charitable and voluntary support.)

Consumer satisfaction studies could take many different forms: patients' and their relatives' views obtained by interviews, formal questionnaires, and composite approaches. The areas which could be researched include satisfaction with drug treatments and interventions such as radiotherapy, nerve blocks, physiotherapy, art therapy; satisfaction with services such as community-based nursing teams or hospital support teams; satisfaction with the fabric of hospice buildings, out-patient departments, food, facilities for visiting, access to pet animals, and other features of hospice philosophy which can make existence more 'dignified' than in hospital.

In palliative care this methodology is relatively new and untested. In Dublin (where modern European hospice care began) an interview-based study identified the needs and problems of hospice in-patients, and the extent to which they were met after admission.[46] The interviews were informal and unstructured but were tape-recorded and subsequently assessed and rated for content "on (1) patients' awareness of dying and (2) opinions of their care". The interviews were conducted on the day before admission and repeated 8 days after admission. The study showed surprisingly that one day before being admitted, less than half of the patients showed awareness of dying and over half seemed unaware that they were going to a hospice. After admission, nearly all patients were satisfied that the hospice had met their needs. Of the 91 consecutive patients to be admitted who were eligible for this study, 41 were excluded from the first interview and of the 50 eligible after 1 week, a further 19 were excluded. The reasons for exclusion were given as 'confusion', 'too ill or weak to carry on conversation', 'not within the Dublin area on the day prior to admission', 'refusal by the patient/doctor of family' and 'not first admission'. By the second interview 8 days after admission, 14 patients had died. These figures illustrate the extraordinary difficulties which face researchers who wish to study patients in this very late stage of life.

In an English hospice Dand et al.[47] have conducted a more formal 'consumer satisfaction' study which used a structured interview. This was based on a schedule of items covering a wide range of topics, including physical symptoms, psychological distress, nursing needs, views of community staff before admission and of hospice staff 1 week after admission, and of the hospice fabric and facilities. The items had pre-defined categories for the scoring the the patients' verbal responses. Another aspect of this study was the interview with the patient's main carer (closest relative or friend), which was done usually on the same day as the patient's, and covered similar ground. The results from this study have yet to be published in full, but they may throw further light on the previously noted discrepancies between patients' and carers' perception of the same illness.[48]

V. PROBLEMS OF QUALITY-OF-LIFE RESEARCH

To understand the noticeable lack of controlled prospective studies of quality of life in palliative care, it is useful to examine the practical difficulties that may obstruct the mounting of such research. The problems arise in the areas of research methodology, philosophical/ethical issues, and staff resistance.

Some of the methodological problems have already been alluded to. Most of the quality-of-life instruments in current use were developed for cancer clinical trials. The inclusion of questions about hair loss, for example, which is appropriate for chemotherapy studies, may seem at best irrelevant or at worst offensive to advanced cancer patients. Again, the increasing use of patient self-rated forms may strike some hospice staff as being over-intrusive for very sick patients. They would also be inappropriate when patients are unable to speak, or hold a pen. The lack of accurate translations of English-language questionnaires is another obstacle in many European countries. These deficiencies have to be tackled and rectified, rather than being used as excuses to persist solely with observer-rated scoring systems such as the Karnofsky index.

In cancer trials, there are clear pointers to the timing of quality-of-life assessments: for example, pre-chemotherapy baseline, after each pulse, and at regular follow-ups. The frequency and timing of assessments in palliative care is equally critical, but not so clear. Should the baseline be at diagnosis, or when a patient is referred, or accepted by a hospice team? Palliative medical regimens are not usually pulsed like chemotherapy cycles, so how often and when should repeat measures be done?

Somewhat more contentious are the 'philosophical' and ethical difficulties.[49] Even if hospice staff (and their management boards, which in the U.K. often have a majority of lay members) agree to the use of a quality-of-life evaluation, they may balk at a full-scale controlled clinical trial to assess the value of a new treatment. The use of randomization is especially likely to arouse ethical objections (although paradoxically, it is only by randomization that certain 'grey' areas in medical decision making may be resolved).

Again within clinical trials, the description of one group as a 'control', and particularly if its allocated treatment is a 'placebo', can prove to be an ethical stumbling block. Yet another example is a protocol's need for 'invasive' tests such as a blood count, when some of the patients may have already expressed a dislike of such investigations in the past. Finally, there appears to be no consensus in Europe over the question of 'informed consent' in clinical trials.[50] In studies involving very sick or dying subjects, the idea of requesting consent which may involve written permission could strike many palliative care staff or hospice Ethics Committees as objectionable.

The third, and perhaps the most serious obstacle to conducting quality-of-life research in palliative care, is the resistance — usually born, one regretfully suspects, of ignorance or inexperience — from the clinical staff directly involved with the families. Some staff members may even have come into palliative care in order to turn their back on what they see as unwarranted experimentation on sick patients. Others may approve of research, but adopt too strenuously the role of 'patient advocate'. Many of the 'ethical' objections raised above may be quoted by staff seeking to defend their patients from what they perceive as a 'final indignity'.

It is not always easy to refute these arguments against conducting research in the terminally ill. Indeed it is a proud achievement of palliative care that these objectives are fairly heard and nearly always heeded, in the interests of the patients. It is more appropriate to point out examples where simple, noninvasive quality-of-life studies have shown clear benefit to patients, when traditional issues such as 'response' and 'survival' are irrelevant. One area where recent studies have started to challenge traditional attitudes about the appropriateness of 'aggressive' palliative measures is that of malignant disease in the elderly.[51]

With a consistently aging but more health-conscious population in Western countries, the distinctions between 'middle-age' and 'elderly' are becoming blurred. Studies are now showing that older people can tolerate similar or slightly modified chemotherapy regimes as younger adults,[52,53] and the criteria for palliative surgical intervention have also been reviewed.[54]

VI. FUTURE OF QUALITY-OF-LIFE RESEARCH IN PALLIATIVE CARE

The purpose of this chapter is not to cast a shadow of despondency over the paucity of quality-of-life research results in the palliative care setting. On the contrary, the exciting rapid emergence and divergence of palliative care systems through Europe should be seen as a cause for celebration of the patient's right to have a quality of life at all. Research is now urgently needed, preferably on a cooperative multicenter basis, to demonstrate or refute the benefits of new trends, and to show ways of improving and making them more cost effective.

There are two directions in which the clinical research methodology in this area must develop. The first is the identification of appropriate, feasible, and reliable measures of quality of life, which have been validated for this population. These may be questionnaires or interview based, as either could be more relevant for specific settings. With questionnaire-based studies, it is crucial that patients participate actively in the rating. Given the family orientation of palliative care, it is important for quality of life of relatives and other carers to be assessed as well. For example, the most practical and cost-effective methods for assisting 'anticipatory grief' and providing bereavement support have yet to be established.

When quality-of-life tools are applied in palliative care, they should cover some areas of common interest with those of patients who are not seen as 'advanced' or 'terminally ill', so that these groups are not always regarded as separate species of cancer sufferers: rather, as the same travelers at different stages of the same journey.

It would seem to make sense, therefore, for some common measures to be tested and introduced into palliative care which have credibility in 'curative' oncology. The EORTC approach,[55] with a 'Core' questionnaire and 'Modules' which are specific for different settings may fall into this category. The benefits and costs of new therapies for terminally ill cancer patients could thus be compared meaningfully with those with early disease. Comparative research such as this could help to answer some of the difficult questions about when to stop certain 'radical' treatments, and when to initiate certain palliative services.[11]

The second major hurdle to be crossed in the European health care community is producing valid translations of good instruments. There may be merit in having some purely uninational forms, which can be sensitive to differences between countries in the attitudes of staff and public towards the diagnosis of cancer.[56] However, it would be better if quality-of-life questionnaires had international applicability. This will have the obvious advantage of enabling larger multicenter studies across European boundaries. It will also give us the opportunity of studying the fascinating differences between the cultural influences of nations on the quality of life of their advanced cancer patients.

REFERENCES

1. Saunders, C., What's in a name?, *Palliat. Med.*, 1, 57, 1987.
2. Ventafridda, V., Palliative medicine: a new approach, *J. Palliat. Care*, 4, 15, 1988.
3. Stedeford, A., Couples facing death, *Br. Med. J.*, 283, 1033, 1981.
4. Johnson, I. S., Rogers, C., Biswas, B., and Ahmedzai, S., What do hospices do? A survey of hospices in the United Kingdom and Eire, *Br. Med. J.*, 300, 791, 1989.
5. Ahmedzai, S. and Wilkes, E., Dying with dignity: a British view, in *Cost Versus Benefit in Cancer Care*, Stoll, B. A., Ed., Macmillan, Basingstoke, 1988, 73.
6. McCann, B. A., A profile of the evolution of hospice programs in the United States, in *The Care of the Dying*, Health Services Manpower Review, Keele, 1987, 17.
7. Toscani, F. and Mancini, C., Inadequacies of care in far advanced cancer patients: a comparison between home and hospital in Italy, *Palliat. Med.*, 4, 31, 1989.
8. Clench, P., The Dorothy House Foundation, Managing to care, in *Community Services for the Terminally Ill*, Clench, P., Ed., Patten Press, Richmond, 1984, chap. 2.
9. Dunlop, R. J., Davies, R. J., and Hockley, J. M., Preferred versus actual place of death: a hospital palliative care support team experience, *Palliat. Med.*, 3, 1971, 1989.
10. Mount, B. M. and Scott, J. F., Whither hospice evaluation, *J. Chronic Dis.*, 36, 731, 1983.
11. Stoll, B. A., Saying no is difficult in cancer, in *Cost Versus Benefit in Cancer Care*, Stoll, B. A., Ed., Macmillan, Oxford, 1988, 97.
12. Ahmedzai, S., Measuring quality of life in hospice care, *Oncology*, 4, 115, 1990.
13. Wachtel, T., Masterson-Allen, S., Reuben, D., Goldberg, R., and Mor, V., The end stage cancer patient: terminal common pathway, *Hospice J.*, 4, 43, 1988.
14. Twycross, R. G., *The Edinburgh Symposium on Pain Control and Medical Education*, Royal Society of Medicine Services Ltd, London, 1989.
15. McIllmurray, M. B. and Warren, M. R., Evaluation of a new hospice: the relief of symptoms in cancer patients in the first year, *Palliat. Med.*, 3, 135, 1989.
16. Lipton, S., Pain relief in active patients with cancer: the early use of nerve blocks improves the quality of life, *Br. Med. J.*, 298, 37, 1989.
17. Moinpour Mcmillen, C., Feigl, P., Metch, B., Hayden, K. A., Meyskens, F. L., and Crowley, J., Quality of life end points in cancer clinical trials: review and recommendations, *J. Natl. Cancer Inst.*, 81, 485, 1989.
18. Mosley, J. G., Progression of disease, in *Palliation in Malignant Disease*, Churchill Livingstone, Edinburgh, 1988, chap. 1.
19. Fearon, K. C. H. and Carter, D. C., What's new in general surgery. Cancer cachexia, *Ann. Surg.*, 208, 1, 1988.
20. Taylor, M. B., Moran, B. J., and Jackson, A. A., Nutritional problems and care of patients with far-advanced disease, *Palliat. Med.*, 3, 31, 1989.
21. Tchekmedyian, N. S., Tait, N., Moody, M., Greco, F. A., and Aisner, J., Appetite stimulation with megestrol acetate in cachectic cancer patients, *Semin. Oncol.*, 13, 37, 1986.
22. Ralston, S. H., Gallacher, S. J., Patel, U., Dryburgh, F. J., Fraser, W. D., Cowan, R. A., and Boyle, I. T., Comparison of three intravenous bisphosphonates in cancer-associated hypercalcaemia, *Lancet*, 1180, 1989.
23. Oxman, T. E. and Silberfarb, P. M., Psychiatric aspects of cancer in the aged, *Cancer Surv.*, 6, 511, 1987.
24. Hughes, J. and Lee, D., Depression among cancer patients admitted for hospice care, in *Psychosocial Oncology*, Watson, M., Greer, S., and Thomas, C., Eds., Pergamon Press, Oxford, 1988, 193.
25. Hetzel, M. R., Laser palliation of tracheobronchial tumours: a review, *Palliat. Med.*, 2, 134, 1988.
26. McGowan, I., Barr, H., and Krasner, N., Palliative laser therapy for inoperable rectal cancer — does it work?, *Cancer*, 63, 967, 1988.
27. Simonds, A. K., Iriving, J. D., Clarke, S. W., and Dick. R., Use of expandable metal stents in the treatment of bronchial obstruction, *Thorax*, 44, 680, 1989.
28. McNeil, B. J., Weichselbaum, R., and Pauker, S. G., Tradeoffs between quality and quantity of life in laryngeal cancer, *N. Engl. J. Med.*, 982, 1981.
29. De Haes, J. C. J. M., Quality of life: conceptual and theoretical considerations, in *Psychosocial Oncology*, Watson, M., Greer, S., and Thomas, C., Eds., Pergamon Press, Oxford, 1988, 61.
30. Twycross, R. G., Quality before quantity — a note of caution, *Palliat. Med.*, 1, 65, 1987.
31. Hinton, J., Comparison of places and policies for terminal care, *Lancet*, 29, 1979.
32. Greer, D. S., Mor, V., Sherwood, S., Morris, J. N., and Birnbaum, H., National hospice study analysis plan, *J. Chronic Dis.*, 36, 737, 1983.
33. Higginson, I. and McCarthy, M., Evaluation of palliative care: steps to quality assurance?, *Palliat. Med.*, 3, 267, 1989.

34. Spitzer, W. O., Dobson, A. J., Hall, J., Chesterman, E., Levi, J., Shepherd, R., Battista, R. N., and Catchlove, B. R., Measuring the quality of life of cancer patients. A concise QL-index for use by physicians, *J. Chronic Dis.*, 34, 585, 1981.

35. Mor, V., Laliberte, L., Morris, J. N., and Wiemann, M., The Karnofsky performance status scale, *Cancer*, 53, 2002, 1984.

36. MacAdam, D. B. and Smith, M., An initial assessment of suffering in terminal illness, *Palliat. Med.*, 1, 37, 1987.

37. Cella, D. F., Lee-Riordan, D., Silberman, M., Andrianopoulos, G., Gray, G., Puri, S., and Tulsky, D., Quality of life (QL) in advanced cancer: three new disease-specific measures, *Proc. Ann. Meet. Am. Soc. Clin. Oncol.*, 1989, 315.

38. Fowlie, M., Berkely, J., and Dingwall-Fordyce, I., Quality of life in advanced cancer: the benefits of asking the patient, *Palliat. Med.*, 3, 55, 1989.

39. Higginson, I., Wade, A., and McCarthy, M., A comparison of four outcome measures of terminal care, in *A Safer Death*, Plenum Press, London, 1988, 205.

40. Ward, A. W. M., *Home care services for the terminally ill*, a report for the Nuffield Foundation, Univ. Sheffield Printing Unit, Sheffield, 1985, 33.

41. Selby, P. and Robertson, B., Measurement of quality of life in patients with cancer, *Cancer Surv.*, 6, 523, 1987.

42. Beck-Friis, B., Strang, P., and Eklund, G., Physical dependence of cancer patients at home, *Palliat. Med.*, 3, 281, 1989.

43. Katz, S. and Akpom, C. A., A measure of primary sociobiological functions, *Int. J. Health Serv.*, 6, 493, 1976.

44. Biswas, B. A., Mitchell, S., and Ahmedzai, S., Measuring nursing dependency in a hospice, presented at Recent Advances in Palliation and Terminal Care Conf., Leicester, England, November 25, 1988 (abstr.).

45. Luck, M., Lawrence, B., Pocock, B., and Reilly, K., *Consumer and Market Research in Health Care*, Chapman and Hall, London, 1988.

46. McDonnell, M. M., Patients' perceptions of their care at Our Lady's Hospice, Dublin, *Palliat. Med.*, 3, 47, 1989.

47. Field, D., Measuring the satisfaction of patients and relatives with hospice care, presented at Annu. Conf. Eur. Soc. Psychosoc. Oncol., London, September 1, 1989.

48. Ahmedzai, S., Morton, A., Reid, J. T., and Stevenson, R. D., Quality of death from lung cancer: patients' reports and relatives' retrospective opinions, in *Psychosocial Oncology*, Watson, M., Greer, S., and Thomas, C., Eds., Pergamon Press, Oxford, 1986, 1987.

49. Downie, R. S. and Calman, K. C., A question of dying, in *Healthy Respect: Ethics in Health Care*, Faber and Faber, London, 1987, 206.

50. Rees, G. J. G., What is best for the patient? A European view, in *Cost vs Benefit in Cancer Care*, Stoll, B. A. Ed., Macmillan, Oxford, 1988, 31.

51. Mosley, J. G., Special problems for patients at the extremes of life, *Palliation in Malignant Disease*, Churchill Livingstone, Edinburgh, 1988, 139.

52. Sella, A., Logothetis, C. J., Dexeus, F. H., Amato, R., Fitz, K., and Finn, L., Cisplatin combination chemotherapy in elderly patients, *Proc. Annu. Meet. Am. Soc. Clin. Oncol.*, 1989, 315.

53. Smit, E. F., Carney, D. N., Harford, P., Sleijfer, D. T., and Postmus, P. E., A phase II study of oral etoposide in elderly patients with small cell lung cancer, *Thorax*, 44, 631, 1989.

54. Lewis, A. A. M. and Khoury, G. A., Resection for colorectal cancer in the very old: are the risks too high?, *Br. Med. J.*, 296, 459, 1988.

55. Aaronson, N. K., Bullinger, M., and Ahmedzai, S., A modular approach to quality of life assessment in cancer clinical trials, *Cancer Res.*, 111, 231, 1988.

56. Bracarda, S., Roila, F., Basurto, C., Picciafucco, M., Ballatori, E., Soldani, M., Crino, L., Del Favero, A., and Tonato, M., Quality of life of Italian lung cancer patients (pts): reproducibility and validation of a new questionnaire, *Proc. Annu. Meet. Am. Soc. Clin. Oncol.*, 1989, 240.

Chapter 24

QUALITY-OF-LIFE RESEARCH IN HOSPICE CARE

Susan Masterson-Allen and Vincent Mor

TABLE OF CONTENTS

I. INTRODUCTION

The shift in disease burden from acute to chronic illness which characterizes contemporary industrialized nations has resulted in a quest for appropriate measures by which to evaluate methods of health care delivery, as well as patient status. Terminal cancer patients present a particular challenge in this regard. Since "state of science" treatment is often administered without arresting the progress of disease, the goal of curing must be replaced by one of caring, and the medical model must be expanded to include considerations of psychosocial as well as disease-related factors. Maximizing the patient's quality of life as death approaches replaces disease improvement as a realistic goal for health care providers.

Recognizing that the acute care model upon which the modern health care system was founded did not fit well with the needs of terminally ill patients,[1] a new model of care called "hospice" originated in England in the late 1960s and emerged in the U.S. and Canada in the mid-1970s. Hospice care is characterized by palliative rather than curative care, by treating the patient and family, rather than just the patient, as the unit of care, and by the administration of care by an interdisciplinary team whose members are geared toward meeting the unique needs of terminally ill patients and their families. Hospice's growth in the decade and a half since its introduction to North America is testimony to the public's perceived need for an alternate system of care for the dying cancer patient. Recent estimates suggest that over 200 palliative care services in Canada, and over 1500 hospices in the U.S. are currently in operation.[2] As of this writing, hospice's acceptance into the medical mainstream is virtually complete.

The purpose of this paper is to review hospice research which focuses on quality-of-life outcomes. We will first consider several issues that are germane to the hospice context, including the operationalization of quality of life as it is consistent with hospice goals. We also discuss the extent to which hospice organizational arrangement contributes to variation in outcome, and review the methodological challenges facing researchers and health care providers interested in measuring the quality of life of hospice patients and their families.

II. QUALITY-OF-LIFE ISSUES IN HOSPICE CARE

Quality of life is a multidimensional construct, the components of which differ considerably between a healthy and a medically ill population. While the ability to care for oneself and fill social roles may be taken for granted in good health, it is this very ability to "live fully" that is of paramount importance in the presence of disease. While living fully implies social and psychological aspects of well-being, as well as physical, it is the patient's physical condition which constrains or facilitates social interaction, and which has implications for emotional health or distress. Thus, physiological parameters are central to the concept of quality of life in sick populations.[3]

The components of quality of life are simplified for the terminally ill patient: "For those who are dying, life takes on a new shape: it narrows, sometimes to a single room; work and running a household are no longer part of it. Friends and family are seen in a new way. Values change. What was once important may seem insignificant, while things once ignored have great weight".[4]

Despite this simplification of life as death approaches, there is still the potential for variation in outcomes which may determine the extent to which a patient's last days are comfortable and serene. Hospice care is designed to address those aspects of quality of life which are most relevant to the terminal cancer patient population. Thus, hospice's emphasis on palliation is intended to minimize pain and other symptoms, and in so doing, to maximize physical functioning and the independent performance of daily activities.

Emphasis on the patient and family as the unit of care encourages continued interaction with loved ones. Furthermore, the family is not "abandoned" after the patient's death but is offered bereavement counseling to assist the family through the inevitable grieving and adjustment phase which follows the death of a loved one.

Success in symptom control, in maintaining the highest degree of physical functioning possible given the patient's condition, and in fostering patient and family interaction is expected to positively affect the patient's mood state, and to be reflected in high levels of satisfaction with care, by both the patient and the family.

Finally, although not specifically cited as a direct goal of hospice care, the hospice orientation toward providing care in a home-like environment has frequently been interpreted to mean the patient's home. This orientation is applied most appropriately to the home-based hospice tradition which predominates within the U.S., rather than the hospital-based model which characterizes England and Canada, although home care hospices are increasing in prevalence in these countries, as well.

III. HOSPITAL-BASED VS. HOME CARE HOSPICES

Whether or not a hospice has inpatient beds may affect specific quality-of-life outcomes. For example, pain control may be more efficacious in hospital-based hospices, given the combination of a high priority placed on palliation and increased ability to provide continuity of care within a self-contained hospice facility, as opposed to a patient's home. While family members may be well intentioned, they may find compliance with a continuous pain control regimen administered at home to be difficult, or may not be sensitive to indications of the need to increase medication in order to alleviate distress.[5]

On the other hand, patients cared for in hospital-based hospices may have less involvement with their significant others than patients cared for in a home care hospice, given that a high level of support by family members is necessary for the terminally ill patient to be able to stay at home.[5] Powers and Burger,[6] using data from the National Hospice Study, found that patients who selected a home-care hospice were less likely to live alone than patients choosing a hospital-based hospice or conventional care, and that the primary caregivers of home-care hospice patients reported being able to depend on a greater number of people for help. Finally, as may be expected, those patients and families who express a preference for the hospice patient to die at home may have a better chance of having this preference realized in a home-care hospice.

Given the differences in organizational arrangement that are labeled "hospice", it seems reasonable to consider hospice as more of a philosophical approach to care provision than as an institutional entity. However, the locus of care is bound to make a difference, regardless of uniformity in philosophical approach. As both England and Canada move toward more heterogeneity in hospice organizational arrangements, rather than the strictly hospital-based palliative care service model, these likely differences in outcome should be considered carefully and expectations adjusted accordingly.

IV. METHODOLOGICAL ISSUES

Quality-of-life measurement is beset by the difficulties inherent in defining and measuring any outcome of a subjective nature. However, the unique characteristics of a terminal population present further obstacles to reliable and valid measurement. Four challenges to quality-of-life assessment in the context of hospice care are discussed below.

There is a lack of standardized scales which have been validated for the cancer patient population. For example, the use of standardized indices of depression that rely heavily on the contribution of somatic symptoms consistently overestimate depression in medically ill samples such as the terminally ill cancer patient.[7] Plumb and Holland[8] separated the physical and nonphysical components of the Beck Depression Inventory and found that while cancer patients resembled persons who had attempted suicide on the physical dimensions of depression, they resembled healthy next-of-kin on the nonphysical components. Similarly, administration of a psychometrically shortened nonsomatic version of the Profile of Mood States[9,10] to a population of cancer patients and their informal caregivers revealed approximately equal levels of positive and negative affect among cancer patients and their healthy caregivers.[11]

Not only is there a problem of confounding disturbed mood state with the physiological sequelae of disease among cancer patients, but the psychometric properties of scales developed for very different populations can make their application problematic. For example, the Profile of Mood States (POMS), often used in cancer patient populations, was standardized on psychiatric patients.[9] Average level of mood state among cancer patients reported in the literature are almost uniformly lower than those reported by the authors of the tests.[12] The relatively high standard deviations observed in cancer patient populations also suggest that there is considerable skew in the distribution of responses, with most respondents reporting little or no mood disturbance on any of the nonsomatic dimensions of the scale.

A second caveat to the measurement of psychosocial outcomes in a hospice population is the high probability of substantial nonresponse by patients as they approach death. Data from the National Hospice Study (NHS) indicate that patients are typically in their last weeks of life at entry into hospice (median length of stay for 15,000 NHS patients was 30 days).[13] Nonresponse may be attributable to a loss of cognitive clarity, due to brain metastases or medication side effects. Excessive symptoms such as pain, nausea, and shortness of breath can also diminish the patient's capacity to undertake the interviewing process. Finally, a depressed mood state or anxious condition may disincline a patient to agree to interview. All of these factors contribute to a questionable representativeness of subjective measure results.

Proxied interviews unavoidably reflect the perceptions of the proxy, rather than the patient. Proxies for the terminally ill are generally caretaking staff or families. Staff members serving as proxies may have a vested interest in minimizing the unresolved problems experienced by the patient, especially if they view negative patient outcomes as reflecting on the system of patient care.

Since family members are major providers of care, their assessments of the patient might reflect their own need to minimize the pain and problems that their loved one experiences. Alternatively, the patient's experience may be viewed from a strong emotional standpoint, resulting in an overestimate of the patient's difficulties.[14] Finally, a proxy might misinterpret what is most salient to the patient in his/her terminal phase of illness. For example, a comparison of ratings by 23 pairs of patient and primary caregivers on multiple quality-of-life indicators revealed that caregivers overestimated the patient's experience of pain, nausea, and vomiting, and underestimated the impact of illness on the extent to which the patient experienced sexual satisfaction and "fun".[15] Similarly, NHS data indicate that patient and primary caregiver ratings of the patient's pain were only moderately correlated.[4]

Finally, the brief period of time which characterizes most hospice patients' length of stay and thus their "exposure" to hospice, challenges researchers to construct measures that are sensitive to variation in those aspects of physical and psychosocial well-being which are amenable to the hospice intervention.[14] Nearly one quarter of NHS patients died within 10 days of admission,[4] implying that the opportunity of hospice staff to operationalize an intensive, personalized intervention was extremely limited. This challenge is further complicated by the inexorable decline of functioning and mental awareness and the increase in the number and complexity of symptoms as death approaches.[16] These parameters of the hospice population force us to consider, how large a difference can the intervention reasonably be expected to make? If patients deteriorate at a given rate, can we expect hospice to affect that rate?

With the conceptual and methodological issues enumerated above in mind, we will now turn to an overview of research conducted in the hospice arena to date which investigates quality-of-life outcomes in hospice care. Our focus is primarily on research that compares hospice to "conventional" care for the terminally ill, i.e., care on a nonhospice ward of an acute care hospital. In particular, we draw heavily from the two most comprehensive hospice evaluation projects conducted to date: the National Hospice Study, a nonrandomized, multisite investigation of the impact of hospice on costs and quality of life outcomes,[17] and a randomized clinical trial of patients admitted to a hospice unit in a Veterans Administration Hospital affiliated with the UCLA School of Medicine.[18]

V. PHYSIOLOGICAL OUTCOMES: PAIN, SYMPTOMS, AND PHYSICAL FUNCTIONING

Pain control is one of the central objectives of hospice care. A review of research suggests that the prevalence of pain in the terminally ill is between 30 and 60%.[13] Evaluation studies demonstrate that hospice does not result in patients experiencing more pain. Indeed, the National Hospice Study reports that hospice may achieve small but significant positive differences in achieving pain control. However, this effect may be confined to the hospital-based model of hospice care.[4,19]

NHS analyses examined patients' experience of pain as death approached across three settings: conventional hospital care, hospital-based hospice care, and home hospice care. The measure used was a rating of pain experienced by the patient, as judged by the patient's principal care person (PCP). Patients served in a hospital-based hospice were significantly less likely to be in "persistent severe pain" than patients served in a conventional hospital setting at both 3 weeks (3 vs. 14%; p <0.05) and 1 week (5 vs. 22%; p <0.05) prior to death. Fewer patients in a hospital-based hospice were reported to be in persistent severe pain than patients served in a home care hospice, although this difference was not significant. NHS medications data indicate that hospital-based hospice patients had the highest level of analgesic use administered on a regular basis, which may account for the difference in observed pain levels.[19]

NHS patients were also asked to report on their experience of pain, using the Melzack self report pain index. However, only 62% of the 1087 patients included in this analysis were able to respond on the self report measures at three weeks before death, and this proportion declined as death approached. Correlations between the self-report item and PCP judgment were 0.43, which indicate moderate but not strong agreement on the patient's experience.

Analyses of the symptom experience of NHS patients indicates that the prevalence of symptoms is high at 6 weeks before death, and increases as death approaches such that virtually no one was asymptomatic at the final measure before death.[16] Analyses of the number of symptoms patients experience again indicate a benefit for patients served by hospital-based hospices over patients served in either a conventional hospital setting or home care hospice.[19]

In contrast to NHS findings, Kane and colleagues found no differences in pain and symptom experience between patients served in the hospice program and those served on a conventional hospice ward.[18] However, critics of this study point out that no attempt was made to compare pain and symptom levels at comparable time periods. Therefore, patients very close to death and those further away were averaged together. If there were differences attributable to hospice care, the methodology utilized to measure outcomes may have masked these differences.[20] Furthermore, since measures were based on self-report, it could not have been possible to include the experience of all patients, particularly those who were most symptomatic and those who were closest to death. Substantial nonreporting may also cloud differences between one mode of care and an alternative.

Finally, neither of the evaluation studies found significant differences in physical functioning between hospice and nonhospice groups, measured by the Karnofsky Performance Status scale in the NHS and Katz' Activities of Daily Living scale in the UCLA Veteran's Administration Study. Although both studies concur that symptoms escalate and functioning declines as death approaches, whether or not the hospice intervention is able to ameliorate pain and symptomatology in the last days of life is not clear. The methodological difficulties inherent in measuring these parameters preclude a definitive answer, but indications thus far are that hospital-based hospices may have greater success in symptom control than either home-care hospices or conventional hospital care.

VI. PATIENT MOOD STATE

Despite the fact that hospice has few structured protocols that are specifically intended to either identify or ward off patient depression, anxiety, or dysphoric mood, hospice advocates nevertheless argue that the hospice approach to caring for the whole person, rather than merely the patient's disease, should indirectly affect mood state. Additionally, the ambiance of the hospice care model, in both in-patient and home settings, should be less anxiety provoking than the impersonality of conventional methods of care for the terminally ill. Finally, the availability of pastoral and other forms of counseling should directly affect patients' level of depression, anxiety, and sense of hopelessness.

In contrast to hospice advocates' expectations, neither the National Hospice Study nor the UCLA Veterans Administration Hospice study found differences between hospice and conventional care with regard to mood state outcomes. Kane and colleagues[21] found no difference in depression (measured by the CES-D) or anxiety (measured by the Ware anxiety scale) between patients randomized to either hospice or conventional care. The National Hospice Study[19] found similar results using a rating of emotional state made by the patient's caretaker. NHS interviewers also administered the depression subscale of the Profile of Mood States to patients, as well as a subset of items from the Rosenberg Self-Esteem Scale. However, only 60% of patients were able to respond for themselves at the baseline interview, and this proportion was reduced to 44% of those still alive by the seventh interview, conducted 14 weeks after baseline.[14] Thus, the sickest patients, precisely those expected to report the highest levels of mood disturbance, are not represented by these results. Patient nonresponse may account for the relatively low levels of mood disturbance observed in these studies.

It is in this area of psychosocial measurement that methodological complications are most difficult to circumvent. Finding a measure that will adequately capture variation in "what is possible" regarding the mood state of dying cancer patients is difficult in and of itself. Further, while it seems unacceptable to ask a proxy's opinion of the patient's mood, the inevitability of patient nonresponse in this population makes a self-report approach equally untenable. Findings of "no difference" in mood state between patients served by hospice and those served by conventional care must be considered with these substantial caveats in mind.

VII. SITE OF DEATH

Although not specifically designated as a desired outcome of hospice care, death at home is nevertheless associated with the hospice concept. Indeed, many patients and families may consider the hospice option specifically because it increases the chances that the patient will remain at home with loved ones until death. Among all the possible psychosocial outcomes that can be investigated in relation to hospice care, this is the most straightforward, uncomplicated by methodological difficulties.

The base rate of home deaths for cancer patients in the U.S. today appears to be between 15 and 20% of the population. The proportion of hospice deaths occurring at home can be compared to this national rate. Bass and colleagues[22] found that 57% of patients served in a home care hospice died at home. Similarly, Bonham and colleagues[23] found that 63% of 937 hospice patients died at their own or a relative's home, and Hadlock[24] reported that 67% of 327 patients served by a home care hospice program died at home. Data from the National Hospice Study reveal that 62% of patients served by home care hospices died at home, vs. 27% of hospital based hospice patients and only 13% of conventional care patients.[19]

It is clear that patients and families who prefer home death to death in an institution are more likely to have their preferences realized in the hospice model of care. The fact that patients in hospices that have inpatient beds are less likely than home care hospice patients to die at home may be partially accounted for by the necessarily stronger informal support systems of home care patients such that remaining at home until death is facilitated. However, the difference in proportion of hospice home deaths may also be driven by organizational arrangement per se, i.e., the presence of inpatient beds increases the likelihood that they will be utilized.

VIII. FAMILY BEREAVEMENT OUTCOMES

The hospice philosophy treats patients and families as the unit of care and the target of services. The hospice model of intervention can have a positive impact upon the families of hospice patients both while the patient is alive and after the patient has died. Hospice advocates feel that the emphasis on family involvement in caretaking should yield positive benefits to family members. Furthermore, when family involvement is combined with the hospice emphasis on bereavement counseling, we should expect long-term benefits for the family, potentially mitigating some of the deleterious effects of bereavement.[25]

Cameron and Parkes[26] examined the next of kin of patients who were treated by a palliative care unit in Royal Victoria Hospital, Montreal and next of kin of patients who died in a hospital. Over 1 year after the patient's death, palliative care unit patients' families showed less deterioration in health, required fewer sedatives, and were less angry than were comparison families. In an uncontrolled study of hospice bereavement programs' effectiveness, Barzelai[27] also found substantial decrease in reported anxiety that was attributed to the hospice intervention.

The National Hospice Study found no significant differences between hospice and non-hospice primary care persons in terms of any of the following outcomes measured an average 4 months after the death of the patient: hospitalization, number of physician visits, increased alcohol use, use of medication for anxiety, or thoughts of suicide. Hospital-based primary care persons reported depression and severe grief reaction significantly less often than home-care hospice caregivers, probably due to the proximity and intense physical and emotional involvement inherent in the situation of personally caring for a loved one in the terminal stage of illness. However, no significant differences were observed between hospice primary caregivers and the family members of patients cared for in conventional settings.[13]

Kane and colleagues[28] compared family members of hospice patients with family members of control patients and found decreases in depression and anxiety in both groups by 18 months post-patient death. However, there were no significant differences between the groups in depression or anxiety, or in more concrete indicators such as bed days, physician visits, contacts with friends and relatives, or smoking or drinking behaviors.

The mixed results in the area of bereavement counseling may be attributable to the fact that a high proportion of persons not in need of services are included in the studies. It may be that relatively few family members are in actual need of bereavement counseling, and that services should be targeted to this group. Second, the variability of programs labeled "bereavement services" is considerable, ranging from telephone and post card contact to in-person contact with a professional counselor over several months.

IX. SATISFACTION WITH CARE

The one area in which hospice care appears to have a clear advantage over conventional care of the terminally ill is in patient and family satisfaction with care. This is in spite of the fact that satisfaction scales are notoriously skewed in the direction of patients being satisfied with their care, regardless of the model of care delivery.

Naylor[29] compared hospice family members' satisfaction with patients' care with that of nonhospice family members and found highly significant benefits associated with being served by the hospital-based hospice program. McCusker[30] reports significantly higher satisfaction with care among those randomly assigned to an intensive home care treatment, as compared with controls. The NHS[19] also found hospice had a positive effect on satisfaction. No differences were found in the level of satisfaction among patients (which was over 90% across all settings); but family members of patients served in hospital-based hospices reported greater satisfaction with health care. Kane and colleagues'[21] randomized trial of hospice care found that patients were significantly more satisfied with hospice care, while families were somewhat more satisfied.

Given the fact that variation in satisfaction with the delivery of medical care has historically been difficult to measure, the consistency of results across studies which indicate a benefit for hospice care has significant implications. Failure to find differences in other parameters relevant to the hospice model may be of less importance than the finding of greater satisfaction on the part of patients and their families. As one investigator of hospice care comments: "One might ask whether any differences in areas other than satisfaction were really necessary. If indeed we are looking at a service provided to terminally ill individuals, is it not sufficient that they experience a more satisfactory service during their last days?.[31]

X. SUMMARY

We have reviewed research findings comparing the hospice model of care for the terminally ill with conventional hospital care on those parameters of quality of life deemed to be most relevant to the hospice intervention. As we have seen, there are substantial methodological difficulties inherent in measuring the psychosocial status of the terminally ill which may obscure differences between the outcomes of one mode of service delivery and an alternative. The most important of these methodological difficulties reviewed here are the lack of standardized scales developed specifically for a terminally ill population, patient nonresponse, proxied responses, and the lack of sensitivity of existing measures to capturing variation in patient outcome during the last weeks of life.

Ironically, it is that parameter — satisfaction with care — that is most often criticized for its lack of variability in patient populations that has been found to empirically detect an effect of the hospice intervention. We should take our cue from these findings in terms of further quality-of-life measurement development for hospice patients. It may be that the aspects of hospice care that do not lend themselves well to measurement, e.g., continued interaction with loved ones, comfort and familiarity, and the absence of alienation and impersonality often induced by traditional institutional settings, all contribute to a general feeling captured by the concept of patient and family "satisfaction with care". Increase in symptomatology and decline in functioning appear to be inevitable in the terminal phase, and as such any health-related quality-of-life measure that is predicated on these constructs will be unable to detect the effect of psychosocial and even health care interventions. On the other hand, hospice may induce in patients and families the feeling that they chose the best route to manage one of the most difficult of all human experiences.

ACKNOWLEDGMENT

This research is supported in part by National Cancer Institute grants #CA41020, CA46331, and CA36560.

REFERENCES

1. **Saunders, C.**, Hospice care, *Am. J. Med.*, 65, 726, 1978.
2. **Lamers, W. M.**, Hospice care in North America, in *Cancer, Stress and Death*, Day, S. B., Ed., Plenum Press, New York, 1986, 133.
3. **Mor, V.**, Cancer patients' quality of life over the disease course: lessons from the real world, *J. Chronic Dis.*, 40, 535, 1987.
4. **Morris, J. N., Suissa, S., Sherwood, S., Wright, S. M., and Greer, D.**, Last days: a study of the quality of life of terminally ill cancer patients, *J. Chronic Dis.*, 39, 47, 1986.
5. **Morris, J. N., Sherwood, S., Wright, S. M., and Gutkin, C. E.**, The last weeks of life: does hospice care make a difference?, in *The Hospice Experiment*, Mor, V., Greer, D. S., and Kastenbaum, R., Eds., The Johns Hopkins University Press, Baltimore, 1988, 109.
6. **Powers, J. S. and Burger, M. C.**, Terminal care preferences: hospice placement and severity of disease, *Public Health Rep.*, 102, 445, 1987.
7. **Craig, W. G. and Abeloff, M. D.**, Psychiatric symptomatology among hospitalized cancer patients, *Am. J. Psychiatry*, 131, 1323, 1974.
8. **Plumb, M. M. and Holland, J.**, Comparative studies of psychological function in patients with advanced cancer: self reported depressive symptoms, *Psychosom. Med.*, 39, 264, 1977.
9. **McNair, D. M., Lorr, M., and Droppleman, L. F.**, *EITS Manual for the Profile of Mood States*, Educational and Industrial Testing Services, San Diego, 1981.
10. **Guadagnoli, E. and Mor, V.**, Measuring cancer patients' affect: revision and psychometric properties of the Profile of Mood States (POMS), *J. Consult. Clin. Psychol.*, 1, 150, 1989.
11. **Mor, V. and Masterson-Allen, S.**, unpublished data, 1990.
12. **Cassileth, B. R., Lusk, E. J., Strouse, T. B., Miller, D. S., Brown, L. L., and Cross, P. A.**, A psychological analysis of cancer patients and their next-of-kin, *Cancer*, 55, 72, 1985.
13. **Mor, V. and Masterson-Allen, S.**, *Hospice Care Systems: Structure, Process, Costs and Outcomes*, Springer-Verlag, New York, 1987.
14. **Mor, V.**, Assessing patient outcomes in hospice: what to measure?, in *Psychosocial Assessment in Terminal Care*, Dush, D. M., Cassileth, B. R., and Turk, D. C., Eds., Haworth, New York, 1986.
15. **Curtis, A. E. and Fernsler, J. I.**, Quality of life of oncology hospice patients: a comparison of patient and primary caregiver reports, *Oncol. Nurs. Forum*, 16, 49, 1989.
16. **Wachtel, T., Allen, S., Reuben, P., Goldberg, R., and Mor, V.**, The end stage cancer patients: terminal common pathway, *Hospice J.*, 4, 43, 1988.
17. **Mor, V., Greer, D. S., and Kastenbaum, R., Eds.**, *The Hospice Experiment*, The Johns Hopkins University Press, Baltimore, 1988.
18. **Kane, R. L., Bernstein, L., Wales, J., Leibowitz, A., and Kaplan, S.**, A randomized controlled trial of hospice care, *Lancet*, 1, 890, 1984.
19. **Greer, D. S., Mor, V., Morris, J. N., Sherwood, S., Kidder, D., and Birnbaum, H.**, An alternative in terminal care: results of the National Hospice Study, *J. Chronic Dis.*, 39, 9, 1986.
20. **Cassileth, B. R.**, Major Hospice Research Projects Review and Evaluation, National Hospice Organization, Arlington, VA, 1984.
21. **Kane, R. L., Klein, S. J., Bernstein, L., Rothenberg, R., and Wales, J.**, Hospice role in alleviating the emotional stress of terminal patients and their families, *Med. Care*, 23, 189, 1985.
22. **Bass, D. M., Pestello, E. P., and Garland, T. N.**, Experiences with home hospice care: determinants of place of death, *Death Educ.*, 8, 199, 1984.
23. **Bonham, G. S., Gochman, D. S., Burgess, L., and Fream, A. M.**, The Hospice Decision: Multiple Determinants, Final Rep., University of Louisville, Louisville, KY, 1986.
24. **Hadlock, D. C.**, The hospice intensive care of a different kind, *Semin. Oncol.*, 12, 357, 1985.
25. **Osterwies, M., Solomon, F., and Green, M., Eds.**, *Bereavement: Reactions, Consequences, and Care*, National Academy Press, Washington, D.C., 1984.
26. **Cameron, J. and Parkes, C. M.**, Terminal care: evaluation of effects on surviving family of care before and after bereavement, *Postgrad. Med. J.*, 59, 73, 1983.

27. **Barzelai, L. P.,** Evaluation of a home based hospice, *J. Fam. Practice,* 12, 241, 1981.
28. **Kane, R. L., Klein, S. J., Bernstein, L., and Rothenberg, R.,** The role of hospice in reducing the impact of bereavement, *J. Chronic Dis.,* 39, 735, 1986.
29. **Naylor, D. B.,** Quality of Life as an Outcome of Hospice Care, Ph.D. dissertation, University of Akron, 1983.
30. **McCusker, J.,** Development of scales to measure satisfaction and preferences regarding long term and terminal care, *Med. Care,* 22, 476, 1984.
31. **Kane, F. L.,** Lessons from hospice evaluations, in *Psychosocial Assessment in Terminal Care,* Dush, D. M., Cassileth, B. R. E., and Turk, D. C., Eds., Haworth, New York, 1986, 3.

INDEX

Printed and bound by CPI Group (UK) Ltd, Croydon, CR0 4YY

23/10/2024

01778245-0011